Handbook of Pediatric and Neonatal Surgery

Handbook of Pediatric and Neonatal Surgery

Editor: Selena Hudson

MURPHY & MOORE
www.murphy-moorepublishing.com

www.murphy-moorepublishing.com

MURPHY & MOORE

Cataloging-in-Publication Data

Handbook of pediatric and neonatal surgery / edited by Selena Hudson.
p. cm.
Includes bibliographical references and index.
ISBN 978-1-63987-293-0
1. Children--Surgery. 2. Newborn infants--Surgery. 3. Children--Diseases--Treatment. 4. Pediatrics. I. Hudson, Selena.
RD137 .H36 2022
617.98--dc23

Murphy & Moore Publishing,
1 Rockefeller Plaza,
New York City, NY 10020, USA

ISBN 978-1-63987-293-0 (Hardback)

Contents

Preface

Pediatric surgery is a subspecialty of surgery that involves the surgery of infants, fetuses, children, young adults and adolescents. A few of its subspecialties are fetal surgery and neonatal surgery. Technologic developments such as computed tomography, sophisticated ventilators, ultrasound and advances in parental nutrition have revolutionized the diagnosis and treatment of disorders in newborns. This has reduced morbidity and mortality of infants who suffer from major surgical and medical issues. Common pediatric diseases that may require pediatric surgery are abdominal wall defects such as gastroschisis, omphalocele and hernias, congenital malformations such as cleft lip and palate, intestinal atresia, and meconium plugs. Chest wall deformities such as pectus excavatum and childhood tumors such as neuroblastoma, liver tumors and kidney tumors are also treated within this field. Pediatric and neonatal surgery is an upcoming field of science that has undergone rapid development over the past few decades. This book explores all the important aspects of this field in the present day scenario. It is a vital tool for all researching and studying this field.

Significant researches are present in this book. Intensive efforts have been employed by authors to make this book an outstanding discourse. This book contains the enlightening chapters which have been written on the basis of significant researches done by the experts.

Finally, I would also like to thank all the members involved in this book for being a team and meeting all the deadlines for the submission of their respective works. I would also like to thank my friends and family for being supportive in my efforts.

Editor

Preface

1

Caustic Ingestion

Abdulkerim Temiz

Abstract

Caustic ingestion with resultant esophagitis and gastritis is still an important social and medical problem due to early and long-term complications. This injury is seen frequently as an accidental event and may also lead to psychosocial impacts, including antisocial behavior, suicide attempts, criminal incarceration, and educational delinquency. It often occurs as a result of uncontrolled and unsafe storage of materials used in household cleaning. Despite the various treatment proposals, optimal management of the patients remains controversial. The presentation of the depth and extent of injury with endoscopy plays a key role in treatment planning. In the absence of life-threatening complications, the general approach is conservative management in the acute period. The most common complications are esophageal stricture and gastric outlet obstruction. Different treatment methods such as bougienage, stent application, balloon dilation, or esophageal replacement are used in the treatment of the caustic esophageal strictures. The decision of the least invasive method for the treatment of complications will reduce the potential hazardous results.

Keywords: caustic, esophagitis, esophageal stenosis, pyloric stenosis

1. Introduction

Caustic ingestion, which can cause severe morbidity and mortality, is still an important problem worldwide, especially in developing countries, which have an uncontrolled market selling cheap cleaning solutions of unknown composition. Despite several educational and public health initiatives to prevent caustic ingestion in children, in the United States (US), an estimated 5000–15,000 cases of caustic ingestion (incidence 1.08 per 100,000) occur each year [1]. Caustic ingestion also imposes a severe economic burden in terms of medical costs, as children with caustic injuries incurred hospital charges greater than $22 million US dollars in 2009. It is thought that the total costs exceed these amounts when indirect costs such as parental lost income or lodging for parents during hospitalization of children are factored in. These injuries may also lead to psychosocial impacts, including antisocial behavior, suicide attempts, criminal incarceration, and educational delinquency, as well as domestic problems such as family break-up, relocation, or loss of employment. De Jong et al. reported that 50% of children who ingested a caustic substance developed behavioral or educational problems [2]. Moreover, 25% of the families of severely affected children developed domestic problems [2]. Caustic injury may occur via accidental ingestion or as a suicide attempt. Caustic injury is usually more serious inpatients who attempted suicide as compared with accidental ingestion [3]. These cases usually occur in low income and poorly educated families [4]. The age distribution of caustic injury shows a bimodal pattern [1]. The first peak is seen in children between 1 and 5 years of age. In this period, injuries always occur due to accidental ingestion. De Jong et al. reported caustic injured patients aged as young as 1 month [2]. This usually occurs due to incorrect preparation of baby food with a liquid caustic substance accidentally in infancy or the neonatal period [2, 5]. The second peak of distribution is seen during and after the pubertal period; the majority of the cases are suicide attempts [6]. The type of ingested substances varies by geography. While alkaline ingestion is usually seen in more developed countries, acidic ingestion is seen usually in developing countries.

2. Etiology and pathophysiology

Caustic ingestion often occurs as a result of uncontrolled and unsafe storage of materials used in household cleaning. The extent and outcome of caustic ingestion depends on the identity of the caustic substance, as well as the concentration, the pH, the duration of contact between the substance and tissue, and the physical form of the substance. Increased free oxygen radical production, which arises due to ischemia and direct injury, leads to excessive tissue damage in addition to direct injury from the substance. Increased tissue or blood levels of free oxygen radicals have been demonstrated in different experimental studies [7–9]. Ischemic injury occurs during the first 1–4 days, which is defined as the acute necrotic phase. Severe inflammation, necrosis, edema, and hemorrhage are observed during this period. The second period is the subacute phase, usually observed between 4 and 15 days of injury. Mucosal sloughing, bacterial invasion, mucosal ulcer with fibrin crusts and increased granulation tissue due to fibroplasia and increased collagen deposition are the main findings in the second period. Because the aforementioned healing tissue is quite fragile, esophageal perforation or complications of endoscopy may occur during this period. Thus, endoscopy is only recommended in the first 24–48 hours or 2 weeks after the injury. The chronic or cicatrization phase begins at the end of the second week and may continue for several months.

The majority of reported cases are alkaline ingestions. Alkaline ingestion causes liquefaction necrosis, saponification of fats, penetration into the deeper layers, denaturation of proteins, emulsification of cellular membranes, and thrombosis of blood vessels [10]. Because of the greater viscosity of alkaline substances compared to acidic substances, prolonged contact with the substance often occurs in alkaline ingestion. Traditionally, alkaline substances cause tissue damage at pH levels higher than 11.5. It has been reported that a 30% solution of sodium hydroxide is able to induce a full thickness injury in 1 second. Additionally, caustic injury may occur with a lower concentration but a longer contact time. Mattos et al. demonstrated that the level of macroscopic and microscopic injury mainly depends on the concentration used as the aggressiveness of injuries gradually increases. Even a caustic soda solution at a concentration of 1.83% is able to induce epithelial necrosis in 1 hour [11]. However, they concluded that solution concentration revealed to be most important determinant in injury. Acidic injury causes coagulation necrosis; this results in the formation of an eschar, which limits the depth of penetration and injury. Injury related to acidic ingestion usually occurs with substances with a pH <2. Because of protective effects of eschar formation and rapid transit to the stomach due to low viscosity, acidic ingestion results in more gastric injury than alkaline ingestion. Commonly, gastric injury and complications occur in patients who have ingested an acidic substance, while alkaline ingestion is associated with esophageal injury and complications. Although Temiz et al. diagnosed severe gastric injury in 40.27% of acid-ingesting patients and in 10.71% of alkaline-ingesting patients, there was no difference in the rate of esophageal stricture development between these patients [5]. However, Ciftci et al. reported that the gastric outlet obstruction rate is higher with alkaline ingestion than acidic ingestion [12].

Caustic ingestion may also cause airway injury, resulting in laryngeal and lower airway edema and respiratory distress [5, 6]. Additionally, fibroblast proliferation occurs as a result of caustic injury due to alkaline or acid ingestion, resulting in circular and longitudinal contraction in the submucosal and muscular layers. The clinical manifestations are esophageal stricture, gastric outlet obstruction, gastroesophageal reflux, and hiatal hernia [10].

3. Clinical presentation

Caustic ingestion is seen frequently as an accidental event in children, especially in low income families. It usually occurs between 1 and 3 years of age [2]. The male/female ratio shows a male predominance. Clinical presentations of caustic ingestion vary from no injury to fatal complications. The outcomes and clinical findings depend on the properties of the caustic substance such as type, amount, physical form and depth, and extent of injury. Solid substances may adhere to the mucosa and be difficult to swallow. Therefore, solid substances commonly cause upper level damage, such as upper respiratory, oral cavity, or pharynx injury. Liquid substances may be swallowed easily. Thus, injury to the lower levels such as the esophagus or the stomach occurs more frequently with liquid substances. In the early stage, patients may refer with vomiting, excessive salivation, refusal to drink, apparent oral mucosal findings that vary from mild hyperemia to severe edema and diffuse fibrin sheets on lips, oral, or oropharyngeal mucosa [5, 13, 14]. Respiratory distress, stridor, hoarseness, aphonia, and dyspnea indicate respiratory tract injury. Drooling, dysphagia, odynophagia, and chest or abdominal pain usually observed in severely injured patients. Nausea or hematemesis also may occur. Gaudreault et al. reported severe esophageal burns in only 18–33% of patients with specific clinical signs and symptoms of caustic injury [13]. They concluded that positive clinical signs or symptoms cannot predict esophageal injury. Although they recommended endoscopic evaluation in symptomatic patients, they did not suggest endoscopy for asymptomatic patients, especially those with a questionable history [13]. Temiz et al. reported severe esophageal injury in 19.3% of patients with no symptoms whereas nearly 60% of their patients with significant physical findings had no or mild esophageal injury [5]. Boskovic and Stankovic reported that 6.03% of patients with normal clinical findings had severe esophageal injuries, whereas 66.6% of patients with positive clinical findings had no or mild esophageal findings [15]. Additionally, severe gastric injury was seen in 6.8% of caustic ingestion patients; 1.7% of them had no clinical signs whereas 5.1% of them had positive clinical findings. These results show that the sensitivity and specificity of clinical findings regarding esophageal injury are 74 and 73%, respectively, with a positive predictive value of 0.33 and a negative predictive value of 0.66. They calculated these values as sensitivity 75%, specificity 68%, positive predictive value 0.15, and negative predictive value 0.97 for gastric injury [15]. Temiz et al. observed severe gastric injury in 18.5% of all caustic ingestion patients; 3.9% of these patients had normal physical findings whereas 14.6% of them had positive clinical findings [5]. Fifty percent of patients who developed gastric outlet obstruction did not have physical findings [5]. They calculated the sensitivity and specificity of clinical findings regarding severe esophageal injury as 80.6 and 32.8%, respectively. Also, they reported the sensitivity and specificity of clinical findings regarding severe gastric injury as 75.7 and 29%, respectively. Severe complications, including severe esophageal or gastric injury (especially transmural necrosis or perforation), should be considered in patients with abdominal/chest pain and hematemesis. More serious and fatal presentations secondary to caustic ingestion, such as disseminate intravascular coagulation, tracheoesophageal fistula, brachiocephalic fistula, paralyzed vocal cords, and acute pancreatitis have been reported [16, 17].

Button battery ingestion seems to cause the most severe injuries. Button battery tends to become lodged at areas of physiological narrowing in the gastrointestinal tract, such as the pharyngoesophageal junction, gastroesophageal junction, pylorus, ligament of Treitz, Meckel diverticulum or ileocecal valve (**Figure 1a** and **b**). Larger batteries usually tend to be affixed in the esophagus, whereas smaller batteries pass into the stomach and intestine [18]. Especially, button batteries with a diameter of 20 mm or larger can become lodged in the esophagus in children [19]. The complications associated with button battery ingestion are the result of a combination of four mechanisms, including leakage of the alkaline substance, absorption of the toxic substance, and necrosis secondary to either direct pressure from the battery or electrical discharge [18]. Votteler et al. demonstrated that mucosal necrosis occurred within 1 hour and ulceration within 2 hours of battery placement in an experimental study [20]. Litovitz et al. reported that batteries become lodged within 4 hours of ingestion, and esophageal perforation occurs 6 hours after ingestion [21]. These results are related to the site at which the battery is lodged, the contact time and the possibility of heavy metal absorption [18, 20, 22]. The complications of esophageal impactions are more severe than those of lower gastrointestinal impactions. The most dangerous complications, such as esophageal or aortic perforation, trachea-esophageal fistula, hemorrhagic shock, severe esophageal bleeding, and vocal cord paralysis, have been observed in patients with esophageal button battery impactions [19]. Fatal aorto esophageal fistula and perforation of the brachiocephalic artery secondary to button battery ingestion have been reported in children [23, 24].

The clinical complaints of late presenting patients are slightly different. Generally, after 3 weeks, the patients may admit with dysphagia, vomiting, or respiratory problems [25]. These complaints

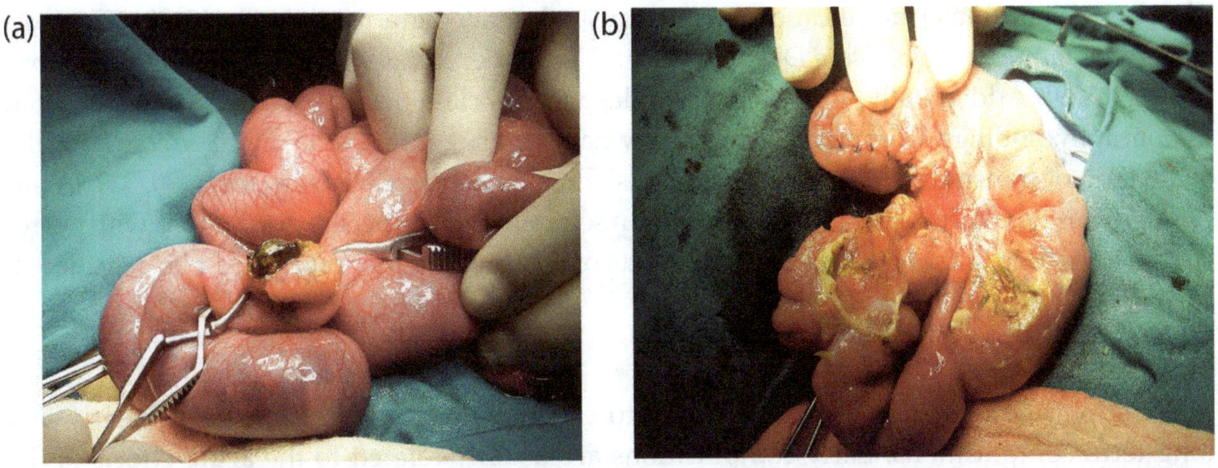

Figure 1. Perforation of Meckel's diverticulum by button battery (a) and caustic injury of adjacent intestinal segments (b).

indicate late complications such as esophageal stricture, gastric outlet obstruction, or gastroesophageal reflux. Late complications especially esophageal strictures or gastric outlet obstructions cause dysphagia, insufficient oral intake or vomiting. Malnutrition, growth retardation, feeding intolerance, dehydration or liquid and electrolyte imbalance may develop secondary to these symptoms and complications. Obstructive complications usually occur at the level of physiological narrowing of the gastrointestinal tract, especially at three esophageal narrowing and the pylorus.

3.1. Staging

Staging is important to separate severely injured patients from mildly injured or healthy children. The classification of patients allows for the identification of patients at risk of developing early or late complications. Several different grading systems have been described and suggested in previous studies [26, 27]. The modification of the method of Di Costanzo grading system is summarized in **Table 1** [5, 28]. All classifications based on endoscopic findings have been prepared on the basis of mucosal findings, mucosal involvement, and the depth of injury.

Grade	Findings
0	Normal
1	Mucosal edema Hyperemia
2a	Hemorrhagic mucosa Bullous mucosa Exudates Fibrinous membranes Superficial ulceration
2b	Circumferential ulceration (addition to the grade 2a)
3	Scattered small necrotic area Hemorrhagic black or brown mucosa

Table 1. Modify Di Costanzo classification [5, 28].

Most researchers make modifications to previously described grading systems [3, 28]. The most preferred staging systems were Di Costanzo and Zargar grading system or their modifications [3, 10, 26–29]. Additionally, Ryu et al. have described a classification according to computed tomography findings. Computed tomography has been suggested to be more effective for the evaluation of transmural injuries to esophagus and stomach as well as necrosis [30, 31]. In our opinion, this type of imaging is advantageous in selected cases, especially in patients with necrosis or perforation, although the radiation effects of computed tomography must be considered.

3.2. Complications

The complications that develop secondary to caustic ingestion are divided into early and long-term complications. Early complications are usually related to the acute effects of the caustic substance, which generally manifest as tissue necrosis. Chemical pneumonitis, atelectasis, aspiration pneumonia, and dysphagia are some of early complications due to the acute effects of ingestion [2]. Tracheoesophageal fistula is another early stage complication. Poley et al. detected severe systemic complications more frequently among patients who ingested acidic substances than those who drank alkaline substances in their report on adolescent and adult patients [28]. They reported renal insufficiently, hepatic dysfunction, diffuse intravascular coagulation, and hemolysis as systemic complications [28]. These authors reported 16% overall mortality. They showed a worse death rate with the ingestion of acidic substances compared with alkaline substances (14 vs. 2%); 11% of overall mortality was related to systemic complications [28]. Early complications may also have catastrophic consequences, and some complications can result in death [23]. Ulceration, edema, gastrointestinal hemorrhage, total loss of the vocal cord, vocal cord paresis, denuded epiglottis, aorta esophageal fistula, esophageal perforation, perforation of Meckel's diverticulum, and perforation of the brachiocephalic artery are early stage complications that have been reported previously [18, 19, 24, 32–37]. Acute pancreatitis has been reported as an early complication secondary to accidental caustic ingestion in a young adult [16]. Skin injuries are seen in some cases (**Figure 2a** and **b**).

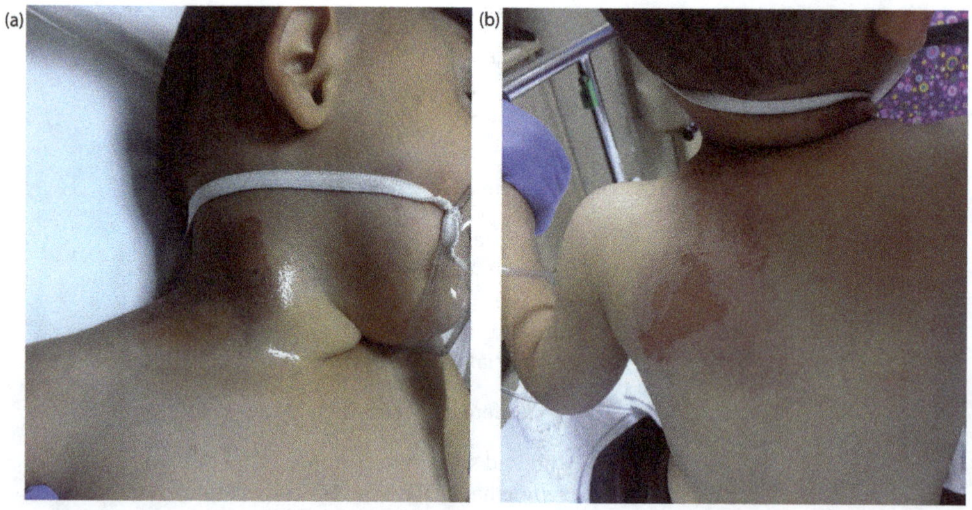

Figure 2. Injury of the neck (a) and back (b) resulting from casting onto the skin during caustic ingestion.

Long-term complications usually develop 3 weeks after the injury. Most commonly, strictures occur due to increased fibrosis in the injured area. The esophagus is the most severely affected gastrointestinal segment in most caustic ingestion patients. Therefore, the majority of upper gastrointestinal strictures secondary to caustic ingestion develop in the esophagus. Esophageal strictures may involve a short segment (usually accepted as shorter than two vertebral bodies in length) or a long segment (described as more than two vertebral bodies in length), or even the whole esophagus [38, 39] (**Figure 3a–d**). The rate of esophageal stricture has been reported to be between 2 and 63% in different series [2, 13, 29, 40–42]. Baskin et al. reported that 4.7% of grade-2a injured patients and 26% of grade 2b injured patients

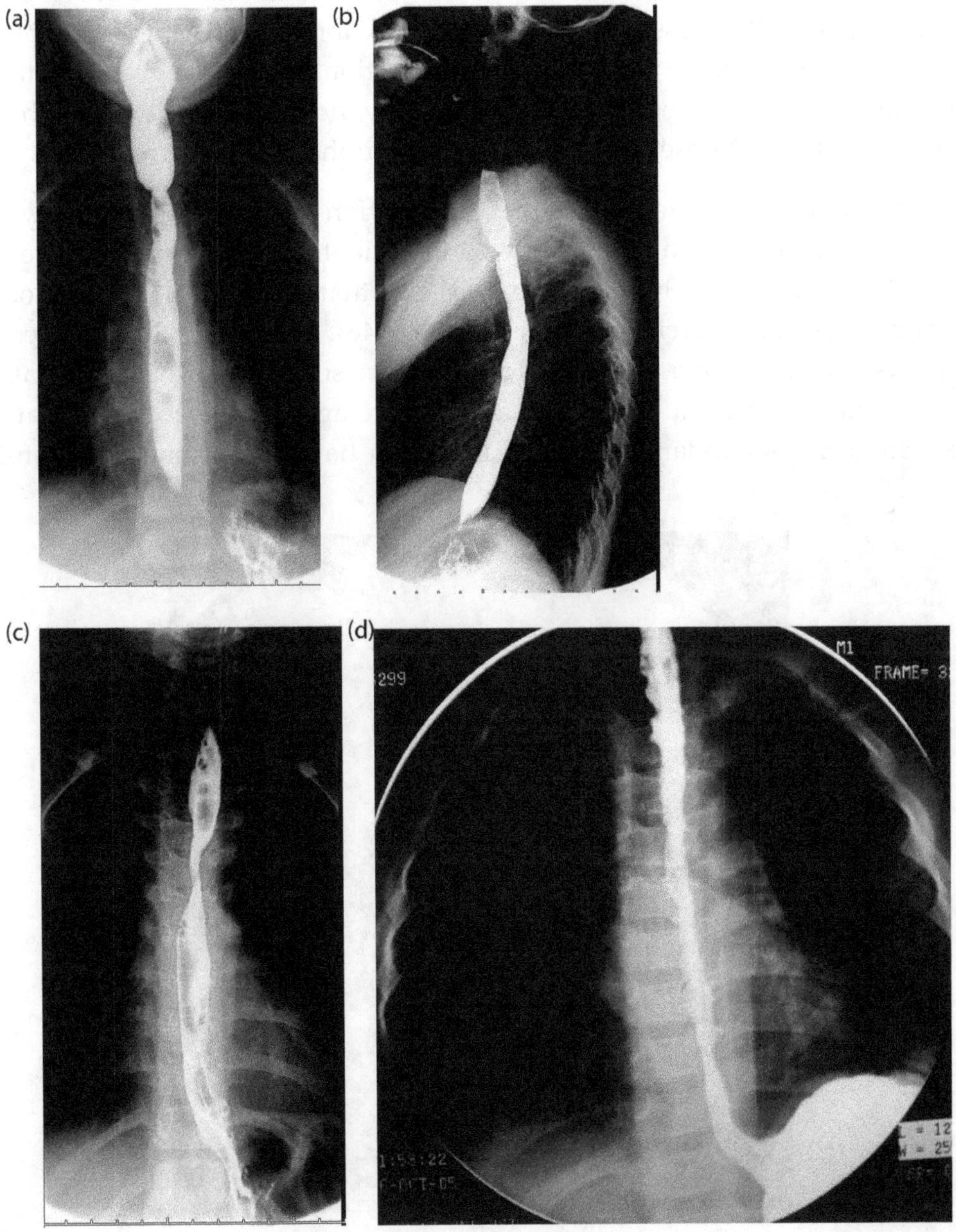

Figure 3. Barium meal studies reveal short segment (a and b) and long segment (c and d) stricture of esophagus in 7 years old boy and 15 years old girl respectively.

develop esophageal strictures [29]. Huang et al. reported that all grade 2 and 3 injured patients develop esophageal strictures [40]. Temiz et al. showed an esophageal stricture rate of 32.1 and 100%, respectively, in patients with grade 2b and 3 injuries [5]. The second most common level of upper gastrointestinal stricture due to caustic ingestion is the pylorus (**Figure 4**). This usually occurs due to accumulation of the ingested substance at the antrum or pylorus level. Several studies have reported that the overall incidence of gastric outlet obstruction is between 5 and 10% [12, 43–45]. Temiz et al. showed a pyloric obstruction rate of 15.7% in patients with severe gastric injury [5]. Gastric outlet obstruction may present with gastroesophageal reflux symptoms. The third long-term complication of caustic ingestion is gastroesophageal reflux and hiatal hernia (**Figure 5**). It occurs as a result of esophageal shortening and retraction due to the inflammation and fibrosis that develop secondary to the ingestion injury. Progressive inflammation and fibrosis may cause disruption of His' angle and even a hiatal hernia. This clinical presentation may cause growth retardation or the inability to eat. Also, gastroesophageal reflux may increase the rate of esophageal stricture and influence the response to the treatment of esophageal stricture.

Esophageal carcinoma is another long-term complication [46–48]. This is usually squamous cell carcinoma. Appelqvist and Salmo showed in patients that had ingested lye (the mean age of patients at the time of lye ingestion was 6.2) that the mean latent period between ingestion and esophageal carcinoma was 41 years [46]. Moreover, 84% of these patients had squamous cell carcinoma at the middle part of esophagus. Kochhar et al. reported two patients with esophageal carcinoma after acidic agent ingestion [49]. Patients with esophageal strictures secondary to caustic ingestion have more than a 1000-fold risk of

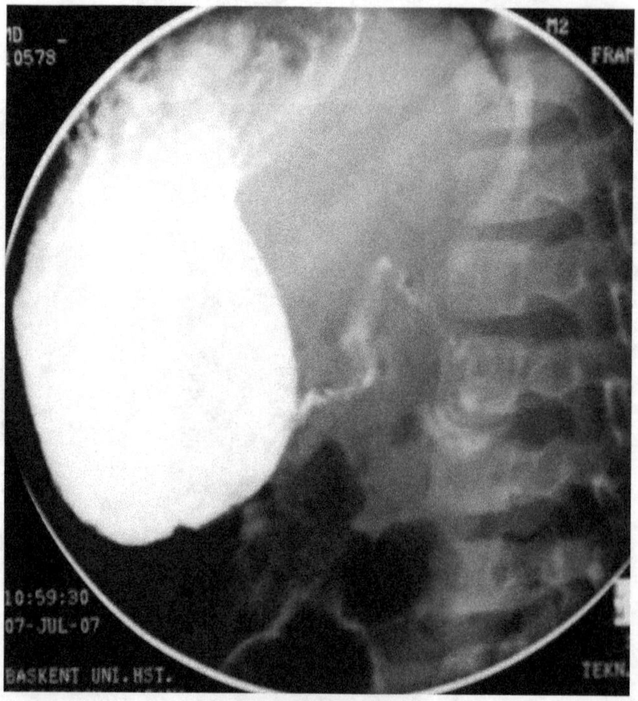

Figure 4. Barium meal study reveals pyloric stenosis secondary to the acidic substance ingestion.

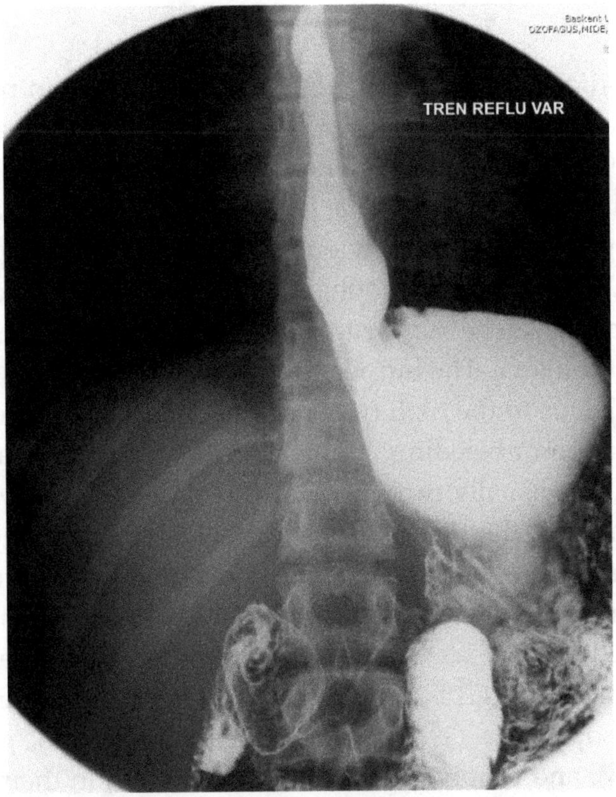

Figure 5. Gastroesophageal reflux and sliding type of hiatal hernia is presented by contrast study.

developing esophageal carcinoma [49]. Appelqvist et al. reviewed a total of 2414 patients with esophageal carcinoma and found that 2.6% of them had a history of caustic injury of the esophagus [46].

4. Diagnostic methods

Several techniques and methods, including laboratory tests, radiological studies, scintigraphy, and endoscopy, are used to determine the severity and depth of injury.

4.1. Laboratory

White blood cell count, C-reactive protein, plasma creatinine level, aspartate aminotransferase (AST), alanine aminotransferase (ALT), and blood gases are usually assessed in serious cases. These tests can be used both in diagnosis and in management to define whether the patient has developed complications. High white blood cell counts (>20,000 cells/mm^3), low arterial pH (<7.22), and low base excess (< −12) are considered signs of serious esophageal injury in adults [50, 51]. However there is no clinical study that examined the relation of laboratory findings and caustic injury level. Laboratory tests are also used for the detection and monitoring of systemic and metabolic complications such as liver damage or renal insufficiency [28].

4.2. Endoscopy

Several studies have indicated that clinical signs are not helpful in predicting the degree of injury and late complications. However, the necessity for endoscopy has been discussed in the literature previously; esophagogastroduodenoscopy is still the most preferred and effective diagnostic practice and approach [4, 5, 28, 53] It is based on direct visualization and staging of injury according to the grading system previously described. It can be performed using a rigid or flexible endoscope. While only the esophagus can be seen by rigid endoscopes, both the esophagus and the stomach can be seen with a flexible endoscope. It is recommended within the first 24–48 hours after injury. The burned area of the esophagus is weakest between days 7 and 21 after injury [2]. Due to the high frequency of complications related with endoscopy, such as fistulas, perforation or bleeding, it is not recommended in patients with high grade injuries [2]. Moreover, it is usually recommended to stop endoscopy at the first severe circumferential burn because of the risk of complications [2, 52]. Poley et al. reported that the esophagus was the most severely affected segment of the upper gastrointestinal tract in 79% of their patients [28]. Injury to the stomach, especially the fundus and body, was relatively common. They observed damage to the duodenum only in 6% of their patients [28]. Doğan et al. observed gastric injury in 17.1% of patients [53]. Urgancı et al. reported normal or mild injury (57%), severe esophagitis (19.1%), erosive gastritis (4.3%), gastric necrosis (0.3%), esophagogastritis (3.7%), and esophagogastroduodenitis (4%) in their series [4]. Temiz et al. reported that 18.4% of patients with severe esophageal injury likewise had severe gastric injury (**Figure 6a–d**). Also, 3.4% of their patients had more severe damage to the stomach than to the esophagus [5]. They performed complete upper gastrointestinal endoscopy to avoid overlooking a gastric injury, even in patients with severe esophageal damage. They reported that there were no complications due to late or complete endoscopy, even in severely damaged patients [5]. There are many articles about esophageal endoscopic findings, but there are limited studies providing gastric findings after caustic ingestion in children [5, 28]. Poley reported that normal findings or mild esophageal injury was found in 40% of patients, while this value was 80% in a study by Boskovic [15, 28]. Doğan et al. reported normal or mild injury in 47.5% of patients [53]. Temiz et al. reported that 43.2% of their patients had normal or mild esophagitis demonstrated by endoscopy, while they all presented with positive clinical findings [5]. In this way, unnecessary hospitalization was prevented by endoscopy [5, 15, 28]. Also, endoscopy can be used for planning the treatment of possible complications such as early dilation of the esophagus in severely injured patients [5, 54]. Radiologically suspected or proven gastrointestinal perforations, severe respiratory injury with distress, poor general condition or metabolic imbalance are accepted as contraindications of endoscopy. However, endoscopy can be performed under sedation within a short period of time. The rate of complications related to endoscopy is very low. Bleeding, perforation, and mucosal tears are complications of endoscopy. Iqbal et al. reported a 0.06% rate of complications in all endoscopy procedures, regardless of the indication [55]. Although Doğan et al. reported that esophageal perforation occurred after endoscopy in one patient (0.21%), most of the articles which examined the results of endoscopy in caustic ingestion patients reported no complications [5, 15, 28, 53]. Although many articles have emphasized the importance of early endoscopy in planning the treatment strategy, some centers do not offer early endoscopic examination, claiming that

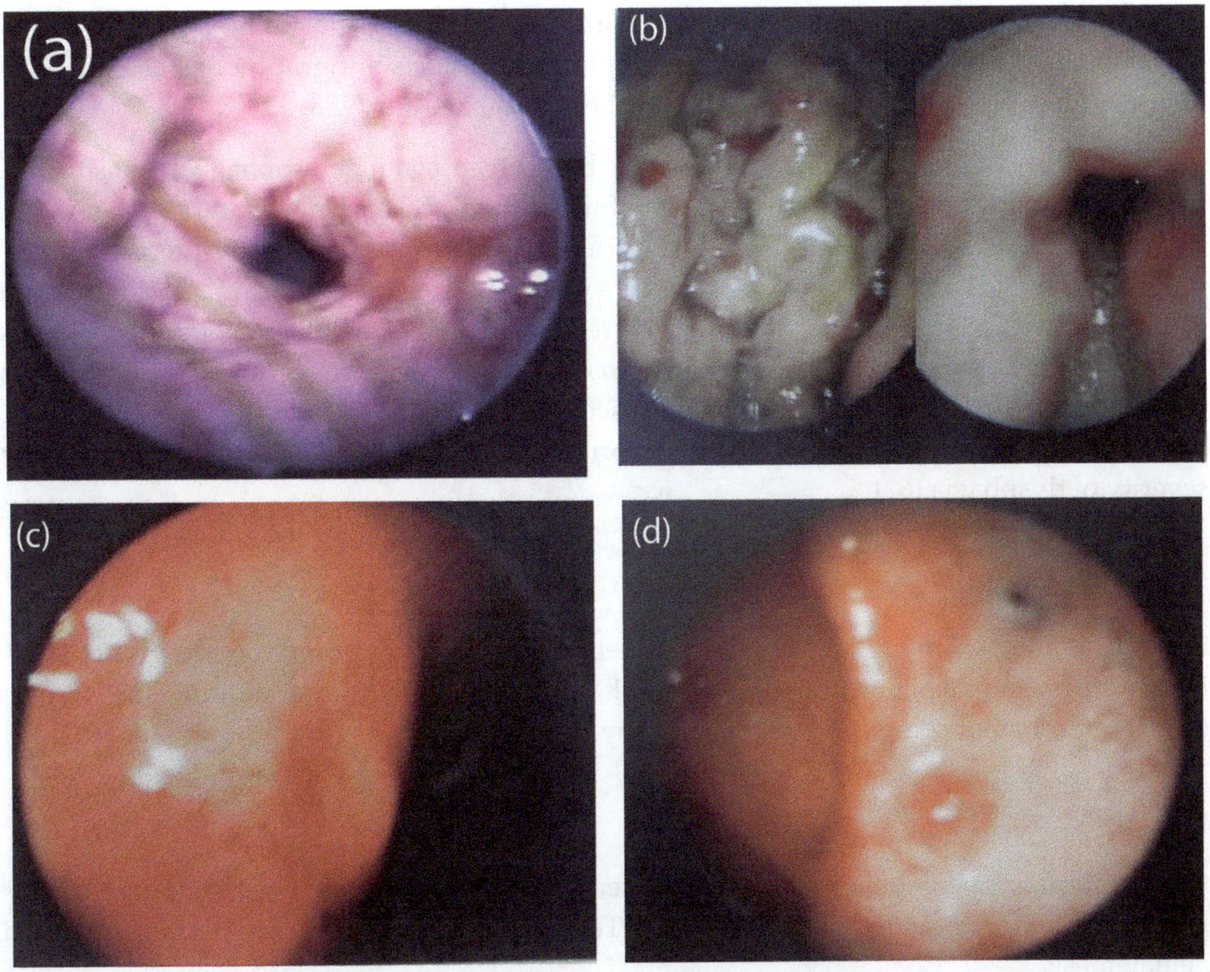

Figure 6. Endoscopy demonstrated the severe caustic injury in the esophagus (a) antrum and pylorus (b). Pylorus narrowing was observed in the control endoscopy (c). A pint point appearance of pylorus in a patient admitted during the past period (d).

endoscopic findings do not change treatment strategies [14, 42, 56]. Additionally, the risk of general anesthesia and the complications of endoscopy are avoided using these protocols [42]. Lamireau et al. reported that the absence of symptoms was always associated with no or minimal lesions in their patients. Therefore, they did not recommend endoscopy in asymptomatic patients, especially in developed countries [14]. In the same way, Gupta et al. reported that all patients with clinically significant injuries were symptomatic. Also, all asymptomatic patients had normal findings on endoscopic examinations [56].

4.3. Scintigraphy

In the last two decades, clinical and experimental studies have been performed assessing the value of scintigraphic evaluation and detection of caustic injury of the esophagus [57, 58]. Millar et al. performed a prospective clinical study to assess whether sucralfate has an affinity for the chemically injured esophagus and to assess the accuracy of radiolabeled sucralfate as an indicator of the presence and extent of esophageal injury [57]. They found that technetium-99m scintigraphy is an accurate diagnostic method to assess caustic esophageal injury [57]. Technetium-99m pyrophosphate scintigraphy has been used in diagnostic studies on the detection of caustic esophageal injury [58, 59].

In the late period, scintigraphic studies may be used to evaluate esophageal transit time, gastric emptying and gastroesophageal reflux, which are common complications [60]. Technetium-99m sulfur colloid in milk or formula is often used for gastrointestinal scintigraphic studies [61]. Kochhar et al. performed a study to assess esophageal motor dysfunction in patients with corrosive esophageal stricture. They used segmental and total esophagus transit time. They found that esophageal transit time is prolonged in one-third of patients with corrosive injury-induced esophageal strictures despite adequate esophageal dilatation. They also reported that these findings were correlated with the length of the stricture and the severity of dysphagia [62].

4.4. Radiology

Several radiological modalities are used to define early and late complications. These studies vary from simple plain chest or abdominal X-ray to complex contrast studies such as cine esophagography or computerized tomography.

4.4.1. Chest X-ray, erect abdominal X-ray

Pneumothorax, pneumomediastinum, or pneumoperitoneum, which are signs of esophageal or gastric perforation, can be observed. These methods are often used in patients with hematemesis.

4.4.2. Esophagogastrography

This is useful for the demonstration of early or late complications. Esophageal stenosis, hiatal hernia, gastroesophageal reflux, pyloric stenosis, esophageal perforation, gastric perforation or tracheoesophageal fistula can be demonstrated with contrast studies. Traditional esophagography may not show pathology in some cases. In these situations, cine esophagography may be helpful (**Figure 7**). In suspected patients, the uses of water-soluble substances, which are less irritant than barium, are preferred for the demonstration of esophageal or gastric perforation (**Figure 8**). However, more radiologic details with better images are obtained with barium meal studies. Contrast studies are also used to determine the location and length of the esophageal stricture (**Figure 9a** and **b**).

4.4.3. Ultrasonography (US)

There have been some studies that focused on the utility of endoscopic esophageal or gastric miniprobe US to predict of outcomes of caustic injury [63–66]. The basis for this method is to evaluate the integrity of the mucosa and deeper muscle layers or to assess gastric wall thickness. Endoscopic ultrasonographic findings are classified as grade-1 when involving only the mucosal edema and grade-2 and grade-3 with destruction of the muscular layers. Grades 2

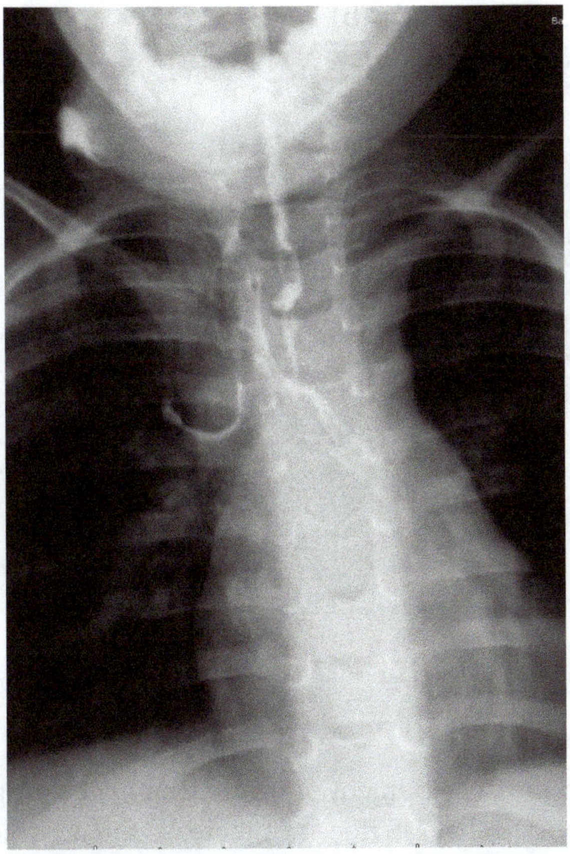

Figure 7. Tracheoesophageal fistula was described by cine esophagography.

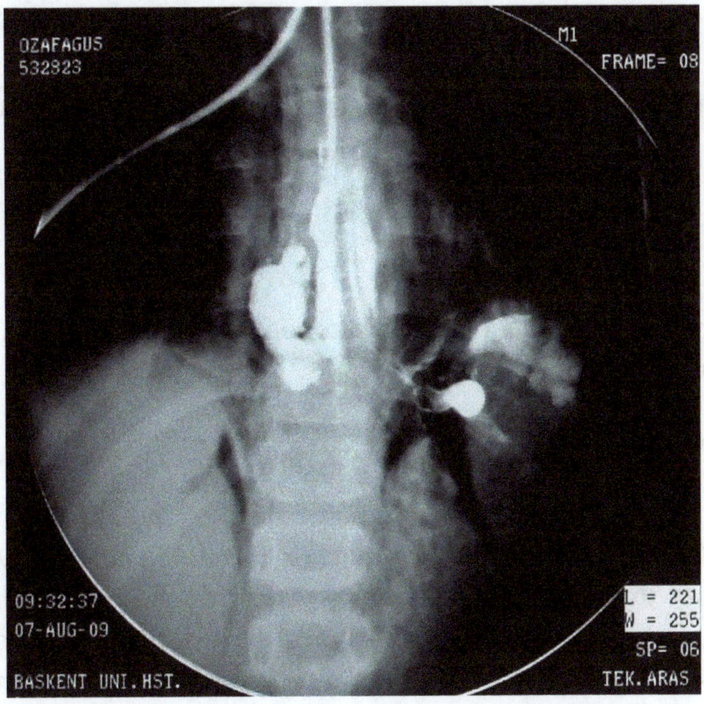

Figure 8. Contrast meal study revealed esophageal perforation after dilatation session.

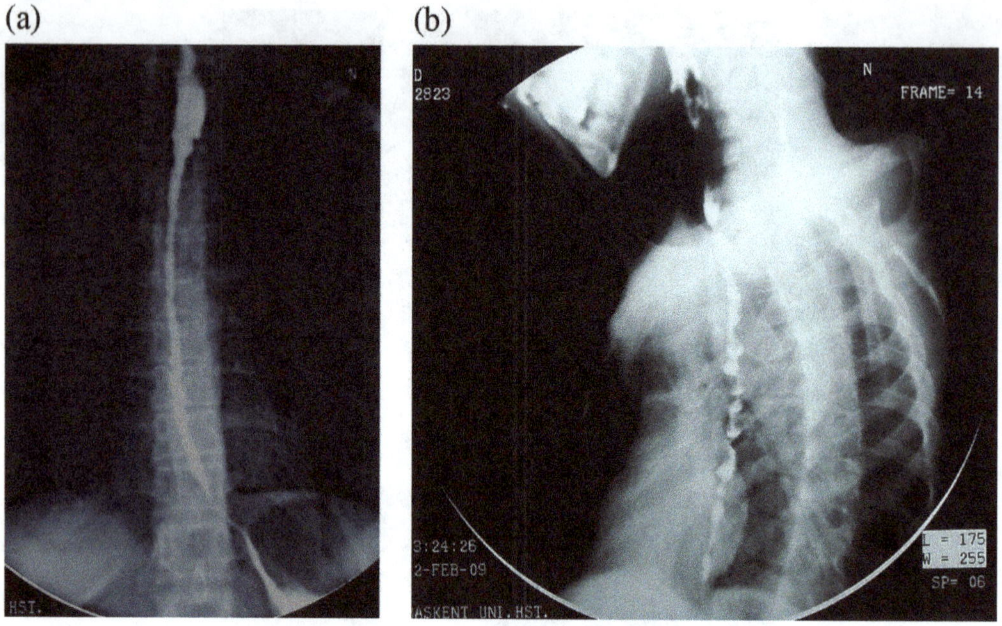

Figure 9. (a) and (b) Multiple and long segment strictures of esophagus were showed by esophagography.

and 3 are associated with the development of future esophageal or gastric strictures [63–66]. However, Chiu et al. reported that US does not increase the accuracy of predicting early or late complications when used in conjunction with conventional endoscopic observation [66].

4.4.4. Computerized tomography (CT)

CT is usually used to define transmural injury and the extent of necrosis in patients with complications such as esophageal or gastric perforations due to caustic ingestion. Ryu et al. recently described a grading system to predict late complications after caustic ingestion [30].

5. Treatment

The treatment approach to caustic ingestion can be divided into two stages: acute management and the treatment of complications.

5.1. Acute management

The acute management of caustic ingestion is based on the general principles of acute trauma life support guidelines. The aim of this approach is the stabilization of vital functions. This includes continuity of the airway and respiratory function and controlling the circulation. Hemodynamic and respiratory stabilization should be priority aims. Endotracheal intubation may be necessary in patients with severe airway caustic injury. Intubation can be difficult in patients with a severely affected airway. Fiber optic laryngoscopy may provide direct visualization and safe intubation. Thus, the complications that occur secondary to blind intubation may be prevented [6, 10]. Oral feeding is discontinued and adequate intravenous fluid replacement should be provided [10, 31]. A detailed history and identification and measurement of the pH level of the ingested caustic substance will provide information about the severity of the injury. Chest and erect abdominal X-ray should be performed to look for pneumomediastinum, pneumothorax, and pneumoperitoneum, which indicate esophageal or gastric perforation. pH neutralization is not recommended, because it can increase damage by direct effects on the mucosa. This may also cause emesis and vomiting, which may cause recurrent injury to the esophagus [10]. Nasogastric decompression is recommended to prevent vomiting and to provide gastric decompression. However, the benefits have not been conclusively shown. It may be used as a stent in severe circumferential injury. The placement of nasogastric tubes is recommended under endoscopic visualization to prevent esophageal perforation. Oral feeding is still controversial. The authors who believe in the necessity of endoscopy recommend feeding after endoscopy if the findings are normal or mild [5, 53]. In patients with severe esophagitis, enteral nutrition may be applied via a nasogastric tube. However, some authors prefer enteral nutrition without endoscopy for patients who are able to swallow their saliva easily [42]. They perform barium contrast esophagography after 3 weeks. In cases of esophageal or gastric stricture, endoscopy and dilatation are performed [42]. Total parenteral nutrition is preferred in patients with severe gastric injury or who are intolerant to enteral nutrition with normal gastroscopic findings [5, 42]. Proton pump inhibitors or H_2 antagonists are usually recommended to prevent possible gastroesophageal injury or stress ulcers [25, 29, 31]. However, the beneficial effects of agents that reduce gastric pH levels remain unclear. Broad spectrum antibiotics are preferred by many authors, especially in patients with airway injury [5, 6, 25]. However, there is no evidence that antibiotics reduce infections of the injured area or the rate of stricture formation. The benefits of corticosteroids are still controversial. Two different studies that presented a meta-analysis of the literature regarding the use of corticosteroids in caustic injury showed that steroids do not have beneficial effects [67, 68]. Anderson et al. found that there is no benefit from the use of steroids in caustic injured patients regarding the rate of stricture formation [69]. However, there are also studies presenting the opposite opinion. Mamede et al. found that antibiotics combined with corticosteroids reduced the incidence of stenosis [70]. These authors reported infection and gastrointestinal bleeding as side effects of corticosteroids, especially in patients who had ingested large amounts of a caustic substance. Bautista et al. also reported that dexamethasone had better effects than prednisone [71]. Usta et al. investigated the effects of a high dose methylprednisolone (1 g/1.73 m^2) on caustic esophageal burns [72]. They found that the stricture development rate and the duration of total parenteral nutrition were statistically significantly low in the methylprednisolone group [72]. Boukthir et al. reported that high dose methylprednisolone seems to improve the prognosis and prevent stricture formation in grade-2b injured patients [73]. Another situation is the treatment of metabolic complications of caustic injury including renal insufficiency, hepatic dysfunction, diffuse intravascular coagulation, and hemolysis or acute pancreatitis. Supportive care and medication are important [28]. Blood and blood product replacement, hemodialysis and other medications are arranged depending on the clinical and laboratory findings of the patient.

5.2. Treatment of complications

5.2.1. Acute complications

The most severe acute complications are esophageal and gastric perforations. These complications are diagnosed by regular chest or abdominal X-ray. Esophageal perforation is commonly described in adult patients. Aggressive surgical interventions such as esophagectomy or esophagostomy are recommended in adults with esophageal perforation [74, 75]. It is known that more conservative treatment modalities are preferred in several diseases in children. Tube thoracostomy into the pleural space or mediastinum may be performed. However, gastric perforation due to caustic ingestion is more often reported than esophageal perforation in children [76–78]. It is diagnosed by a pneumoperitoneum under the diaphragm and requires immediate surgery. Partial or total gastrectomy with roux-n-y gastrojejunostomy or esophagojejunostomy or different gastrointestinal reconstruction procedures may required.

5.2.2. Esophageal stricture

Esophageal stricture is most serious complication of caustic ingestion. It usually occurs in patients with grade 2a and more severe injury. Various treatment approaches ranging from minimally invasive methods such as balloon dilatation to aggressive surgery such as colonic transposition have been described.

5.2.2.1. Dilatation

Bougienage has traditionally been used as a first step in the treatment of esophageal stricture. Bougienage can be performed both antegradely by using Savary-Gilliard dilatators over a guide wire and retrogradely via gastrostomy. Balloon dilatation has recently become the most common and preferred method of dilatation [38, 79–81]. The dilatation force is applied equally and radially at the esophageal wall with balloon dilatation; rigid dilatators induce axial, radial, and shearing force [80, 82]. Balloon dilation can be performed easily with low complication rates in experienced hands. Esophageal perforation is the most serious complication of esophageal balloon dilatation and has been reported to occur in 0.33–45% of balloon dilatation sessions in previous studies [38, 80, 83, 84]. Esophageal perforations usually occur in patients with delayed treatment or with long segment strictures that have become fibrotic. Esophageal perforations that occur secondary to dilatation are almost always treated with a conservative approach [38, 76, 79]. Respiratory distress, fever, or severe chest pain could cause a perforation after dilatation. Chest X-ray may reveal pneumothorax or pneumomediastinum. Treatment with broad spectrum antibiotics and the interruption of feeding are the initial treatment steps. Chest tube insertion may be required in respiratory distress or in the presence of pleural effusion. However, complication rates can be reduced by using a staged dilatation, i.e., gradually increasing the diameter over consecutive sessions to the required balloon diameter with experienced hands [38, 79]. It is known as remodeling time; stabilization of the esophageal stricture requires between 6 months and 3 years. In light of this information, long-term dilatation may be required in severe cases [38, 85]. Gündoğdu et al. reported that the success rate of conservative approach was higher in patients younger than 8 years of age, and in strictures due to caustics other than lye involving upper third portion and less than 5 cm of length [85]. Repeated hospitalization and general anesthesia are accepted as disadvantages of long-term dilatation. Doo et al. reported a 91% technical success rate and a 64% clinical success rate [84]. Kim et al. obtained a 100% technical success rate and a 46% clinical success rate in their patients [39]. However, Alshammari et al. reported a 33% failure rates for balloon dilatation of caustic esophageal strictures [86]. Temiz et al. reported the results of long-term dilatation up to 4 years; full recovery occurred with long-term dilatation [38]. The author suggested that balloon dilatation is a safe and effective method and that the dilatation program should be carried out for at least 2 years before deciding that dilatation has failed [38]. Tiryaki et al. reported their experience with early prophylactic bougienage methods. They found that the strictures had resolved after 6 months of dilatation in patients initially treated prophylactically with early bougienage, whereas stricture resolution did not occur for more than 1 year in patients in whom dilatation began after stricture development [54]. Uygun et al. evaluated their early and late dilatation results in patients with short and long segments caustic esophageal strictures [79]. They reported a 100% success rate. Also, they reported that treatment with early balloon dilatation was significantly faster and shorter than that in the late dilatation group, and short stricture treatment was also of significantly shorter duration than long stricture treatment [79]. However, there are no controlled data to support the use of early dilatation, which could increase the risk of perforation [87].

Balloon dilatation is usually performed as one dilatation every 3 weeks for the first 3 months with subsequent modifications as required thereafter [88]. However, the patient's complaints and clinical condition are the most influential factor on the frequency of sessions. Temiz et al. reported that dilatations were performed weekly initially [38]. Eventually, balloon dilatation will be accepted as a safe and effective treatment modality with a low rate of complications for caustic esophageal strictures [38, 42, 79, 89].

5.2.2.1.1. Balloon dilatation technique

This operation is performed under general anesthesia. The radiopaque guide wire is introduced fluoroscopically or endoscopically to the stomach. The balloon catheter is pushed over the wire and placed in the stricture. Then, the balloon is inflated with radiocontrast solution. The balloon is inflated until a flattening of the hourglass deformity of the stricture observed for 2–4 minutes [38, 42] (**Figure 10a–c**). The same procedure is applied at each location for multiple or long segment strictures. The first dilatation starts with the smallest balloon even 4 or 6 mm diameter. The balloon sizes are increased to the appropriate diameter equal to the patient's esophageal diameter, defined by the thumb rule, i.e., the esophageal diameter is equal to the diameter of the patient's own thumb [42, 90].

5.2.2.2. Stenting

Intraluminal esophageal stenting is an option in cases of intractable strictures. It should be mentioned that stenting should be continued until complete esophageal healing. Therefore, stenting is a long-term treatment strategy. Mutaf reported outcomes with polytetrafluorethylene stents

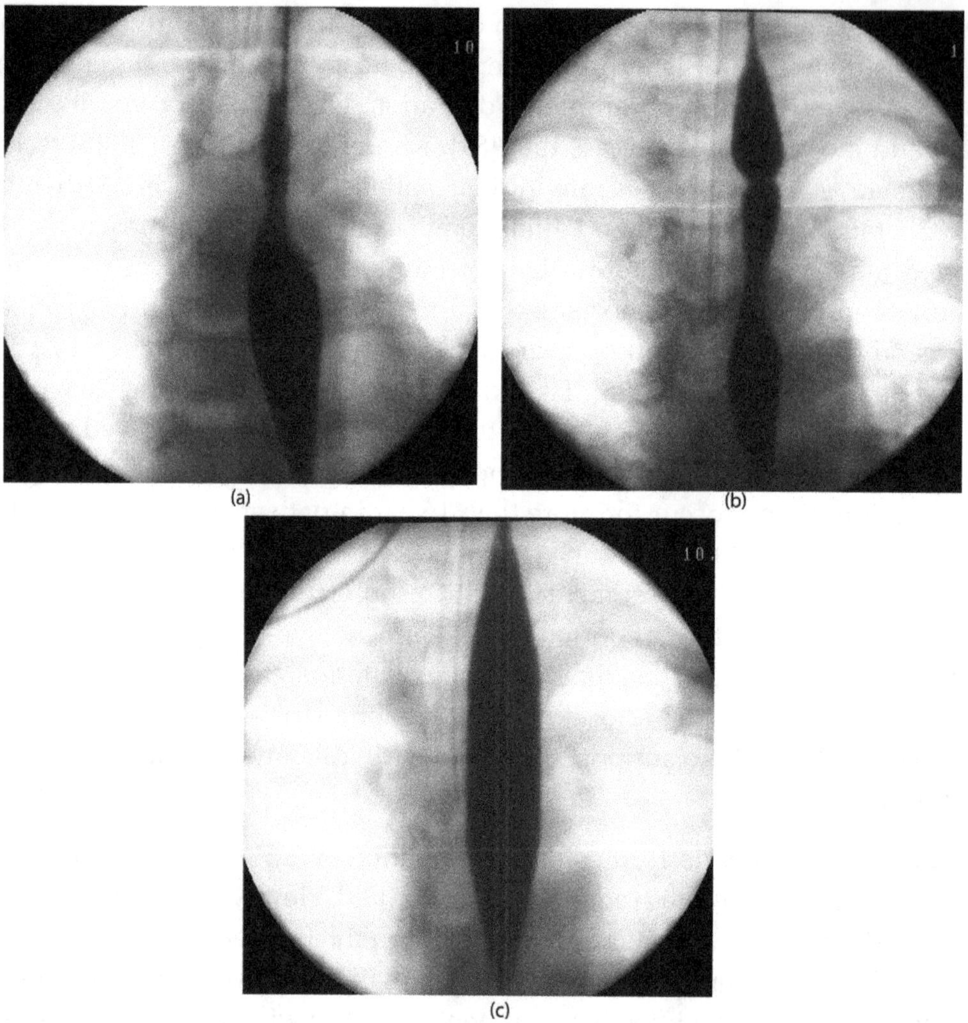

Figure 10. (a)–(c) The balloon catheter is pushed over the wire and placed in the stricture. Then, the balloon is inflated with radiocontrast solution until a flattening of the hourglass deformity.

5 mm in diameter or larger [88]. The stent was replaced with a 1 mm larger stent every third week, and was left in place for 1 year after a stent diameter of 10 mm was reached. However, stent placement is usually applied after dilatation session in different series [91–93]. Using this method, a success rate of 68% was reported. Atabek et al. also reported that 72.7% of their patients resumed normal feeding after 9–14 months of stenting. So, long-term stenting is an effective method to reduce the necessity for major surgical intervention for recalcitrant esophageal strictures [91]. Foschia et al. reported an 86.6% success rate with dynamic stents. They claimed that stenting reduces the necessity of dilatation sessions [92]. Gastroesophageal reflux and poor patient compliance are the most commonly encountered causes of stenting failure [88]. However, stents can worsen esophagitis by increasing reflux. The migration of stents, sialorrhea, retching, esophageal subclavian fistula, stent dislocation and perforation, soft plate injury, swallowing difficulties, chest pain, and vomiting are the reported complications [88, 91, 93]. Zhang et al. reported complete improvement in all their limited number of patients with self-expanding stents without serious complications [94]. Recently, self-expandable, biodegradable stents have become available and usable for the treatment of esophageal strictures. Stent integ-

rity and a radial force that continues for 6–8 weeks are seen as the advantages of the approach [87]. However, there have been no controlled trials yet on these stents.

5.2.2.3. Topical mitomycin C and steroid treatment

These options are based on their antifibroblastic properties, with a preventive effect on collagen synthesis and chronic scarring [42, 95–97]. El-Asmar et al. performed a double-blinded, randomized, placebo-controlled trial on the effects of topical mitomycin C application in patients with caustic esophageal strictures [98]. They found that topical mitomycin C application statistically significantly reduced the number of dilatation sessions. Mitomycin C is usually recommended at a dose of 0.4 mg/ml, which is applied with cotton or a pledget via a rigid endoscope [98, 99]. Additionally, submucosal application of triamcinolone acetonide, a member of the steroid family, has been used in patients with refractory caustic strictures. It can be applied together with endoscopic dilation [42, 97]. In the treatment approach, 2 ml (40 mg/ml) of triamcinolone acetonide is injected into quadrant 3 or 4 of the esophageal stricture at intervals of 2 or 3 weeks until full recovery [42].

5.2.2.4. Surgery

It is well established that the child's own esophagus is the ideal option and the esophagus should be preserved without any replacement for native esophagus [100–103]. The ideal organ to be used for replacement is expected to deliver food efficiently from the mouth to the intestinal system, to be resistant to stomach acid, grow parallel to the child, preserving cardiac and respiratory functions [101, 102]. The indication of esophageal replacement in patients with caustic stricture is failure of normal swallowing [100] (**Figure 11a** and **b**). Although multiple strictures, longer than 5-cm stricture and tortuous strictures, which do not allow to passage of the guidewire are the contraindications of esophageal dilatation, it is still controversial

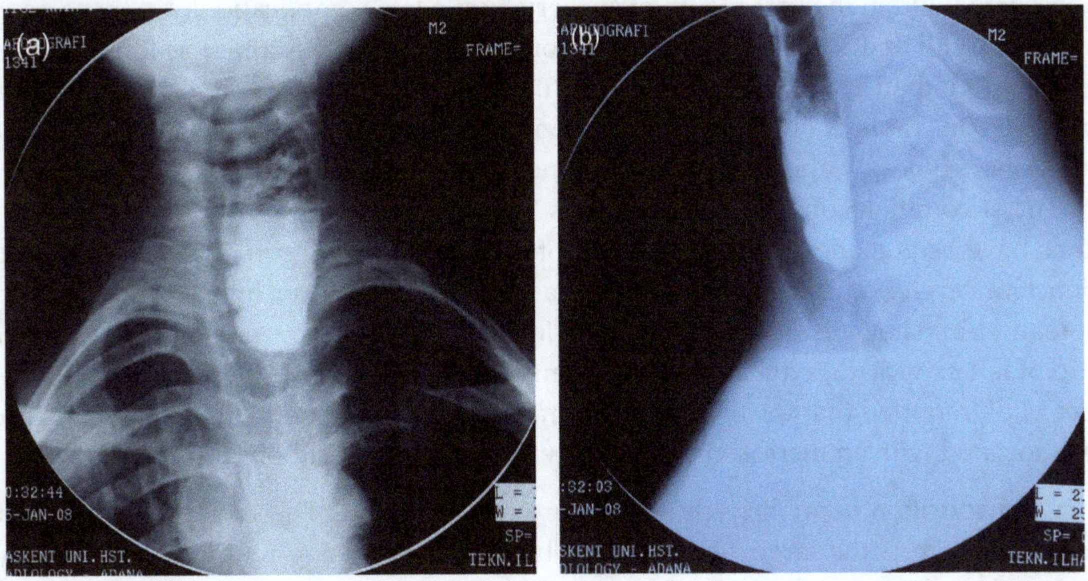

Figure 11. Complete obstruction of the cervical esophagus prevents oral feeding. Posterior-anterior (a) and lateral (b) frame of obstruction.

[38, 100]. Psychological problems may also occur secondary to prolonged dilatation, which required repeated anesthesia are other indications for esophageal replacement [100]. Spitz reported that necessity of regular dilatation for 6–12 months following the ingestion constituted an indication for esophageal replacement in caustic esophageal injury [104]. Gundoğdu et al. suggested that difficulty to swallow saliva, total or nearly total obliteration of the lumen involving more than 3 cm of an esophagus at admittance, difficulty in swallowing within one-month period following the recent dilation after completion of one-year dilation program were the main indications of esophageal replacement [105]. Social and psychological problems due to the lack of normal feeding or swallow, interrupted schooling and domestic family problems secondary to prolonged and multiple hospital admissions may be also considered other reasons of esophageal substations [102].

Surgical techniques include resection and end-to-end anastomosis, colonic or jejunal interposition, reversed gastric tube, or gastric transposition have been described for esophageal replacement in patients with resistant strictures [100, 104, 106]. Although the colon is the most commonly used intestinal component, progressively increased gastric transposition has been reported in recent years. Colonic interposition can be performed in the posterior mediastinum with transhiatal esophagectomy. It can be also done retrosternally by leaving the native esophagus.

Various segments of the colon can be used depending on the discretion of the surgeon [107, 108]. Ergün et al. used the left colon in 75% of their patients, while Bothereau et al. performed right colonic interposition in 87% of their patients [107, 108]. However, the latter authors reported no statistically significant difference in the complication rates [108]. Complications of colonic transposition are also frequently seen. Hamza et al. reported 1% mortality due to postoperative respiratory problems or sepsis [100]. Bothereau et al. reported 4% mortality secondary to complications [108]. Complications are classified under three main titles as early, late, and long-term complications. Early complications are defined as those occurred within the first month of surgery, while late complications are those occurred between 1 month and 1 year after surgery. Complications are described as long-term, while occurring more than 1 year after operation [109]. Complications of colonic interposition are summarized in **Table 2** [100, 107–112]. Cervical anastomotic leakage, adhesive intestinal obstructions, coloesophageal stricture, redundancy, gastrocolic reflux, and graft necrosis are the most common complications (**Figures 12** and **13a** and **b**). Furthermore, several suggestions have been made to reduce the rate of complications. Ergün et al. reported that the incidence of cervical anastomotic stricture was significantly lower by two-stage procedure. Bothereau et al. showed the upper thoracic inlet enlargement by resection of manubrium and tip of left clavicle to reduce the rate of complications in colonic interposition [108]. Also, Chirica et al. reported that the absence of thoracic inlet enlargement, delayed reconstruction were associated with an increased risk of early and late complications in adults [113].

Gastric transposition is another choice of surgical treatment. The method popularized by Spitz et al. which is the largest-scale study, has been increasingly utilized in recent years [103]. It is based on the good blood supply of the stomach. The right gastric and gastroepiploic vessels are preserved, and the left gastric and left gastroepiploic vessels are ligated. After the stomach is fully mobilized and passed transhiatal, posterior mediastinally, fundus

Intraoperative complication	Pneumothorax
	Tracheal injury
	Major bleeding
	Recurrent laryngeal injury
Early complications	Death
	Greft necrosis
	Respiratory failure
	Gstrocolic reflux
	Sepsis
	Fistula
	Cervical anastomotic stricture
	Cologastric anastomosis stricture
	Dehiscence of colocolic anastomosis
	Dehiscence of cologastric anastomosis
	Dumping syndrome
	Intussusception
	Enterocutaneous fistula
	Biliary reflux
Late complications	Anastomotic stricture
	Reflux
	Redundancy
	Ulceration
	Greft hernia into the pleura
	Intestinal obstruction
	Aspiration pneumonia
	Incisional hernia
	Postprandial neck bulge
Long-term complication	Relux
	Dysphagia
	Pain
	Nocturnal regurgitation
	Redundancy
	Anastomotic stricture
	Ulceration
	Scoliosis
	Malnutrition

Table 2. Complications of colonic interposition [100, 107–112].

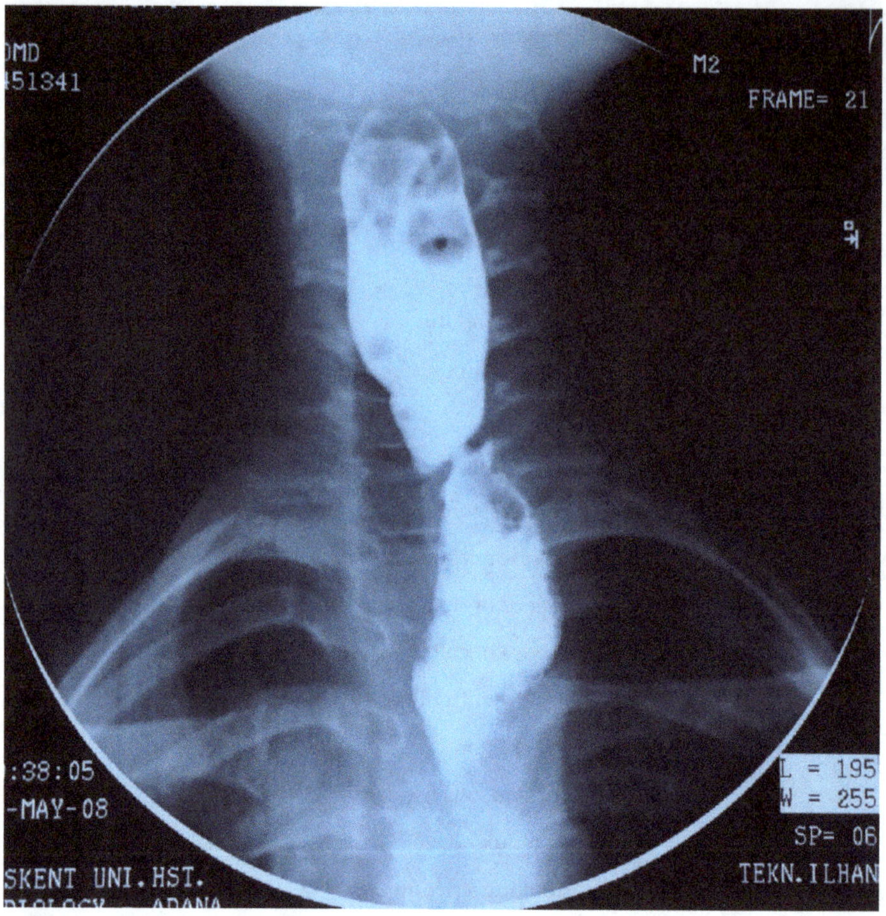

Figure 12. Coloesophageal stricture in a 14 years old girl underwent colonic interposition.

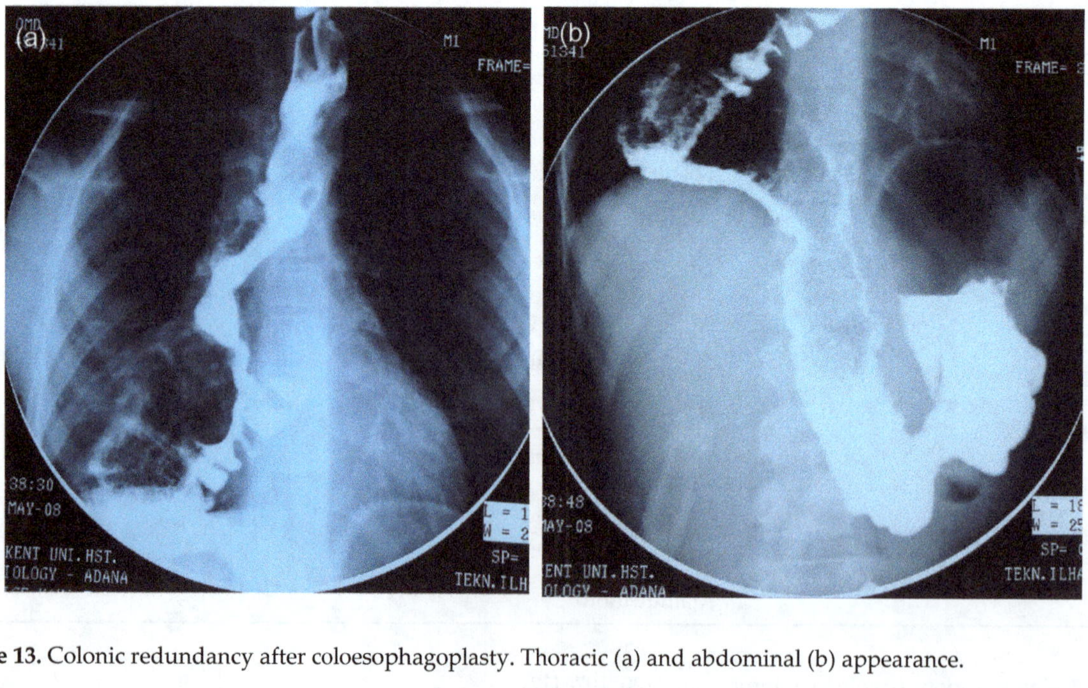

Figure 13. Colonic redundancy after coloesophagoplasty. Thoracic (a) and abdominal (b) appearance.

is pulled up from the cervical incision. Anastomosis between the stomach and esophagus is performed between the gastric fundus, which is easily mobilized and has a good blood supply and the cervical esophagus. Pyloroplasty or pyloromyotomy is carried out with the aim of facilitating gastric emptying [101, 102, 104]. Gastric transposition can usually be performed without thoracotomy. Spitz et al. performed thoracotomy in selected patients, due to dense fibrous tissues [114]. The most common complications of total gastric transposition up are the anastomotic leakage, stenosis, swallowing disorders, delayed gastric emptying, and mortality [101, 103, 114, 115]. Anastomotic leakage usually resolves spontaneously, while it requires surgical correction in a few cases [114, 115]. Stenosis usually improves with a number of dilatation sessions [114, 115]. Spitz reported that 94% of patients with swallowing difficulties experienced major swallowing problems before the gastric transposition. Severe gastric emptying problem may require converting to the pyloroplasty or Roux-en-Y gastrojejunostomy [103]. Spitz found the result of gastric transpositions to be good to excellent in terms of absence of swallowing difficulties or other gastrointestinal symptoms in 90% of their patients [114]. In another study, Marujo reported excellent and good results in 85 and 15% of patients, respectively [115]. In addition, Angotti et al. reported that all patients had gain weight and height postoperatively [101]. Davenport et al. also reported the long-term results of gastric transposition and showed that gastric transposition allowed satisfactory growth and nutrition for the majority of children [116]. The authors also observed respiratory symptoms in a number of patients and suggested that respiratory symptoms were related to small lung volume, rather than an increased airway resistance. In another study, Tannuri et al. compared esophagocoloplasty and gastric transposition in terms of early complications and mortality [117]. The authors reported that minor complications were statistically significantly higher in colonic transposition, while the rate of major complications was statistically significantly higher in gastric transposition. However, they found no significant difference in the mortality rates between the groups. Hence, they recommended esophagocoloplasty based on their experiences.

5.2.3. Gastric outlet obstruction

Gastric injury is less encountered than esophageal injury in caustic ingestion. Gastric outlet obstruction may develop as early as 3 weeks or as late as 10 weeks [118]. Endoscopy is recommended to diagnose the gastric injury and to tailor the treatment modality. There are two different approaches including minimal invasive technique, endoscopic balloon dilatation of the obstruction, and surgical intervention to resolve the obstructions [43, 45, 119, 120].

5.2.3.1. Endoscopic dilatation

On the other hand, there is limited experience on endoscopic treatment of gastric outlet obstruction secondary to the caustic ingestion in children. Treem et al. reported successful treatment outcomes of pyloric obstruction secondary to caustic ingestion with endoscopy-guided balloon dilatation before three decades. Nasr et al. also reported two patients who underwent endoscopic dilatation; one of them improved only with dilatation. Dehghani et al. reported a patient with pyloric stenosis treated with balloon dilatation [118]. The authors achieved normal pyloric canal after four dilatation sessions. In another study, Temiz et al. attempted endoscopic dilatation in seven patients with corrosive stricture, and performed successful dilatation in five of them [119]. However, symptoms of pyloric obstruction recurred in three patients. Due to the inability to pass the guidewire through the pylorus, they were unable to reperform dilatation. Despite low successful rates, the authors recommended endoscopic balloon dilatation before a surgical intervention.

5.2.3.2. *Technique of balloon dilatation*

Endoscopy is performed under general anesthesia. After focusing on the pylorus, a radiopaque guidewire is inserted through the pylorus under the guidance of endoscopy. A balloon catheter is passed over the guidewire and through the pylorus. The location of the balloon is monitored endoscopically. Then, the balloon is inflated with a radiopaque solution under fluoroscopic guidance. Inflation is performed for at least 2 minutes after the expansion of hourglass deformity of the obstruction [119] (**Figure 14a–c**).

5.2.3.3. *Surgical options*

To date, several surgical techniques including Heicke-Mikulicz pyloroplasty, Finney pyloroplasty, Jabulay pyloroplasty, gastrojejunostomy, and Billroth-I procedure have been described for the treatment of acquired gastric outlet obstructions [12, 119, 120]. The preference may vary depending on the discretion of the surgeon. Ozcan et al. performed retrocolic gastrojejunostomy in all patients, while Ozokutan et al. performed gastroduodenostomy and Billroth-I procedure [45, 120]. However, the timing of surgery is of utmost importance for the method to be selected. Surgical intervention is recommended at the end of cicatrization period of caustic injury [44, 119, 121]. Due to anastomotic stricture, secondary to the progressive inflammatory process may develop in early operated patients. Temiz et al. reported anastomotic stricture in a case that underwent gastrojejunostomy after 6 weeks of injury. Endoscopic dilatation may help to solve this problem [119] (**Figure 15a** and **b**). Dumping syndrome is another postoperative clinical condition. Ozcan suggested an anastomosis not exceeding 2 cm to prevent postoperative dumping syndrome [45].

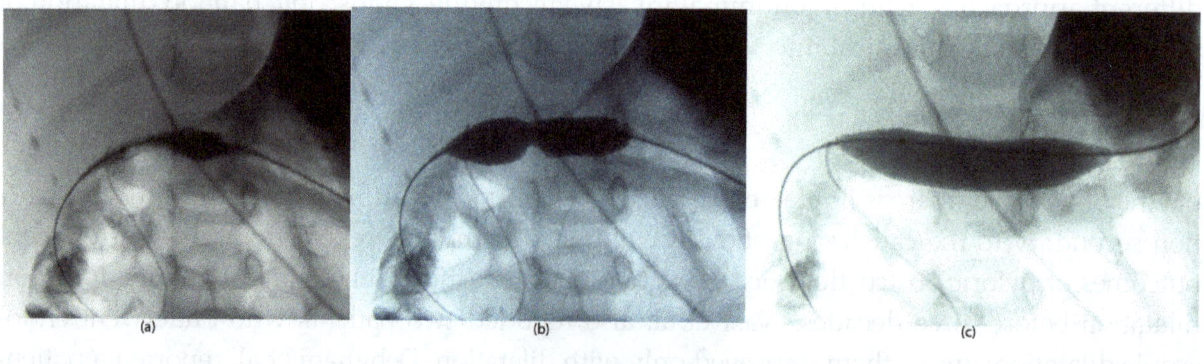

Figure 14. (a)–(c) After placement of guide wire under endoscopic guidance through the pyloric stenosis, a balloon catheter is passed over the guidewire and inflated with radiocontrast solution until a flattening of the hourglass deformity.

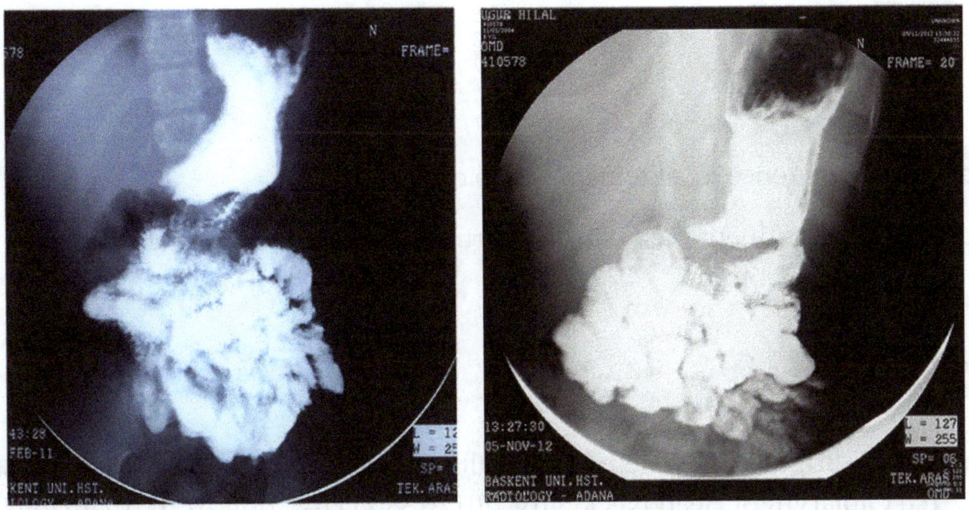

Figure 15. Anastomotic stricture was revealed by gstrography (a), after ballon dilatation easy flow from gastrojejunostomy is seen (b).

5.2.4. Gastroesophageal reflux

Caustic esophageal injury results with narrowed and also shortened esophagus [122]. This process alters the lower esophageal sphincter function, which leads to gastroesophageal reflux. As a consequence, reflux can adversely affect the development of stenosis and response to treatment of the stenosis. Mutaf et al. recommended that patients with caustic esophageal burn should be screened for gastroesophageal reflux during the treatment period [122]. The most preferred surgical procedures for gastroesophageal reflux disease include the Nissen, Thal, and BoixOchoa procedures. However, all these procedures have a significant recurrence rate in the patients, particularly with a shortened esophagus. In addition, Collis gastroplasty with partial or complete fundoplication can be used as alternative surgical techniques in the treatment of a shortened esophagus (**Figure 16a** and **b**).

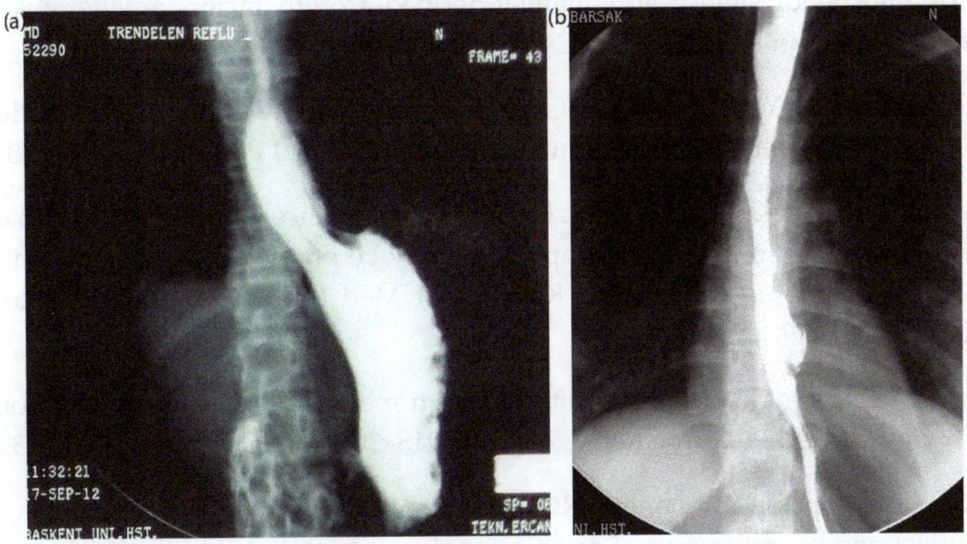

Figure 16. The sliding type of hiatal hernia (a) was ameliorated with Collis gatsroplasty (b).

Author details

Abdulkerim Temiz

Address all correspondence to: aktemiz@yahoo.com

Başkent University, Faculty of Medicine, Department of Pediatric Surgery, Turkey

References

[1] Johnson CM, Brigger MT: The public health impact of pediatric caustic ingestion injuries. Arch Otolaryngol Head Neck Surg. 2012;138:1111–5. doi: 10.1001/jamaoto.2013.672.

[2] de Jong AL, Macdonald R, Ein S, Forte V, Turner A: Corrosive esophagitis in children: a 30-year review. Int J Pediatr Otorhinolaryngol. 2001;57:203–11.

[3] Arévalo-Silva C, Eliashar R, Wohlgelernter J, Elidan J, Gross M: Ingestion of caustic substances: a 15-year experience. Laryngoscope. 2006;116:1422–6.

[4] Urgancı N, Usta M, Kalyoncu D, Demirel E: Corrosive substance ingestion in children. Indian J Pediatr. 2014;81:675–9. doi: 10.1007/s12098-013-1170-0.

[5] Temiz A, Oguzkurt P, Ezer SS, Ince E, Hicsonmez A: Predictability of outcome of caustic ingestion by esophagogastroduodenoscopy in children. World J Gastroenterol. 2012;18:1098–103. doi: 10.3748/wjg.v18.i10.1098.

[6] Lupa M, Magne J, Guarisco JL, Amedee R: Update on the diagnosis and treatment of caustic ingestion. Ochsner J. 2009;9:54–9.

[7] Somuncu S, Cakmak M, Erdogan S, Caglayan O, Akman H, Kaya M: Trapidil, an inhibitor for phosphodiesterase and platelet-derived-growth factor, ameliorates corrosive esophageal burn in rats. Tohoku J Exp Med. 2005;207:203–8.

[8] Ozel SK, Dagli TE, Yuksel M, Kiyan G, Kotiloglu E: The roles of free oxygen radicals, nitric oxide, and endothelin in caustic injury of rat esophagus. J Pediatr Surg. 2004;39:1381–5.

[9] Temiz A, Ünal B, Koçer NE, Oğuzkurt P, Ezer SS, İnce E, Yalçın HS, Hiçsönmez A: Late complications of corrosive esophagitis may be predicted using biochemical methods: preliminary report. Türkiye Klinikleri J Med Sci. 2012;32:193–200. doi:10.5336/medsci.2011-25229.

[10] Contini S, Scarpignato C: Caustic injury of the upper gastrointestinal tract: a comprehensive review. World J Gastroenterol. 2013;19:3918–30. doi:10.3748/wjg.v19.i25.3918.

[11] Mattos GM, Lopes DD, Mamede RC, Ricz H, Mello-Filho FV, Neto JB: Effects of time of contact and concentration of caustic agent on generation of injuries. Laryngoscope. 2006;116:456–60.

[12] Ciftci AO, Senocak ME, Büyükpamukçu N, Hiçsönmez A: Gastric outlet obstruction due to corrosive ingestion: incidence and outcome. Pediatr Surg Int. 1999;15:88–91.

[13] Gaudreault P, Parent M, McGuigan MA, Chicoine L, Lovejoy FH: Predictability of esophageal injury from signs and symptoms: a study of caustic ingestion in 378 children. Pediatrics. 1983;71: 767–70.

[14] Lamireau T, Rebouissoux L, Denis D, Lancelin F, Vergnes P, Fayon M: Accidental caustic ingestion in children: is endoscopy always mandatory? J Pediatr Gastroenterol Nutr. 2001;33:81–4.

[15] Boskovic A, Stankovic I: Predictability of gastroesophageal caustic injury from clinical findings: is endoscopy mandatory in children? Eur J Gastroenterol Hepatol. 2014;26:499–503. doi: 10.1097/MEG.0000000000000060.

[16] Nijhawan S, Jain P: Acute pancreatitis as an unusual complication of corrosive ingestion. J Gastrointestin Liver Dis. 2007;16:345–6.

[17] Gupta V, Kurdia KC, Sharma A, Mishra AK, Yadav TD, Kochhar R: Tracheoesophageal fistula in adults due to corrosive ingestion: challenges in management. Updates Surg. 2015;67:75–81. doi: 10.1007/s13304-015-0292-5.

[18] Samad L, Ali M, Ramzi H: Button battery ingestion: hazards of esophageal impaction. J Pediatr Surg. 1999;34:1527–31.

[19] Marom T, Goldfarb A, Russo E, Roth Y: Battery ingestion in children. Int J Pediatr Otorhinolaryngol. 2010;74:849–54. doi: 10.1016/j.ijporl.2010.05.019.

[20] Votteler TP, Nash JC, Rutledge JC: The hazard of ingested alkaline disk batteries in children. JAMA. 1983;249:2504–6.

[21] Litovitz T, Schmitz BF: Ingestion of cylindrical and button batteries: an analysis of 2382 cases. Pediatrics. 1992;89:747–57.

[22] Bass DH, Millar AJ: Mercury absorption following button battery ingestion. J Pediatr Surg. 1992;27:1541–2.

[23] Hamilton JM, Schraff SA, Notrica DM: Severe injuries from coin cell battery ingestions: 2 case reports. J Pediatr Surg. 2009;44:644–7. doi: 10.1016/j.jpedsurg.2008.10.110.

[24] Loots DP, du Toit-Prinsloo L, Saayman G: Disk battery ingestion: a rare cause of perforation of the brachiocephalic artery. Forensic Sci Med Pathol. 2015;11:614–7. doi: 10.1007/s12024-015-9706-4.

[25] Stiff G, Alwafi A, Rees BI, Lari J: Corrosive injuries of the oesophagus and stomach: experience in management at a regional paediatric centre. Ann R Coll Surg Engl. 1996;78:119–23.

[26] Di Costanzo J, Noirclerc M, Jouglard J, Escoffier JM, Cano N, Martin J, Gauthier A: New therapeutic approach to corrosive burns of the upper gastrointestinal tract. Gut. 1980;21:370–75.

[27] Zargar SA, Kochhar R, Mehta S, Mehta SK: The role of fiberoptic endoscopy in the management of corrosive ingestion and modified endoscopic classification of burns. Gastrointest Endosc. 1991;37:165–9.

[28] Poley JW, Steyerberg EW, Kuipers EJ, Dees J, Hartmans R, Tilanus HW, Siersema PD: Ingestion of acid and alkaline agents: outcome and prognostic value of early upper endoscopy. Gastrointest Endosc. 2004;60:372–7.

[29] Baskin D, Urganci N, Abbasoğlu L, Alkim C, Yalçin M, Karadağ C, Sever N: A standardised protocol for the acute management of corrosive ingestion in children. Pediatr Surg Int. 2004;20:824–8.

[30] Ryu HH, Jeung KW, Lee BK, Uhm JH, Park YH, Shin MH, Kim HL, Heo T, Min YI: Caustic injury: can CT grading system enable prediction of esophageal stricture? Clin Toxicol (Phila). 2010;48:137–42. doi: 10.3109/15563650903585929.

[31] Keh SM, Onyekwelu N, McManus K, McGuigan J: Corrosive injury to upper gastrointestinal tract: still a major surgical dilemma. World J Gastroenterol. 2006;12:5223–8.

[32] Kua K, Jonas N, O'Donnell R: The larynx and caustic soda ingestion. Arch Dis Child. 2015;100:570. doi: 10.1136/archdischild-2014-307588.

[33] Shabino CL, Feinberg A: Esophageal perforation secondary to alkaline battery ingestion. JACEP. 1979;8:360–3.

[34] Chiang MC, Chen YS: Tracheoesophageal fistula secondary to disc battery ingestion. Am J Otolaryngol. 2000;21:333–6.

[35] Anand TS, Kumar S, Wadhwa V, Dhawan R: Rare case of spontaneous closure of tracheo-esophageal fistula secondary to disc battery ingestion. Int J Pediatr Otorhinolaryngol. 2002;63:57–9.

[36] Grisel JJ, Richter GT, Casper KA, Thompson DM: Acquired tracheoesophageal fistula following disc-battery ingestion: can we watch and wait? Int J Pediatr Otorhinolaryngol. 2008;72:699–706. doi: 10.1016/j.ijporl.2008.01.015.

[37] Okuyama H, Kubota A, Oue T, Kuroda S, Nara K, Takahashi T: Primary repair of tracheoesophageal fistula secondary to disc battery ingestion: a case report. J Pediatr Surg. 2004;39:243–4.

[38] Temiz A, Oguzkurt P, Ezer SS, Ince E, Hicsonmez A: Long-term management of corrosive esophageal stricture with balloon dilation in children. Surg Endosc. 2010;24:2287–92. doi: 10.1007/s00464-010-0953-x.

[39] Kim JH, Song HY, Kim HC, Shin JH, Kim KR, Park SW, Jung HY, Lee GH, Park SI: Corrosive esophageal strictures: Long-term effectiveness of balloon dilation in 117 patients. J Vasc Interv Radiol. 2008;19:736–41.

[40] Huang YC, Ni YH, Lai HS, Chang MH: Corrosive esophagitis in children: Pediatr Surg Int. 2004;20:207–10.

[41] Broto J, Asensio M, Jorro CS, Marhuenda C, Vernet JM, Acosta D, Ochoa JB: Conservative treatment of caustic esophageal injuries in children: 20 years of experience. Pediatr Surg Int. 1999;15:323–5.

[42] Bicakci U, Tander B, Deveci G, Rizalar R, Ariturk E, Bernay F: Minimally invasive management of children with caustic ingestion: less pain for patients. Pediatr Surg Int. 2010;26:251–5. doi: 10.1007/s00383-009-2525-5.

[43] Tekant G, Eroğlu E, Erdoğan E, Yeşildağ E, Emir H, Büyükünal C, Yeker D: Corrosive injury-induced gastric outlet obstruction: a changing spectrum of agents and treatment. J Pediatr Surg. 2001;36:1004–7.

[44] Kaushik R, Singh R, Sharma R, Attri AK, Bawa AS: Corrosive-induced gastric outlet obstruction. Yonsei Med J. 2003;44:991–4.

[45] Ozcan C, Ergün O, Sen T, Mutaf O: Gastric outlet obstruction secondary to acid ingestion in children. J Pediatr Surg. 2004;39:1651–3.

[46] Appelqvist P, Salmo M: Lye corrosion carcinoma of the esophagus: a review of 63 cases. Cancer. 1980;45:2655–8.

[47] Kozarek RA, Sanowski RA: Caustic cicatrization of the pharynx associated with dysphagia and premalignant mucosal changes. Am J Gastroenterol. 1982;77:5–8.

[48] Zhang X, Wang M, Han H, Xu Y, Shi Z, Ma G: Corrosive induced carcinoma of esophagus after 58 years. Ann Thorac Surg. 2012;94:2103–5. doi: 10.1016/j.athoracsur.2012.03.110.

[49] Kochhar R, Sethy PK, Kochhar S, Nagi B, Gupta NM: Corrosive induced carcinoma of esophagus: report of three patients and review of literature. J Gastroenterol Hepatol. 2006;21:777–80. doi: 10.1111/j.1440-1746.2006.03211.x.

[50] Rigo GP, Camellini L, Azzolini F, Guazzetti S, Bedogni G, Merighi A, Bellis L, Scarcelli A, Manenti F: What is the utility of selected clinical and endoscopic parameters in predicting the risk of death after caustic ingestion? Endoscopy. 2002;34:304–10.

[51] Cheng YJ, Kao EL: Arterial blood gas analysis in acute caustic ingestion injuries. Surg Today. 2003;33:483–5.

[52] Thompson JN: Corrosive esophageal injuries. I. A study of nine cases of concurrent accidental caustic ingestion. Laryngoscope. 1987;97:1060–8.

[53] Doğan Y, Erkan T, Cokuğraş FC, Kutlu T: Caustic gastroesophageal lesions in childhood: an analysis of 473 cases. Clin Pediatr (Phila). 2006;45:435–8.

[54] Tiryaki T, Livanelioğlu Z, Atayurt H: Early bougienage for relief of stricture formation following caustic esophageal burns. Pediatr Surg Int. 2005;21:78–80.

[55] Iqbal CW, Askegard-Giesmann JR, Pham TH, Ishitani MB, Moir CR: Pediatric endoscopic injuries: incidence, management, and outcomes. J Pediatr Surg. 2008;43:911–5. doi: 10.1016/j.jpedsurg.2007.12.036.

[56] Gupta SK, Croffie JM, Fitzgerald JF: Is esophagogastroduodenoscopy necessary in all caustic ingestions? J Pediatr Gastroenterol Nutr. 2001;32:50–3.

[57] Millar AJ, Numanoglu A, Mann M, Marven S, Rode H: Detection of caustic oesophageal injury with technetium 99m-labelled sucralfate. J Pediatr Surg. 2001;36:262–5.

[58] Çiftçi ÖD, Gül SS, Açıksarı K, Maman A, Çavuşoğlu T, Bademci R, Taskiran D, Erbaş O: The diagnostic utility of scintigraphy in esophageal burn: a rat model. J Surg Res. 2016;200: 495–500. doi: 10.1016/j.jss.2015.09.006.

[59] Aksu B, Durmus-Altun G, Ustun F, Torun N, Kanter M, Umit H, Sut N: A new imaging modality in detection of caustic oesophageal injury: technetium-99m pyrophosphate scintigraphy. Int J Pediatr Otorhinolaryngol. 2009;73:409–15. doi:10.1016/j.ijporl. 2008.11.008.

[60] Maurer AH, Parkman HP: Update on gastrointestinal scintigraphy. Semin Nucl Med. 2006;36:110–8.

[61] Warrington JC, Charron M: Pediatric gastrointestinal nuclear medicine. Semin Nucl Med. 2007;37:269–85.

[62] Kochhar R, Mittal BR, Kumar S, Bhattacharya A, Sethy PK, Dutta U: Segmental and total oesophageal transit time in patients with corrosive-induced oesophageal stricture. Nucl Med Commun. 2007;28:920–3.

[63] Kamijo Y, Kondo I, Soma K, Imaizumi H, Ohwada T: Alkaline esophagitis evaluated by endoscopic ultrasound. J Toxicol Clin Toxicol. 2001;39:623–5.

[64] Kamijo Y, Kondo I, Kokuto M, Kataoka Y, Soma K: Miniprobe ultrasonography for determining prognosis in corrosive esophagitis. Am J Gastroenterol. 2004;99:851–4.

[65] Kamijo Y, Kondo I, Watanabe M, Kan'o T, Ide A, Soma K: Gastric stenosis in severe corrosive gastritis: prognostic evaluation by endoscopic ultrasonography. Clin Toxicol (Phila). 2007;45:284–6.

[66] Chiu HM, Lin JT, Huang SP, Chen CH, Yang CS, Wang HP: Prediction of bleeding and stricture formation after corrosive ingestion by EUS concurrent with upper endoscopy. Gastrointest Endosc. 2004;60:827–33.

[67] Pelclová D, Navrátil T: Do corticosteroids prevent oesophageal stricture after corrosive ingestion? Toxicol Rev. 2005;24:125–9.

[68] Fulton JA, Hoffman RS: Steroids in second degree caustic burns of the esophagus: a systematic pooled analysis of fifty years of human data: 1956–2006. Clin Toxicol (Phila). 2007;45:402–8.

[69] Anderson KD, Rouse TM, Randolph JG: A controlled trial of corticosteroids in children with corrosive injury of the esophagus. N Engl J Med. 1990;323:637–40.

[70] Mamede RC, De Mello Filho FV: Treatment of caustic ingestion: an analysis of 239 cases. Dis Esophagus. 2002;15:210–3.

[71] Bautista A, Varela R, Villanueva A, Estevez E, Tojo R, Cadranel S: Effects of prednisolone and dexamethasone in children with alkali burns of the oesophagus. Eur J Pediatr Surg. 1996;6:198–203.

[72] Usta M, Erkan T, Cokugras FC, Urganci N, Onal Z, Gulcan M, Kutlu T: High doses of methylprednisolone in the management of caustic esophageal burns. Pediatrics. 2014;133:E1518–24.

[73] Boukthir S, Fetni I, Mrad SM, Mongalgi MA, Debbabi A, Barsaoui S: High doses of steroids in the management of caustic esophageal burns in children. Arch Pediatr. 2004;11:13–7.

[74] Andreoni B, Farina ML, Biffi R, Crosta C: Esophageal perforation and caustic injury: emergency management of caustic ingestion. Dis Esophagus. 1997;10:95–100.

[75] Cattan P, Munoz-Bongrand N, Berney T, Halimi B, Sarfati E, Celerier M: Extensive abdominal surgery after caustic ingestion. Ann Surg. 2000;231:519–23.

[76] Gün F, Abbasoğlu L, Celik A: Acute gastric perforation after acid ingestion. J Pediatr Gastroenterol Nutr. 2002;35:360–2.

[77] Ceylan H, Ozokutan BH, Gündüz F, Gözen A: Gastric perforation after corrosive ingestion. Pediatr Surg Int. 2011;27:649–53. doi:10.1007/s00383-010-2739-6.

[78] Boybeyi O, Karnak I, Tanyel FC, Senocak ME: Management of unusually extensive esophagogastric corrosive injuries: emergency measures and gastric reconstruction. J Pediatr Surg. 2009;44:1022–6. doi:10.1016/j.jpedsurg.2009.02.001.

[79] Uygun I, Arslan MS, Aydogdu B, Okur MH, Otcu S: Fluoroscopic balloon dilatation for caustic esophageal stricture in children: an 8-year experience. J Pediatr Surg. 2013;48:2230–4. doi:10.1016/j.jpedsurg.2013.04.005.

[80] Lan LC, Wong KK, Lin SC, Sprigg A, Clarke S, Johnson PR, Tam PK: Endoscopic balloon dilatation of esophageal strictures in infants and children: 17 years' experience and a literature review. J Pediatr Surg. 2003;38:1712–5.

[81] Pyrtle J, Obando J: Endoscopic management of difficult benign esophageal stricture. Tech Gastrointest Endosc. 2007;9:74–83.

[82] Poddar U, Thapa BR: Benign esophageal strictures in infants and children: results of Savary-Gilliard bougie dilation in 107 Indian children. Gastrointest Endosc. 2001;54:480–4.

[83] Kukkady A, Pease PW: Long-term dilatation of caustic strictures of the oesophagus. Pediatr Surg Int. 2002;18:486–90.

[84] Doo E-Y, Shin JH, Kim JH, Song H-Y: Oesophageal strictures caused by the ingestion of corrosive agents: effectiveness of balloon dilation in children. Clin Radiol. 2009; 64:265–71.

[85] Gündoğdu HZ, Tanyel FC, Büyükpamukçu N, Hiçsönmez A: Conservative treatment of caustic esophageal strictures in children. J Pediatr Surg. 1992;27:767–70.

[86] Alshammari J, Quesnel S, Pierrot S, Couloigner V: Endoscopic balloon dilatation of esophageal strictures in children. Int J Pediatr Otorhinolaryngol. 2011;75:1376–9. doi:10.1016/j.ijporl.2011.07.031.

[87] Vandenplas Y, Hauser B, Devreker T, Urbain D, Reynaert H: A biodegradable esophageal stent in the treatment of a corrosive esophageal stenosis in a child. J Pediatr Gastroenterol Nutr. 2009;49:254–7. doi: 10.1097/MPG.0b013e31819de871.

[88] Mutaf O: Treatment of corrosive esophageal strictures by long-term stenting. J Pediatr Surg. 1996;31:681–5.

[89] Chang CF, Kuo SP, Lin HC, Chuang CC, Tsai TK, Wu SF, Chen AC, Chen W, Peng CT: Endoscopic balloon dilatation for esophageal strictures in children younger than 6 years: experience in a medical center. Pediatr Neonatol. 2011;52:196–202. doi: 10.1016/j.pedneo.2011.05.005.

[90] Tam PKH, Sprigg A, Cudmore RE, Cook RC, Carty H: Endoscopy-guided balloon dilatation of esophageal strictures and anastomotic strictures after esophageal replacement in children. J Pediatr Surg. 1991;26:1101–3.

[91] Atabek C, Surer I, Demirbag S, Caliskan B, Ozturk H, Cetinkursun S: Increasing tendency in caustic esophageal burns and long-term polytetrafluorethylene stenting in severe cases: 10 years' experience. J Pediatr Surg. 2007;42:636–40.

[92] Foschia F, De Angelis P, Torroni F, Romeo E, Caldaro T, di Abriola GF, Pane A, Fiorenza MS, De Peppo F, Dall'Oglio L: Custom dynamic stent for esophageal strictures in children. J Pediatr Surg. 2011;46:848–53. doi: 10.1016/j.jpedsurg.2011.02.014.

[93] Zhang C, Zhou X, Yu L, Ding J, Shi R: Endoscopic therapy in the treatment of caustic esophageal stricture: a retrospective case series study. Dig Endosc. 2013;25:490–5. doi:10.1111/den.12023.

[94] Zhang C, Yu JM, Fan GP, Shi CR, Yu SY, Wang HP, Ge L, Zhong WX: The use of a retrievable self-expanding stent in treating childhood benign esophageal strictures. J Pediatr Surg. 2005;40:501–4.

[95] Heran MK, Baird R, Blair GK, Skarsgard ED: Topical mitomycin-C for recalcitrant esophageal strictures: a novel endoscopic/fluoroscopic technique for safe endoluminal delivery. J Pediatr Surg. 2008;43:815–8. doi: 10.1016/j.jpedsurg.2007.12.017.

[96] El-Asmar KM, Hassan MA, Abdelkader HM, Hamza AF: Topical mitomycin C can effectively alleviate dysphagia in children with long-segment caustic esophageal strictures. Dis Esophagus. 2015;28:422–7. doi: 10.1111/dote.12218.

[97] Kochhar R, Ray JD, Sriram PV, Kumar S, Singh K: Intralesional steroids augment the effects of endoscopic dilation in corrosive esophageal strictures. Gastrointest Endosc. 1999;49:509–13.

[98] El-Asmar KM, Hassan MA, Abdelkader HM, Hamza AF: Topical mitomycin C application is effective in management of localized caustic esophageal stricture: a double-blinded, randomized, placebo-controlled trial. J Pediatr Surg. 2013;48:1621–7. doi: 10.1016/j.jpedsurg.2013.04.014.

[99] Heran MK, Pham TH, Butterworth S, Robinson A: Use of a microporous polytetrafluoroethylene catheter balloon to treat refractory esophageal stricture: a novel technique for delivery of mitomycin C. J Pediatr Surg. 2011;46:776–9. doi: 10.1016/j.jpedsurg.2010.11.030.

[100] Hamza AF, Abdelhay S, Sherif H, Hasan T, Soliman H, Kabesh A, Bassiouny I, Bahnassy AF: Caustic esophageal strictures in children: 30 years' experience. J Pediatr Surg. 2003;38:828–33.

[101] Angotti R, Molinaro F, Noviello C, Cobellis G, Martino A, Del Rossi C, Bianchi A, Messina M: Gastric transposition as a valid surgical option for esophageal replacement in pediatric patients: experience from three Italian medical centers. Gastroenterol Rep (Oxf). 2016;pii: gow012:1–5. doi:10.1093/gastro/gow012.

[102] Arul GS, Parikh D: Oesophageal replacement in children. Ann R Coll Surg Engl. 2008;90:7–12. doi: 10.1308/003588408X242222.

[103] Spitz L, Kiely E, Pierro A: Gastric transposition in children—a 21-year experience. J Pediatr Surg. 2004;39:276–81; discussion 276–81.

[104] Spitz L: Esophageal replacement: overcoming the need. J Pediatr Surg. 2014;49:849–52. doi: 10.1016/j.jpedsurg.2014.01.011.

[105] Gündoğdu HZ, Tanyel FC, Büyükpamukçu N, Hiçsönmez A: Colonic replacement for the treatment of caustic esophageal strictures in children. J Pediatr Surg. 1992;27:771–4.

[106] Ezemba N, Eze JC, Nwafor IA, Etukokwu KC, Orakwe OI: Colon interposition graft for corrosive esophageal stricture: midterm functional outcome. World J Surg. 2014;38:2352–7. doi: 10.1007/s00268-014-2574-3.

[107] Ergün O, Celik A, Mutaf O: Two-stage coloesophagoplasty in children with caustic burns of the esophagus: hemodynamic basis of delayed cervical anastomosis—theory and fact. J Pediatr Surg. 2004;39:545–8.

[108] Bothereau H, Munoz-Bongrand N, Lambert B, Montemagno S, Cattan P, Sarfati E: Esophageal reconstruction after caustic injury: is there still a place for right coloplasty? Am J Surg. 2007;193:660–4.

[109] Coopman S, Michaud L, Halna-Tamine M, Bonnevalle M, Bourgois B, Turck D, Gottrand F: Long-term outcome of colon interposition after esophagectomy in children. J Pediatr Gastroenterol Nutr. 2008;47:458–62. doi: 10.1097/MPG.0b013e31815ce55c.

[110] Boukerrouche A: Left colonic graft in esophageal reconstruction for caustic stricture: mortality and morbidity. Dis Esophagus. 2013;26:788–93. doi: 10.1111/j.1442-2050.2012.01383.x.

[111] Boukerrouche A: Isoperistaltic left colic graft interposition via a retrosternal approach for esophageal reconstruction in patients with a caustic stricture: mortality, morbidity, and functional results. Surg Today. 2014;44:827–33. doi: 10.1007/s00595-013-0758-3.

[112] Raffensperger JG, Luck SR, Reynolds M, Schwartz D: Intestinal bypass of the esophagus. J Pediatr Surg. 1996;31:38–46; discussion 46–7.

[113] Chirica M, Veyrie N, Munoz-Bongrand N, Zohar S, Halimi B, Celerier M, Cattan P, Sarfati E: Late morbidity after colon interposition for corrosive esophageal injury: risk factors, management, and outcome. A 20-years' experience. Ann Surg. 2010;252:271–80. doi: 10.1097/SLA.0b013e3181e8fd40.

[114] Spitz L: Gastric transposition in children. Semin Pediatr Surg. 2009;18:30–3. doi: 10.1053/j.sempedsurg.2008.10.006.

[115] Marujo WC, Tannuri U, Maksoud JG: Total gastric transposition: an alternative to esophageal replacement in children. J Pediatr Surg. 1991;26:676–81.

[116] Davenport M, Hosie GP, Tasker RC, Gordon I, Kiely EM, Spitz L: Long-term effects of gastric transposition in children: a physiological study. J Pediatr Surg. 1996;31:588–93.

[117] Tannuri U, Maksoud-Filho JG, Tannuri AC, Andrade W, Maksoud JG: Which is better for esophageal substitution in children, esophagocoloplasty or gastric transposition? A 27-year experience of a single center. J Pediatr Surg. 2007;42:500–4.

[118] Dehghani SM, Aldaghi M, Javaherizadeh H: Endoscopic pyloroplasty for severe gastric outlet obstruction due to alkali ingestion in a child. Gastroenterol Hepatol Bed Bench. 2016;9:64–7.

[119] Temiz A, Oguzkurt P, Ezer SS, Ince E, Gezer HO, Hicsonmez A: Management of pyloric stricture in children: endoscopic balloon dilatation and surgery. Surg Endosc. 2012;26:1903–8. doi: 10.1007/s00464-011-2124-0.

[120] Ozokutan BH, Ceylan H, Ertaşkin I, Yapici S: Pediatric gastric outlet obstruction following corrosive ingestion. Pediatr Surg Int. 2010;26:615–8. doi: 10.1007/s00383-010-2613-6.

[121] Chaudhary A, Puri AS, Dhar P, Reddy P, Sachdev A, Lahoti D, Kumar N, Broor SL: Elective surgery for corrosive induced gastric injury. World J Surg. 1996;20:703–6

[122] Mutaf O, Genç A, Herek O, Demircan M, Ozcan C, Arikan A: Gastroesophageal reflux: a determinant in the outcome of caustic esophageal burns. J Pediatr Surg. 1996; 31:1494–5.

2

Anesthetic Management of Neonatal Emergency Abdominal Surgery

Esra Caliskan

Abstract

Anesthetic management of neonatal surgical emergencies presents serious difficulties and challenges for the anesthesiologist and is associated with increased risks of morbidity and mortality. Therefore, in these patients, anesthetic assessment should be directed to the patient's current disease and associated anomalies. The provision of safe anesthesia and perioperative management of these cases also depends on a clear understanding of the physiologic and hemodynamic variables of the preterm and term infants and a precise knowledge of the pathophysiology of disease states likely to affect the neonate. This chapter describes physiology and pathophysiology-based view on the neonatal abdominal emergency surgeries. General principles of surgery and anesthetic management of specific neonatal emergencies that include congenital diaphragmatic hernia (CDH), abdominal wall defects, necrotizing enterocolitis, and esophageal atresia are reviewed and discussed.

Keywords: neonatal, emergency abdominal surgery, pediatric anesthesia, neonatal physiology, perioperative anesthetic management

1. Introduction

Advances in obstetrics and neonatology have greatly improved neonatal survival especially for infants with complex anatomical defect and preterm neonates. Most of these anotomical abnormalities to be corrected by surgical interventions after birth, some of them also corrected by intervention before birth [1, 2]. Advances in prenatal diagnosis and survival rate in these patients have resulted in an increase in the anesthetic and surgical approach. Emergency surgical conditions can be life threatening in the neonatal period. Therefore, anesthesiologists must know and better understand the distinctive physiological characteristics of neonates than of adults so that they can have information about response to anesthesia and surgery.

The purpose of this chapter is to provide basic information that will help anesthesiologists to better approach the problems of neonates. The present considerations recommend that to provide safe care these patients are also reviewed.

In this context, anesthetic management will be presented in selected neonatal surgical emergencies including congenital diaphragmatic hernia (CDH), abdominal wall defect (gastroschisis and omphalocele) necrotizing enterocolitis, and esophageal atresia. Clinical presentation and associated anomalies, perioperative approach, surgical stabilization, and postoperative follow-up period are explained and discussed.

2. Physiological features in neonates

2.1. Respiratory system

Lung development can be divided into five stages [3]. In literature and textbook knowledge reviewed, the last stage begins at about 36 weeks' gestation and continues until at least 18 months [4]. Tip II pneumocytes are responsible for surfactant production. These begin to differentiate at 24 weeks' gestation, but surfactant level is not adequate to ensure appropriate pulmonary function until 34–36 weeks of gestation [4, 3]. Therefore, respiratory immaturity and potential for respiratory distress are well-defined entities in the preterm neonate due to a deficiency of surfactant.

One of the characteristics of the fetal circulation is high pulmonary vascular resistance (PVR) [3]. PVR reduces by approximately 10% after labor, but the apparent decrease occurs with the first breath [5]. Pulmonary blood flow and alveolar and arterial PO_2 increase along with the expansion of the lung [5]. These changes are important for modification of the fetal circulation to the adult form of circulation [3, 6]. Over the next 1–2 months, PVR decreases to adult levels.

The differences in the neonatal respiratory system from that of the adult can be summarized as follows:

- Central control of ventilation is not fully developed.
- Response to hypoxia is immature.
- Peripheral feedback mechanisms are not sufficiently mature.
- Neonatal oxygen consumption per kilogram of body weight is twice as much as an adult.
- Lower functional residual capacity (moderate decrease in value of inspired oxygen or ventilation can cause rapid desaturation).

Immature airway and respiratory system can lead to airway obstruction during sedation or mask ventilation. In addition to this, diaphragmatic movement associated with gastric distension can also trigger significant respiratory failure. Infection, airway obstruction, hypoventilation, hypoxemia, and sepsis are among the reasons of apneic episodes [7]. Therewith, anemia may precipitate postoperative apnea and bradycardia in neonate too. Prolonged period of apnea results in hypoxia and hypercapnia. Our current knowledge shows that the risk of postoperative apnea continues in expremature infants until 60 postconceptual weeks [8]. Frequently, preterm infants are victims of respiratory failure due to the immature and sensitive respiratory structures. Many preterm infants needed increased (mechanical ventilatory support or CPAP, supplemental oxygen, etc.) respiratory support to preserve fundamental oxygenation. In hypoxic circumstances, respiratory rates of preterm and newborns decrease paradoxically.

Numerous neonatal emergency abdominal surgeries can be seen associated with respiratory system insufficiency. Respiratory variables, which are mentioned earlier, must be taken into consideration in these cases.

2.2. Cardiovascular system

The circulation of a newborn infant is a transitional characteristic. This means that, a significant decrease in pulmonary vascular resistance after birth. Patent ductus arteriosus (PDA) on the side interventricular shunts and connections are responsible from this circulation.

The fetal circulation is defined by increased PVR, decreased pulmonary blood flow, low systemic vascular resistance, and right-to-left blood flow through ductus arteriosus and foramen ovale [9, 3]. The onset of spontaneous breathing is the main factor that reduces PVR. This reduction of PVR is followed by an increase in systemic vascular resistance and left atrial pressure. Extrauterine circulation changes to a serial type of circulation as an adult.

Physiological closure of ductus arteriosus may take up to first 24 h after birth in healthy infants. However, ductus arteriosus closes anatomically after several days. Different pathological situations may cause shunting of blood via this structure. Anatomic closure of foramen ovale occurs between 3 months and 1 year of age. However, functionally closure takes place immediately. Foramen ovale may persist in 10% of the adult patients.

Reduction of pulmonary blood flow or pulmonary vasoconstriction can cause a return of the fetal circulation characteristics. This circulatory pattern is called persistent fetal circulation (PFC) or persistent pulmonary hypertension of the newborn (PPHN) [10]. Hypoxemia and acidosis can aggravate PFC. In infants with CDH, meconium aspiration and infection may be seen as PFC.

Therefore, neonatal myocardium is less compliant, and newborn's cardiac output is heart-rate dependent. The sympathetic innervation of the developing heart is decreased. In such a case, neonatal heart variable responds to vasoactive drugs.

2.3. Thermoregulation

The newborn baby has a high ratio surface area to body weight and a thin layer of subcutaneous fat tissue. Therefore, they are prone to lose heat more than older children and adults. Heat loss in newborn occurs with four different mechanisms, including evaporation, convection, conduction, and radiation.

Nonshivering thermogenesis is a primary mechanism in heat loss and regulated by brown fat [11]. Brown fat is a located adipose tissue settled in the posterior neck along the interscapular and vertebral areas.

For the reason mentioned earlier, severe temperature changes can be seen in the perioperative period. Hypothermia may trigger myocardial depression, acidosis, and delayed recovery from anesthesia. Maximal precautions should be taken to prevent hypothermia in perioperative period. Applications, which required to be done to prevent heat loss, are listed below.

- Keep the ambient temperature in neutral condition.
- Humidify and warm inspired anesthetic gases.
- Use the heated blanket, radiant warmer, and transport the neonate in a heated incubator.
- Warm blood and intravenous solutions.
- Use heating solution for cleansing the skin.

3. General principles of anesthesia in neonate

Anesthetic management of neonates that require emergency surgery is challenging and may cause serious problems to the anesthesiologist. The identification of patients at high risk for procedure-related morbidity and mortality should be a basic preventive effort. The practice of a safe anesthesia and perioperative management in such patients depends on a clear understanding of the anatomical, physiological, and hemodynamic differences and variables.

Our knowledge about pain perception in newborns has changed in recent years. Unlike the historical information, premature and term infants can feel pain from painful procedures. In recent literatures and studies, it is shown that preterm and term infants have a perception of pain, and these infants give physiological responses (such as autonomic, endocrine, and metabolic) to painful stimuli [12]. These stimulus and stress can increase pulmonary vascular resistance ergo, increase shunting through the foramen ovale, and ductus arteriosus. This phenomenon may result in hypoxemia.

Because of this, a detailed anesthesia plan should be developed for safe patient care, effective pain control, and outcome in perioperative period.

3.1. Effects of anesthetic agents

The effects of anesthetic agents vary with physical growth and changes, organ maturation, development, and coexisting disease in pediatric patient population. Inhalation anesthesia is the commonly used anesthetic technique in children. In infants, minimal alveolar concentration (MAC) is an estimate of anesthetic requirements and changes with age [8, 11]. Infants up to 6 months of age require higher MAC value than older neonates [8]. Volatile anesthetics cause dose-dependent cardiac and respiratory depressant effect in neonates. These effects can cause bradycardia, hypotension, and postoperative apnea. This hypotensive effect is more likely in preterm and term neonates than older children, especially in the induction period.

In contrast, an opioid agent causes fewer hemodynamic changes, but it should be noted that increase the risk of postoperative apnea in preterm and term neonates [2].

In the last 15 years, effects of general anesthetic agents on brain development have made a great progress. The recent animal studies have demonstrated that general anesthetics (especially these acting through the N-methyl-D-aspartate (NMDA) and Gama aminobutyric acid (GABA) receptors) can be responsible from neuronal cell death and deterioration of brain development especially immature brain [13]. It is reported that this effect is to be related to drug dosages and exposure time. Many factors affect brain maturation apart from anesthesia. Dinardo et al. emphasized that neuroanatomic abnormalities preexist in neonatal patients with complex congenital cardiac pathologies. The retardation of brain maturation has been observed in these patients [14]. Long-term neurobehavioral effects of sedative and anesthetic agents should be supported by long-term human studies.

3.2. Monitoring

Basic monitorization should include heart rate-electrocardiograph, pulse oximetry, blood pressure, and temperature in neonates. Two oxygen saturation probes must be plugged (preductal and postductal probes). This approach is intended to evaluate possible PDA-mediated shunt development. Invasive arterial blood pressure and central venous pressure can be monitored in special circumstances such as expected ventilation-perfusion and hemodynamic changes and acid-base imbalance.

Precordial-esophageal stethoscope is a very useful method in neonatal monitoring. With this method, changes in heart rate and respiratory parameters can be identified in the early phase. Although end-tidal carbon monoxide monitorization is a routine application, increase in dead space in the breathing system can cause false and inaccurate measurement in infants.

4. Anesthetic management of special neonatal surgical emergencies

4.1. Congenital diaphragmatic hernia

CDH is one of the complex and compelling anomalies in the neonatal period. CDH occurs in about 1:2400 and 1:3000 live births [8, 15]. Incomplete formation of the diaphragm and the inability of the intestines to return to the abdominal cavity result in CDH. Posterolateral foramen originated hernia (foramen of Bochdalek) constitutes 90% of the cases. In patients with CDH because of the displacement of the abdominal contents until the mediastinum, pulmonary hypoplasia (unilateral or bilateral) and possible mediastinal shift are serious problems. Less than 15% of the remaining lung volume for gas exchange indicates a poor prognosis.

Clinical presentation of CDH includes a scaphoid abdomen, increased anteroposterior diameter of the chest, bowel sounds during chest auscultation, and respiratory distress in variable degrees. Newborn babies with CDH have a 25–30% incidence of cardiac anomalies [11, 15]. Often, gastrointestinal malformations associated with skeletal abnormalities are also possible.

In radiological imaging of the chest, bowel loops in the thoracic cavity and mediastinal shift (due to compression of the lungs) are observed. Therewithal, diagnosis can be made through ultrasongraphy in utero, but this diagnosis should be confirmed in the postpartum period.

4.1.1. Preoperative evaluation

In recent years, one of the strongly highlighted issues in CDH is the timing of surgery. There is considerable argument about this topic. Current approaches, after corrective surgery, are intended to provide cardiopulmonary stabilization. CDH study group reported that only one-third of the patients underwent surgical correction in the first 24 h of life in the mid-1990s. Nowadays, the number of patients who underwent surgery within the 24 h is less than 5% [15, 16]. Because of this, it is recommended that surgical repair should be postponed until after initial resuscitation provides preoperative stabilization.

4.1.2. Preoperative ventilation strategies

The main point in the protective efforts for patients with CDH is minimizing the physiologic instability associated with pulmonary hypoplasia and pulmonary hypertension in the postnatal period. Developing ventilator strategies have played an important role in terms of reducing mortality in the last 20 years.

After delivery (in a neonate who is diagnosed during the intrauterine period) immediate endotracheal intubation (to abstain from positive pressure ventilation and pulmonary barotrauma), ventilation with small tidal volumes, and increased respiratory rates (especially in the presence of pulmonary hypoplasia) are important initial ventilatory maneuvers [8, 15, 16]. Nasogastric tube assists in decompression of gas content of the bowel and protects the lung volume.

Inflating pressures must be kept below 30 cm H_2O with a continuous monitoring of airway pressure [2]. Pulmonary barotrauma may result in serious complications such as pneumothorax, air embolism, pneumomediatinum, and soft tissue emphysema.

In the past years, perioperative management of these patients was intended to maintain adequate oxygenation and prevention of pulmonary hypertension. As hypoxemia and hypercarbia may increase pulmonary vascular pressure, hyperventilation (to lower PCO_2) of high oxygen levels was used. However, to reduce the risk of barotrauma and high mortality incidence, today with a gentle approach, permissive hypercapnia and lower percentage of oxygen are preferred [2, 15].

On this basis, the general approach in preoperative period should include reduction of pulmonary vascular resistance, recovery of pulmonary compliance, minimal ventilatory support, and regression of radiological changes.

4.1.3. *Different presurgical therapy modalities*

4.1.3.1. *Extracorporeal membrane oxygenation*

Some neonates show rapid clinical improvement, if surgery is performed within 48 h. However, some patients may require hemodynamic, respiratory, and medical supportive therapy before definitive surgery. Extracorporeal membrane oxygenation (ECMO) is one of these treatment procedures.

The first reports about ECMO in neonates with CDH were declared in the late 1970s [17]. Oxygenation index (OI)>40, $PaCO_2$ consistently >12, and A-a gradient consistently >600 mmHg were accepted indications for initiation of ECMO in the past [18]. However, nowadays, the indications for ECMO use can be summarized as unresponsiveness to treatment. Currently, more than 30% of CDH neonates are now being managed with ECMO, and it is frequently used in patients with severe reduction of pulmonary volume before surgery [2, 19].

Nonetheless, ECMO should not be used in the presence of different serious clinical cases such as intracranial hemorrhage > Grade I, presence of accompanied congenital anomalies, fatal chromosomal abnormalities, and gestational age <34 weeks [17].

Summarization—ECMO should be considered only on those infants who cannot be treated with conventional medical therapy. So ECMO is used as an additional therapy for patients who have resistant hypoxemia despite inotropic and ventilatory support.

4.1.3.2. *Ex utero intrapartum treatment (EXIT) procedure*

EXIT is an intrauterine treatment procedure in some cases of CDH. In this procedure, after fetal head removal from the uterus, fetus is intubated for assessing oxygenation or connected to the ECMO prior to umbilical cord clamping. In literature, some cases have been reported where fetal gas exchange is supported by ex utero placental circulation for over 60 minutes [2].

4.1.4. *Surgical approach and intraoperative consideration*

In the conventional approach, diaphragmatic defect is repaired via a thoracotomy incision on the ipsilateral side of the hernia. Thoracic approach is preferred in some cases. During the operation, diaphragmatic defect is repaired depending on the size of the defect. Small defects were closed primarily in which large patch graft may be required. After the closure of abdominal viscera, intraabdominal pressure may increase excessively. This clinical situation can worsen respiratory insufficiency and higher ventilation pressure should be required in the intraoperative and postoperative period. But pulmonary barotaruma should be avoided in this period.

4.1.5. Postoperative period

Severity of pulmonary hypoplasia and hypertension is an important factor that affects overall survival. Several factors affect pulmonary compliance after emergency surgery. These factors (such as increased intraabdominal pressure, lung hypoplasia, and postoperative painful stimulus) frequently cause rapid decrease in compliance. Opioids can reduce the stress response and catecholamine release in response to painful stimuli. In addition, opioids provide effective pain control so decrease the pulmonary vasoconstrictor responses to painful stimuli in neonatal intensive care unit (NICU) [2, 16].

4.2. Abdominal wall defect

4.2.1. Gastroschisis and omphalocele

Gastroschisis and omphalocele are characterized by congenital defect in the abdominal wall and herniation or evisceration of abdominal viscera [2, 20, 21]. The incidence of these defects is 1:3000 to 10000 live births [2].

Gastroschisis is defined by the absence of a division in the right abdominal wall if omphalocele is a periumbilical defect of the abdominal wall and a majority in male neonate [2]. Current knowledge supports the fact that omphalocele and gastroschisis arise from separate embryologic processes. Herniation of abdominal contents overlaps with a translucent lamina of peritoneum. The characteristic of the lesion is amniotic membrane. In addition, the intestines, spleen, and liver may be located in a large defect. Both clinical cases should require emergency surgical approach due to rapid and substantial heat and fluid losses by extra abdominal organs (especially bowels). Some congenital anomalies are often associated with omphalocele such as trisomies, congenital cardiac anomalies (e.g., Fallot tetralogy), Bechwith-Wiedemann syndrome, malrotation of the intestine, chromosomal anomalies, and meningocele [21, 2]. Prematurity is an important factor that increases mortality in these patients.

4.2.2. Preoperative period

Although each of the lesions is a different etiology, approaches are similar for both the pathologies. The preoperative fundamental approach to abdominal wall defects primarily includes adequate fluid resuscitation to prevent heat loss and treatment of infection and sepsis to avoid direct trauma to the eviscerated organs [11]. In both the cases for the prevention, the defect (especially large defect) is covered with sterile wet dressing [22].

Dense fluid replacement therapy is required and is vital for these patients. The stomach should be decompressed with a nasogastric tube. This process is intended to reduce regurgitation, aspiration, and bowel distention. Systemic antibiotics should be started primarily. Intense protein loss and translocation of fluid into third space can be seen in ruptured cases. Oncotic pressure is also decreased. Arterial blood gas analysis should be performed.

4.2.3. Intraoperative management

Major issues that we need to pay attention in preoperative approach are also important in the intraoperative period. The maintenance of body temperature and adequate fluid resuscitation should be noted. Because of this, adequate intravenous access must be ensured and invasive monitoring is necessary if an associated cardiac defect is present.

Surgical intervention is required to reduce the bowel back into the abdominal cavity and repair the abdominal wall defect. Different surgical techniques (such as primary closure in the operating room or bedside, placement of a prefabricated silastic silos or fashioning of a hand-sewn silo) are applicable [23]. Silo method is a transition repair procedure. Some infants may remain intubated until final closure in the NICU setting. Nowadays, the sutureless umbilical closure has become a widely accepted technique [24]. In the renewed procedure, herniated viscera are reduced into the abdomen. Umbilical cord is used to pack the abdominal wall defect. This technique may be implemented at the bedside in the neonatal intensive care unit. Nevertheless, in patients with larger defect, surgery should be performed in the operating room. Anesthetic management consists of endotracheal intubation in the awakened patients with gastric decompression after preoxygenation. Anesthesia is maintained with inhalational anesthetics and controlled ventilation. Muscle relaxants may be used to provide optimal surgical circumstances for closure of the defect.

It must be kept in mind that if abdominal defects are closed too tightly, abdominal pressure can increase because of underdeveloped abdominal cavity. This situation can lead to respiratory failure, diminish visceral organ and lower extremity perfusion, and decrease venous return due to caval compression [8]. In this situation, postoperative ventilatory support may be necessary. In patients with associated anomalies, close monitoring (especially airway pressure and central venous pressure) is vital and invasive blood pressure monitorization and arterial blood gas analysis may be useful and observational hemodynamic parameters provide optimal oxygenation and fluid therapy. Respiratory parameters should be monitored closely after surgery. Postoperative mechanical ventilatory support is recommended during 24–48 h in NICU. Prolonged ileus after surgery may cause parenteral nutrition in a longer period.

4.3. Necrotizing enterocolitis

Necrotizing enterocolitis (NEC) is one of the important cause of morbidity and mortality that particularly affects premature infants under 36 weeks of gestational age (usually premature infants fewer than 32 weeks) [2, 16, 21]. The causes of NEC are still unclear. However, the etiology of NEC is considered multifactorial. Prematurity is a definite risk factor mainly affecting premature infants fewer than 32 weeks' gestation and body weight is less than 1500 gr. In addition, hypoxemia, enteral feedings (especially hyperosmolar solutions), cyanotic heart disease, and PDA have been suggested as risk factors. Although the etiology is different, the result is increased mucosal permeability, intestinal ischemia, and sepsis.

Clinical features of these patients are characterized by abdominal distention, retained gastric secretion, bloody stool, and bile-stained aspirates [2, 25]. In some cases, irritability, lethargia, apnea, and temperature instability may accompany this situation. Hypovolemic shock can be seen in cases with generalized peritonitis. A hemorrhagic diathesis with thrombocytopenia may emerge in septic infants. Many of these infants who have developing respiratory insufficiency and hyaline membrane syndrome require intubation and mechanical ventilation support.

It is important to know the risk factors, and early diagnosis and initial treatment in these patients are also necessary. Some cases including less severe ones can be treated with broad-spectrum antibiotics, intravenous fluids, and nasogastric decompression. However, acute phase of NEC required emergency surgery, and pneumoperitoneum is an absolute indication [25, 26]. Positive paracentesis, constant abdominal mass, fixed dilated intestinal loop, and progressive metabolic acidosis are among relative surgical indications [2, 16, 21].

4.3.1. Intraoperative management

Intraoperative approach in patients with NEC should contain close monitoring of invasive arterial and central venous pressure, blood gas, and metabolic analysis. Blood products (such as red blood cells, fresh frozen plasma, and platelets) may be required in infants with coagulaopathies in the early period. In addition, severe hypovolemia is a significant problem in these infants and requires intensive treatment with crystalloid and colloid solutions.

Potent inhalational anesthetics can aggravate a hypovolemic situation. Because of this, frequently inhalational anesthetics are utilized in low concentration to supplement opioids. High-dose opioid (especially fentanyl) is a safe and viable option for balanced anesthesia [8]. Nitrous oxide should not be used. Because of the risk of premature retinopathy, inspired oxygen concentration should be calibrated to keep between an arterial oxygen saturation of 85–90% [16].

Neuromuscular blockers may be used to facilitate surgical intervention. Hemodynamic collapse is often in these newborns. In this regard, despite fluid resuscitation in patients who are not provided adequate perfusion, inotropic agents are often necessary to protect cardiovascular stability. Glucose intolerance is a significant problem particularly in septic patients. Intermittently, arterial blood gas analysis and glucose measurement is an important measurement parameter.

4.3.2. Postoperative consideration

These infants often require postoperative mechanical ventilatory and cardiovascular support. Parenteral nutrition is necessary after sepsis is controlled and metabolic stability is maintained [20].

4.4. Esophageal malformations

4.4.1. Esophageal atresia, tracheoesophageal fistula

Esophageal atresia is the most common esophageal malformation. The incidence reported is at 1 in 2500–3000 live births [27].

Esophageal malformations can manifest in five different forms according to localization of atresia and presence of fistula. The most common defect (80–90%) consists of a blind, upper esophageal pouch with distal tracheoesophageal fistula.

Severe cardiovascular anomalies (such as ventricular septal defect, coarctation of aorta, and Tetralogy of Fallot,) can be associated with esophageal atresia. This anomaly can also be a part of a syndrome known as VATER [vertebra (V) anal (A), tracheoesophageal (TE), renal (R)] or VATER syndrome associated cardiac (C) and limb (L) anomalies called VACTERL syndrome [8, 27]. These associated anomalies worsen the prognosis.

Prenatal diagnosis can be made with the ultrasound. Inability to swallow, choking attacks, aspiration, and abdominal distention should be preoccupying esophageal atresia in the early postnatal period. The disability of the nasogastric tube to pass through the atretic esophagus passage is also seen in the clinical examination.

Definitive diagnosis is made by contrast radiological examination. Pulmonary aspiration, other causes of abdominal distention, and prematurity-dependent problems should be considered in differential diagnosis. Preoperative echocardiography must be performed owing to the associated congenital cardiac anomalies. Concomitant cardiac anomalies and birth weight are among the factors affecting mortality in patients with Tracheoesophageal Fistula (TEF)/EA.

4.4.2. Anesthetic management

The operation of TEF is acceptable and urgent, but not immediate, and the time of surgery is determined by the general condition of the infant. Considering the general condition of the patients, surgical approach can be planned—primary closure of the fistula and anastomosis, gastrostomy before or after definitive surgery, or a delayed primary closure [28]. In patients, who provide clinical improvement, surgery can be carried out within 24–72 h [11]. Antibiotic therapy should be initiated immediately in infants with pulmonary infection. In these cases, surgery may be delayed as much as clinically stability. Despite the intensive, care, support, and antibiotic therapy, if there is continuous clinical worsening and respiratory insufficiency, immediate surgery may be necessary.

However, if the scheduled surgery is delayed, usually fistula is closed, and gastrostomy is performed. Gastrostomy is used to decompress the stomach and decrease regurgitation into the lungs. In addition, gastrostomy provides nutritional support in cases in which definitive surgery is delayed. This process can take 3–6 months.

The basic preoperative anesthetic management in patients undergoing surgical approach includes the following:

- Degree of neonatal age (especially prematurity) and associated congenital anomalies
- Interruption of feeding and intermittent aspiration of the upper esophageal pouch
- Prevent excessive gastric distention due to air intake into the stomach through the fistula

- Evaluation of aspiration pneumonia, if necessary, antibiotic therapy to treat pulmonary infection

Before management of anesthesia, aspiration catheter may be useful to drain secretions in the esophagus. In anesthesia, induction should be administered carefully to prevent abdominal distention and pulmonary aspiration. In general, intubation is performed in awake conditions. Sedation can be administered with titrated dose of fentanyl (0.5–1 $\mu g\ kg^{-1}$) and 25–50 $\mu g\ kg^{-1}$ midazolam [8]. Also deep inhalational anesthesia to induction may be preferable to endotracheal intubation. In this period, maintenance of spontaneous breathing should be noted. Muscle relaxant may be an addition after the ligation of fistula.

The placement of the endotracheal tube (ETT) is important. ETT tip must be above the carina, but it must be placed below the fistula. It may not be easy to find the correct tube localization. Generally, tube is advanced through the right mainstem bronchus and then pulled back slightly until breath sounds are heard bilaterally. Tube localization can be confirmed by flexible fiberoptic bronchoscope [29]. Even with initial optimal position of the ETT, in some patients, ventilation through the fistula still occurs, and this is particularly seen in patients who require high peak airway pressure. In these cases, the use of low inspiratory pressure will prevent gastric distention until the ligation of the fistula.

In appropriate cases, a primary repair can be performed, the fistula is ligated, and esophagus is primary anastomosed. Intraoperatively, retraction of the lung may be required to provide proper exposure intraoperatively. In this period, deterioration of oxygenation is a common problem due to collapsed lung experience by an anesthesiologist. Intermittent ventilation of collapsed lung and close cooperation of surgical team may improve oxygenation.

In addition, precordial stethoscope should be a part of an intraoperative monitorization during repair of the TEF. Precordial stethoscope is placed in the left axilla to assess the adequacy of ventilation in the dependent lung. In infants with associated anomalies such as congenital cardiac defect or hemodynamic instability, invasive arterial monitoring should be performed.

Two oxygen saturation probes may be helpful to evaluate pre- and postductal oxygen saturation and shunt fraction via patent ductus arteriosus.

4.4.3. Postoperative approach

In patients with TEF, significant pathological finding is a reduced amount of tracheal cartilage. Tracheomalacia or defective tracheal wall can cause airway collapse. Therefore, most patients require postoperative ventilatory support in early postoperative period (at least 24–48 h) in NICU. This period may take up 5–7 days in infants who have long gap anastomosis [8, 16, 29]. Intermittent arterial blood gas analysis and chest radiographs will be useful in the postoperative follow-up period.

Opioid infusion is effective in the treatment of postoperative pain and sedation in this period.

Anastomotic leak and strictures are main complications in early postoperative period. Structural and functional abnormalities (such as gastroesophageal reflux and chronic pulmonary disease) are considerable problems that may be encountered in the long-term period [2, 30].

Therefore, it should be noted that EA or TEF is not a small anatomic problem that completely ameliorates by surgical approach.

5. A Special highlight for pediatric spinal anesthesia

In the last 30 decades, pediatric spinal anesthesia has become one of the most attractive and popular topics in anesthesia practice with the increase of our knowledge and experience on this issue. Despite the growing interest, spinal anesthesia requires technical expertise, and it is not still performed in many centers. Notwithstanding, general anesthesia is a standard technique for many pediatric anesthetist.

Spinal anesthesia has become a considerable anesthetic technique for reducing the risk of postoperative apnea in premature and ex-premature infants [31]. Unsupplemented spinal anesthesia may be used in lower abdominal surgery (such as necrotizing enterocolitis, pyloromyotomi, omphalocele, and gastroschisis) in neonatal age group. Abajian et al. in 1984 reported the use of spinal anesthesia in high-risk ex-premature infants and considered regional anesthesia by spinal approach to be safe and effective in these patients [32].

At the same time, spinal anesthesia is characterized by remarkable hemodynamic stability in neonate and infant patients. In reference [33] this physiological characteristic means that minimum or no cardiodepressant effect and is important especially in the neonatal period. Because neonatal heart just after birth is more immature than adult heart and have a lower velocity of contraction and a minimize length-tension correlation.

In infants with limited pulmonary perfusion, it is important to maintain systemic vascular resistance and control of PVR and pulmonary blood flow. Some of these patients require immediate surgical intervention. In these patients, spinal block decreases undesirable adverse effects related to the sympathetic system activity.

Surgical trauma and pain cause a hormonal stress response that is directly related to the severity and urgency of surgery. Spinal anesthesia is an effective pain control technique. Thus, hormonal stress response and catecholamine release reduces in intraoperative and postoperative period [31, 34].

In the previous studies, it has been suggested that when compared with general anesthesia, spinal anesthesia is associated with fewer cardiovascular and respiratory complications, and there is less need for postoperative mechanical ventilation and a shorter hospital stay [35].

Because of these factors, it has to be kept in mind that spinal anesthesia seems reliable and a safe alternative technique in selected cases especially for specific lower abdominal surgery.

6. Summary

Preterm and term neonates may need various surgical interventions, but unfortunately, many of them are urgent. Newborn period is a challenging period for the anesthesiologist. This difficulty is caused by many factors related to neonatal population such as immaturity of physiological processes, organs, and systems, and pathophysiological instability caused by the underlying comorbidities and associated congenital anomalies. For these reasons, anesthesia-associated morbidity and mortality is greater in this group than in older infants and children. A cautious approach to all aspects of perioperative care is vital to minimize the possible side effects. The basics of safe anesthetic management in preterm and term neonates are summarized in this chapter, based on emergency abdominal surgery.

Author details

Esra Caliskan

Address all correspondence to: duru5654@gmail.com

Department of Anesthesiology and Reanimation, Baskent University, Faculty of Medicine, Ankara, Turkey

References

[1] Partridge EA, Flake AW. Maternal-fetal surgery for structural malformations. Best Pract Res Clin Obstet Gynaecol. 2012; 26:669–682. DOI: 10.1016/j.bpobgyn.2012.03.003.

[2] Brusseau R, McCann ME. Anaesthesia for urgent and emergency surgery. Early Hum Dev 2010; 86:703–714. DOI: 10.1016/j.earlhumdev.2010.08.008.

[3] Motoyoma EK, Finder JD. Respiratory physiology in Infants and Children. In: Davis PJ, Cladis FP, Motoyoma EK editors. Smith's Anesthesia for Infants and Children. 8th ed. Philadelphia: Elsevier; 2011. Pp. 23–41. ISBN: 978-0-323-06612-9. ch3.

[4] Joshi S, Kotecha S. Lung growth and development. Early Hum Dev 2007; 83:789–794. DOI: 10.1016/j.earlhumdev.2007.09.007.

[5] Finnemore A, Groves A. Physiology of the fetal and transitional circulation. Semin Fetal Neonatal Med 2015; 20:210–216. DOI: 10.1016/j.siny.2015.04.003.

[6] Souza DD, McDaniel GM, Baum VC. Cardiovascular physiology. In: Davis PJ, Cladis FP, Motoyoma EK editors. Smith's Anesthesia for Infants and Children. 8th ed. Philadelphia: Elsevier; 2011. Pp. 81–115. ISBN: 978-0-323-06612-9. ch4.

[7] Sale SM. Neonatal apnoea. Best Pract Res Clin Anaesthesiol 2010; 24:323–336. DOI: 10.1016/j.bpa.2010.04.002.

[8] Cote CJ. Pediatric anetshesia. In: Miller RD, editor. Miller's Anesthesia. 7th ed. Philadelphia: Churchill Livingstone; 2010. Pp. 2559–2597. ISBN: 978-0-443-06959-8.ch.

[9] Hines MH. Neonatal cardiovascular physiology. Semin Pediatr Surg 2013; 22:174–178. DOI: 10.1053/j.sempedsurg.2013.10.004.

[10] Jain A, McNamara PJ. Persistent pulmonary hypertension of the newborn: advances in diagnosis and treatment. Semin Fetal Neonat Med 2015; 20: 262–271. DOI: 10.1016/j.siny.2015.03.001

[11] Gregory GA, Brett C. Neonatology for anesthesiologist. In: Davis PJ, Cladis FP, Motoyoma EK Editors. Smith's Anesthesia for Infants and Children. 8th ed. Philadelphia: Elsevier; 2011, pp. 513–553. ISBN: 978-0-323-06612-9. ch17.

[12] Anand KJS. Pharmacological approaches to the management of pain in the neonatal intensive care unit. J Perinatol 2007; 27:S4–S111. DOI: 10.1038/sj.jp.7211712.

[13] Sun L. Early childhood general anesthesia exposure and neurocognitive development. Br J Anaesth 2010; 105: i61–i68. DOI: 10.1093/bja/aeq302.

[14] DiNardo JA. Should what we know about neurobehavioral development, complex congenital heart disease, and brain maturation affect the timing of corrective cardiac surgery? Paediatr Anaesth. 2011; 21: 781–6. DOI: 10.1111/j.1460-9592.2010.03429.

[15] Lally KP. Congenital diapragmatic hernia—the past 25(or so) years. J Pediat Surg 2016. Available from http://dx.doi.org/10.1016/j.jpedsurg2016.02.005.

[16] Brett C, Davis PJ. Anesthesia for general surgery in the neonate. In: Davis PJ, Cladis FP, Motoyoma EK editors. Smith's Anesthesia for Infants and Children. 8th ed. Philadelphia: Elsevier; 2011; pp. 554–588. ISBN: 978-0-323-06612-9. ch18.

[17] Harting MT, Lally KP. Surgical management of neonates with congenital diapragmatic hernia. Semin Ped Surg 2007; 16:109–114. DOI: 10.1053/j.sempedsurg.2007.01.007.

[18] Hedrick HL. Evaluation and management of congenital diapragmatic hernia. Pediatr Case Rev 2001; 1:25–36. DOI: 10.1097/00132584-200110000-00004.

[19] Tiruvoipati R, Vinogradova Y, Faulkner G, Sosnowski AW, Firmin RK,Peek GJ. Predictors of outcome in patients with congenital diapragmatic hernia requiring extracorporeal membrane oxygenation. J Pediatr Surg 2007; 42:98–104. DOI: 10. 1016/j.jpedsurg.2007.03.031

[20] Chesley PM, Letbetter DJ, Meehan JJ, Oron AP, Javid PJ. Contemporary trends in the use of primary repair for gastroschisis in surgical infants. Am J Surg 2015; 209: 901–906. DOI: 10.1016/j.amjsurg.2015.01.012.

[21] Dierdorf SF, Krishna G. Anesthetic Management of Neonatal Surgical Emergencies. Anesth Analg 1981; 60: 204–214. ISSN: 0003-2999.

[22] Mann L, Ferguson-Smith MA, Desai M, Gibson AA, Raine PA. Prenatal assessment of anterior abdominal wall defects and their prognosis. Prenat Diagn 1984; 4: 427–435. DOI: 10.1002/pd.1970040606.

[23] Aldrink HJ, Caniano DA, Nwomeh BC. Variability in gastroschisis management: a survey of North American pediatric surgery training programs. J Surg Res 2012; 176:159–163. DOI: 10.1016/j.jss.2011.05.012.

[24] Riboh J, Abrajano C, Garber K, et al. Outcome of sutureless gastroschisis closure. J Pediatr Surg 2009; 44: 1947–1951. DOI: 10.1016/j.jpedsurg.2009.03.027.

[25] Bayley G. Special considerations in the premature and ex-premature infant. Anaesth Intensive Care Med 2014; 15: 107–110. DOI: 10.1016/j.mpaic.2008.01.007.

[26] Pierro A. The surgical management of necrotising enterocolitis. Early Hum Dev 2005; 81(1): 79–85. DOI: 10.1016/j.earlhumdev.2004.10.018.

[27] Natasha Broemling N, Campbell F. Anesthetic management of congenital tracheoesophageal fistula. Pediatr Anesth 2011; 21: 1092–1099. DOI: 10.1111/j.1460-9592.2010.03377.

[28] Andropoulos DB, Rowe RW, Betts JM. Anaesthetic and surgical airway management during trachea-oesophagial fistula repair. Pediatr Anesth 1998; 8:313–319. DOI: 10.1046/j.1460-9592.1998.00734.

[29] Broemling N, Campbell F. Anesthetic management of congenital tracheoesophageal fistula. Pediatr Anesth 2011; 21:1092–1099. DOI: 10.1111/j.1460-9592.2010.03377.

[30] Marseglia L, Manti S, D'Angelo G, Gitto E, Salpietro C, Centorrino A et al. Gastroesophagial reflux and congenital gastrointestinal malformations. World J Gastroenterol 2015; 21: 8508–8515. DOI: 10.3748/wjg.v21.i28.8508.

[31] Bosenberg A. Benefits of regional anesthesia in children. Pediatr Anesth 2012; 22:10–18. DOI: 10.1111/j.1460-9592.2011.03691.

[32] Abajian JC, Mellish RW, Browne AF, Perkins FM, Lambert DH, Mazuzan JE Jr. Spinal anesthesia for surgery in the high-risk infant. Anesth Analg 1984; 63:359-362. ISSN: 0003-2999.

[33] Shenkman Z, Johnson VM, Zurakowski D, et al. Hemodynamic changes during spinal anesthesia in premature infants with congenital heart disease undergoing inguinal hernia correction. Pediatr Anesth 2012; 22:865–870. DOI: 10.1111/j.1460-9592.2012.03873.

[34] Wolf AR, Doyle E, Thomas E. Modifying infant stress responses to major surgery: spinal vs extradural vs opiod analgesia. Pediatr Anesth 1998; 8:305–311. DOI: 10.1046/j.1460-592.1998.00239.

[35] White MC. Approach to managing children with heart disease for noncardiac surgery. Pediatr Anesth 2011; 21:522–529. DOI: 10.1111/j.1460 j.1460-9592.2010.03416.

3

Anesthetic Management of the Newborn Surgical Patient

Marissa Vadi, Chelan Nour, Patrick Leiter and Harmony Carter

Abstract

Providing anesthesia for the newborn requires many considerations beyond what is needed for the older child or adult. This chapter discusses pertinent anesthetic considerations in the care of surgical neonates including preoperative evaluation, intraoperative management and pain management techniques.

Keywords: neonatal anesthesia, anesthetic agents, pain management

1. Introduction

Advances in pediatric anesthesiology have contributed to improved outcomes and survival in newborns requiring surgical intervention. Newborn physiology is characterized by a high metabolic rate, limited cardiopulmonary reserve, and decreased renal function. Multisystem organ immaturity underlies the differences in physiologic response to anesthetics in the neonate when compared to the older child or adult. This chapter discusses physiologic considerations, preoperative evaluation and preparation, intraoperative anesthetic management, and pain management techniques unique to the newborn surgical patient.

2. Physiologic considerations

2.1. Cardiovascular

Fetal cardiac circulation is characterized by two right-to-left shunts: one through the foramen ovale and one through the ductus arteriosus. With the infant's first breaths, the lungs expand, alveolar fluid is cleared, pulmonary vascular resistance markedly decreases, and left atrial pressure increases [1]. These physiologic changes promote functional closure of the fetal cardiac shunts and mark the beginning of the transition from fetal to newborn circulation.

Anatomic closure of the foramen ovale typically occurs within the first year of life, though some studies indicate over one quarter of foramen ovale remain echocardiography probe patent into adulthood [2]. Functional closure of the ductus arteriosus is achieved between 10 and 15 hours of life, and anatomical closure is usually completed by 2 months of age [3]. Neonatal circulation may revert to fetal circulation if the physiological parameters responsible for cardiac shunt closure are not maintained. As such, it is important to avoid factors that increase pulmonary vascular resistance (physiologic stress, hypoxia, hypercarbia, acidosis, and hypothermia) in newborns. Hypervolemia may also promote reopening of the ductus arteriosus and should be avoided.

Maintenance of heart rate is essential in the neonatal period. Cardiac output is dependent on heart rate, as stroke volume is fixed due to decreased compliance of the immature ventricle [4]. Thus, while maintaining preload is important during anesthetic management, increasing preload provides minimal benefit for improving cardiac output. The sympathetic nervous system is also immature in newborns. Bradycardia may occur after stimulating procedures such as laryngoscopy, oropharyngeal suctioning, or gastric tube placement rather than the expected tachycardia seen in patients with mature sympathetic nervous systems. Treatment with anticholinergics may be required.

2.2. Pulmonary

Development of the respiratory system begins during fetal organogenesis and continues throughout childhood. Alveolarization starts at 28 weeks of gestational age, and by 40 weeks, alveoli are present at 20–50% of adult values. Type 2 pneumocytes, the main producers of surfactant, appear at approximately 24 weeks of gestational age but are not fully functional until 34–36 weeks of gestational age [5].

Neonates are an increased risk for respiratory fatigue. High chest wall compliance may cause a paradoxical breathing pattern when large breaths are taken [5]. Newborns have a reduced number of fatigue-resistant high-oxidative diaphragmatic muscle fibers; mature levels are not reached until 8 months of age [6]. Neonatal oxygen requirements are 2–3 times the adult requirement, ranging from 6 to 9 mL/kg/min. Increased oxygen demand is met by increased respiratory rate, as there is a minimal inspiratory reserve to increase tidal volume [7].

Neonatal respiratory drive is determined by pO_2 via peripheral chemoreceptors in the carotid bodies and by pCO_2 influencing central chemoreceptors in the medulla. Respiratory drive is primarily affected by hypoxia, as opposed to hypercarbia in adults. Administration of high oxygen concentrations may depress respiratory drive in the newborn [8].

2.3. Renal

The kidneys are fully developed anatomically by 34–36 weeks of gestational age but continue to develop functionally after birth. The glomerular filtration rate (GFR) is initially decreased in the neonate due to low systemic arterial pressure and high renal vascular resistance but increases during the first several weeks of extrauterine life [9]. As a result of this initial low GFR, there is a decreased ability of the kidneys to maintain electrolyte balance or clear drugs and excess fluids.

2.4. Neurologic risk

The neurologic system is anatomically complete at term, though synaptogenesis and nerve myelination continue throughout childhood. Data from animal studies, as well as retrospective human studies, have raised concern that exposure to anesthetic agents could be detrimental to cognitive development in young children due to effects either on synaptogenesis or apoptosis of the developing brain [10]. The stage of brain development at the time of exposure and the degree of anesthetic exposure, in terms of both exposure frequency and cumulative anesthetic dose, may affect the risk of neurotoxicity.

The SmartTots program, a partnership between the United States Food and Drug Administration and the International Anesthesia Research Society, was established in 2009 to address the growing concern regarding potential adverse consequences of general anesthesia in young children. Two consensus statements, published in 2012 and 2015, counsel that the effect of exposure to anesthetic drugs in young children is unknown. Some, but not all, studies to date have suggested that problems similar to those seen in animals could also occur in infants and toddlers. The benefits of elective procedures must be weighed against the risks associated with anesthesia and surgery [11].

3. Preoperative evaluation and preparation

3.1. History and physical examination

A thorough preanesthetic history and physical examination must be performed with the goals of identifying potential anesthetic complications due to coexisting disease, determining whether further diagnostic studies are required prior to surgery and anticipating postoperative concerns including pain management and level of cardiorespiratory monitoring required.

Factors that should be addressed in the preanesthetic history are outlined in **Table 1**. A review of all organ systems, including identification of genetic syndromes and associated anomalies, should be completed. Examination of previous anesthetic and surgical records may reveal difficulties with airway management, venous access, or anesthetic emergence and assist in planning future anesthetic management.

Physical examination should assess for evidence of coexisting diseases (e.g., craniofacial abnormalities, congenital heart disease, chronic lung disease). Hydration status may be determined by evaluating skin turgor, mucous membranes, fontanelle fullness, and urine output. Existing intravenous catheters should be examined for patency and hypovolemia treated prior to anesthetic induction. Laboratory studies must be reviewed and significant electrolyte abnormalities and/or anemia corrected preoperatively.

The American Society of Anesthesiologists (ASA) physical status classification system is used as a uniform system for describing the degree of patient morbidity prior to an anesthetic (**Table 2**) [12]. The grading system is not intended for use as a measure to predict operative risk.

Factor	Specific concerns
Maternal history during pregnancy	Rh-ABO compatibility
	Diabetes
	Toxemia
	Infection
	Drug or alcohol abuse
Gestational age and weight	Extreme prematurity and/or extremely low birth weight
Significant birth events	Apgar scores
	Neonatal asphyxia
	Meconium aspiration
Perinatal course	Apneas
	Supplemental oxygen requirement
	Need for ventilator support
Medications and medication allergies	Type and severity of adverse medication reaction

Table 1. Factors to address in the preanesthetic history.

Physical score classification*	Definition
ASA I	A normal healthy patient
ASA II	A patient with mild systemic disease
ASA III	A patient with severe systemic disease
ASA IV	A patient with severe systemic disease that is a constant threat to life
ASA V	A moribund patient who is not expected to survive without the operation
ASA VI	A declared brain-dead patient whose organs are being removed for donor purposes

*Emergency cases are designated by the addition of "E" to the classification number.

Table 2. American Society of Anesthesiologists physical status classification system.

3.2. Fasting

Infants are required to fast before procedures requiring sedation and anesthesia in order to minimize the risk of pulmonary aspiration of gastric contents [13]. Fasting times are based on pediatric gastric emptying studies. **Table 3** provides a summary of fasting recommendations by the ASA [14]. Prolonged fasting may lead to hypovolemia and hypoglycemia in infants; glucose-containing intravenous maintenance fluids should be administered prior to the induction of anesthesia.

The majority of pediatric aspiration events occur during anesthetic induction [15]. Risk factors for aspiration in the perianesthetic period include neurologic abnormality, emergency surgery, intestinal obstruction or increased abdominal pressure, light anesthesia, and the skill of the anesthesia provider [16, 17]. Infants and young children are particularly prone to regurgitation and aspiration for a variety of reasons including air swallowing while crying and decreased lower esophageal sphincter incompetence. In one study, almost all cases of pulmonary aspiration occurred in children who gagged or coughed during airway management, either because neuromuscular blockade was not administered or airway manipulation occurred before the child was completely paralyzed [15]. Mortality due to pulmonary aspiration is low, with an estimated incidence between zero and 1:50,000 [15, 16, 18].

Ingested material	Minimum fasting period (hours)
Clear liquids	2
Breast milk	4
Infant formula	6
Nonhuman milk	6
Light meal	6

Table 3. American Society of Anesthesiologists fasting recommendations.

3.3. Postoperative apnea in former premature infants

Postoperative apnea is defined as cessation of breathing or no detectable airflow for 15 seconds or longer, or less than 15 seconds with bradycardia. It has been observed in former premature infants after exposure to all forms of anesthetics (intravenous agents, inhalational agents, and regional anesthesia) [19–21]. The incidence of postoperative apnea varies inversely with gestational age at birth and post-conceptual age at the time of surgery. Apnea risk is greater than 1% until 54 weeks of post-conceptual age or 56 weeks of post-conceptual age in infants with a gestational age of 32 or 35 weeks, respectively [22].

Former preterm infants who are less than 60 weeks of post-conceptual age at the time of surgery should be monitored until free of apnea for at least 12 hours. A monitored bed should be arranged for the postoperative period, and family members should be educated regarding the risk of perianesthesia apnea. Children receiving theophylline or caffeine preoperatively should have these medications continued postoperatively [23]. Caffeine administration does not negate the need for postoperative respiratory monitoring. Factors such as anemia, hypothermia, hypoglycemia, hypocalcemia, acidosis, and hypoxemia may increase the risk of apnea and should be avoided.

4. Intraoperative management

4.1. Monitoring and intravenous access

The ASA's Standards for Basic Anesthetic Monitoring mandates continual evaluation of oxygenation, ventilation, circulation, and temperature during all anesthetics [24]. Placement of both a pre-ductal oxygen saturation monitor on the right upper extremity and a post-ductal oxygen saturation monitor on a lower extremity should be considered in neonates as a means to detect right-to-left shunting across the ductus arteriosus [25]. A nerve stimulator may be used if neuromuscular blocking agents are administered, though the train-of-four response is often diminished in infants less than 2 months old. It is imperative that the operating room be kept warm. Neonates, especially premature infants, are at high risk for heat loss due to an increased surface area to volume ratio when compared to older children and adults [26, 27]. The need for invasive monitoring, including arterial and central venous catheter placement, is determined by the baseline medical condition of the patient and the extensiveness of the planned surgery. Arterial catheters allow for continuous monitoring of heart rate and blood pressure, as well as arterial blood gas sampling [28]. Central venous catheters are utilized when large intravenous access is necessary, central venous pressure monitoring is required, or in hemodynamically unstable conditions likely to require continuous vasopressor infusions. The benefits of placement must always be weighed against the risks associated with use, such as catheter-associated bloodstream infection [29]. A urinary catheter should be considered in surgical cases of prolonged duration or when significant blood loss is expected.

4.2. Anesthetic agents

Most infants arriving as outpatients for surgery may undergo mask induction of anesthesia with inhaled anesthetic agents. Those patients presenting from inpatient hospital wards or the neonatal intensive care unit (NICU) with intravenous access in situ may undergo intravenous induction of general anesthesia [27].

4.2.1. Inhaled anesthetic agents

Inhaled halogenated anesthetics (most commonly sevoflurane, isoflurane, and desflurane) are used for both induction and maintenance of general anesthesia. The minimum alveolar concentration (MAC) is the end-tidal concentration of inhaled anesthetic agent at which 50% of patients do not move in response to a noxious stimulus. MAC values are used to compare the relative potencies of anesthetic agents and vary with age for each particular agent (**Table 4**) [30–32]. Of note, MAC values may differ for preterm neonates depending upon the inhalational agent used and the gestational age of the infant.

Sevoflurane is the halogenated agent most commonly chosen for mask induction of anesthesia; its use is associated with a reduced incidence of breath holding, coughing, laryngospasm, and oxygen desaturation when compared with other inhaled anesthetics [30]. Nitrous oxide, a nonhalogenated agent, may be used in conjunction with halogenated

Characteristic	Sevoflurane	Desflurane	Isoflurane	Nitrous oxide
MAC adult	2.05%	7.0%	1.2%	104%
MAC neonate (full term)	3.2%	9.2%	1.6%	–

Table 4. Minimum alveolar concentration (MAC) values for modern inhalational anesthetics.

inhaled anesthetics to speed inhalational induction ("second-gas effect") or reduce halogenated agent doses during the maintenance phase of anesthesia. Nitrous oxide must be used with caution as it may rapidly diffuse into and expand gas-filled body cavities. Its use should be avoided in laparoscopic surgery and is contraindicated in patients with a pneumothorax [33].

4.2.2. *Intravenous anesthetic agents*

Similar to inhaled halogenated anesthetics, intravenous anesthetic agents may be utilized for both induction and maintenance of anesthesia. Agent choice is commonly based upon the following drug properties: speed of onset, duration of action, cardiovascular stability, and side-effect profile [34].

Propofol is an intravenous agent with sedative-hypnotic properties resulting from gamma-aminobutyric acid (GABA)-mediated inhibitory neurotransmission. Systolic blood pressure falls approximately 15% after propofol administration due to decreases in preload, cardiac contractility, and systemic vascular resistance. Propofol is a potent respiratory depressant, and apnea may occur transiently after bolus administration. Pain on injection may be attenuated with intravenous lidocaine administration.

Ketamine is a phencyclidine derivative that antagonizes N-methyl-D-aspartate (NMDA) receptors. This results in a "dissociative"-type anesthesia and a potential for disturbing dreams or delirium. Ketamine possesses excellent amnestic, analgesic, and bronchodilation properties. Administration is associated with favorable hemodynamic parameters except in catecholamine-depleted patients. The use is limited in patients with a history of seizure disorder and in those in whom increases in intracranial and/or intraocular pressures would be detrimental. Nystagmus, myoclonus, and copious oral secretions are frequent side effects of ketamine use.

Etomidate depresses the reticular activating system and mimics the inhibitory effects of GABA. It possesses minimal effects on the hemodynamic system but can decrease ventilatory drive. Induction doses are known to transiently inhibit enzymes involved in cortisol and aldosterone synthesis with the potential for adrenocortical suppression.

Thiopental is a barbiturate that acts by prolonging the duration of GABA-mediated chloride channel opening. Administration can cause cardiovascular depression that is accentuated in the hypovolemic patient. Compared to other induction agents, acute tolerance to thiopental may develop, and prolonged sedation can be noted after induction doses [35].

4.2.3. Neuromuscular blocking agents

Neuromuscular blocking drugs allow for patient immobility, smooth endotracheal intubation, increased tolerance of mechanical ventilation, and optimal surgical relaxation. They are classified into two groups, depolarizing and non-depolarizing agents, based on activity at the neuromuscular junction [36]. The choice of drug depends on the desired speed of onset, duration of action, route of elimination, and side-effect profile.

Succinylcholine is the only depolarizing agent currently available for clinical use. An increased dose of succinylcholine is necessary in infants due to relative effect resistance at the neuromuscular junction and the larger volume of distribution in the neonate. Succinylcholine is metabolized by circulating pseudocholinesterase. It has a very rapid onset (60 seconds) and short duration of action (5 minutes). Succinylcholine carries an FDA "black box warning" against routine use in children due to risk of hyperkalemic cardiac arrest in patients with undiagnosed neuromuscular disorders [37]. Thus, it is recommended that the use of succinylcholine in children be reserved for emergency intubation or instances where immediate securing of the airway is necessary (e.g., laryngospasm, difficulty airway, full stomach) [38].

Non-depolarizing neuromuscular blocking agents are divided into intermediate (atracurium, cisatracurium, rocuronium, and vecuronium) and long-acting (pancuronium) varieties [26]. Neuromuscular blocking drugs are responsible for over 35% of anesthetic-related hypersensitivity reactions and should be considered as potential causes if anaphylaxis is suspected in the perianesthetic period. The effects of non-depolarizing muscle relaxants may be antagonized by an anticholinesterase (neostigmine or edrophonium) administered in conjunction with an anticholinergic agent (glycopyrrolate or atropine) to minimize parasympathetic side effects. Successful reversal of neuromuscular blockade in infants is demonstrated by adequate return of strong hip and/or arm flexion, abdominal muscle contraction, and return of the train-of-four twitch response to four equal twitches.

Historically, neuromuscular blocking drugs could only be reversed after adequate time had elapsed to demonstrate some natural return of neuromuscular function. Sugammadex, a cyclodextrin oligosaccharide, is a new reversal agent that inactivates steroidal neuromuscular blocking agents such as vecuronium and rocuronium via direct encapsulation. This mechanism allows for rapid and complete reversal of neuromuscular blockade within minutes of administration of a neuromuscular blocking agent. Studies examining sugammadex use in children aged 2–18 years suggest no evidence of higher incidence of adverse effects with sugammadex compared to that with neostigmine or placebo [39]. Data regarding the safety of sugammadex in infants are currently limited.

4.3. Fluid and blood product management

Calculating total intraoperative fluid requirements necessitates considering fluid type, maintenance fluid requirements, evaporative fluid losses, and replacement of intraoperative blood loss.

4.3.1. Glucose requirements

Healthy infants and children can remain euglycemic for up to 17 hours despite fasting. Infants receiving total parenteral nutrition or 10% dextrose in water (D10W) preoperatively require continued glucose replacement intraoperatively [27, 40]. Glucose levels naturally increase intraoperatively secondary to decreased insulin sensitivity from release of surgery-related stress hormones.

4.3.2. Maintenance fluid requirements

Maintenance fluid requirements are determined by accounting for water losses from the renal, pulmonary, and gastrointestinal systems in addition to calculating baseline body weight and calorie usage [40]. While a variety of formulas exist to determine the maintenance fluid requirements of an infant or child, the simplest is the "4-2-1" rule shown in **Table 5** [40, 41].

D5 0.25% normal saline (NS) and D5 0.45% NS are commonly chosen maintenance fluids for children, as they closely accomplish the goal of delivering 3 mEq of sodium, 2 mEq of potassium, 2 mEq of chloride, and 5 g of glucose for every 100 mL of water administered. *Nil per os* (NPO) fluid deficit is calculated by multiplying the hourly maintenance fluid requirement by the number of hours the patient has been NPO. The NPO deficit is typically replaced intraoperatively as follows: half the total volume deficit is administered in the first hour, one quarter in the second hour, and the remaining quarter in the third hour.

Intraoperative evaporative fluid losses may be replenished with isotonic crystalloid or colloid fluids according to the following formula based on the invasiveness of surgery: superficial 1–2 mL/kg/h, moderate/intrathoracic 4–7 mL/kg/h, open intra-abdominal 6–10 mL/kg/h, and neonates with necrotizing enterocolitis >50 mL/kg/h. Current data are limited but do not support specific benefits of human albumin usage over other colloids or crystalloids in neonates [42, 43]. Favored colloid usage is institutional and region specific; many centers in the United States utilize albumin, while institutions in other nations favor hydroxyethyl starches or gelatins [44].

Weight	Hourly	Day
<10 kg	4 mL/kg	100 mL/kg
10–20 kg	40 mL + 2 mL/kg for every kg >10 kg	1 L + 50 mL/kg for every kg >10 kg
>20 kg	60 mL + 1 mL/kg for every kg >20 kg	1.5 L + 20 mL/kg for every kg >20 kg

Table 5. Maintenance fluid requirements by weight.

4.3.3. Blood products

Estimated blood volume is calculated based on the age and weight of the patient (**Table 6**) [45]. Prior to surgery, one may calculate the maximum allowable blood loss (MABL) that would necessitate blood transfusion using the following equation:

$$\text{MABL} = EBV \times \frac{(Hct\ \text{current} - Hct\ \text{min})}{(Hct\ \text{current})} \tag{1}$$

where *Hct current* is the current hematocrit and *Hct min* is the minimum acceptable hematocrit.

Age	Estimated blood volume (mL/kg)
Premature infant (<37 weeks of gestational age)	100
Term infant	90
Toddler	80
School-aged child	75
Adult	65–70

Table 6. Calculating estimated blood volume.

Recommended doses for replacement of blood products are outlined in **Table 7** [46].

Packed red blood cells (PRBCs) have a hematocrit of approximately 55–70%. Fresh frozen plasma (FFP) administration is indicated when there is laboratory evidence of coagulopathy or significant blood loss approaching one blood volume [47]. Intraoperative platelet transfusion is more likely to be necessary with preoperative platelet counts <150,000 per mm^3 or after the loss of two to three blood volumes [41, 48]. Massive blood loss has historically been replaced in a 1:1:1 fashion with PRBCs, FFP, and platelets. Currently, it is recommended that FFP administration begins after one blood volume has been lost or at the first sign of clinical coagulopathy [49]. It is imperative for the surgeon and the anesthesiologist to maintain excellent communication regarding expectations for blood loss and proper preparation of the patient including any necessary laboratory screening tests for blood typing, antibodies, and cross matching.

Product	Dose	Expected increase
Packed red blood cells	10–15 mL/kg	Hemoglobin 2–3 g/dL
Fresh frozen plasma	10–15 mL/kg	Factors 15–25%
Platelets	5–10 mL/kg	Platelets 50–100,000/mm^3
Cryoprecipitate	1–2 units/kg	Fibrinogen 60–100 mg/dL

Table 7. Recommended doses for replacement of blood products.

5. Neonatal pain management

Pain has been defined as "an unpleasant sensory and emotional experience associated with actual or potential tissue damage, or described in terms of such damage" [50]. Accurately defining and quantifying pain in the neonate has challenged the medical community for decades. Neonatal pain pathways are immature and poorly understood; over 40 different pain scales have been developed to assess pain in the term and preterm neonate. Because neonates and infants cannot verbally communicate pain, regrettably their pain may go unrecognized and undertreated.

Historically, it was believed that neonates did not have the same pain perception as older infants and adults. Opioids were known to cause respiratory depression and were considered harmful; thus, postoperative analgesia with opioids was discouraged. This remained the predominant view until as late as in 1987, when research by Anand and colleagues challenged this long-standing tradition by demonstrating that unattenuated noxious or painful stimuli during neonatal cardiac surgery caused a deleterious stress response and increased morbidity. Anand published two landmark papers presenting scientific evidence that neonates experience pain and the medical necessity for treating such pain. Change in practice soon followed, accompanied by a rapid expansion of literature in this area [51–53].

Neonates in the intensive care unit are estimated to undergo as many as 14 invasive procedures associated with pain each day, with analgesia inconsistently provided for many of these procedures (**Table 8**) [54]. This is concerning as research has correlated undertreated pain in the neonatal period with long-term detrimental effects, including behavioral disorders and altered sensitivity to pain later in life [55–59].

5.1. Pain assessment

An ongoing challenge involves appropriately assessing and effectively treating pain in the neonate. The immature dorsal horn circuits predominantly exhibit excitatory tone, with weaker inhibitory GABA and glycine signaling. It is uncertain whether or not this lack of inhibitory processing increases the neonate's perception of pain. Flexion reflexes may be elicited with either tactile or nociceptive touch; conversely, neonates with no behavioral reaction to heel lance showed a strongly activated cortex on EEG in one study, demonstrating the inadequacy of behavioral indicators to reliably detect pain [60].

Distinguishing between pain and agitation is also difficult as there are overlapping behavioral and physiologic manifestations [61]. Facial expression (total facial activity with specific features including brow lowering, eye squeeze, nasolabial furrow, and open mouth) is considered the most sensitive behavioral indicator of acute pain. Other behavior pain indicators include body posture, limb movements, cry, consolability, and sleep/wakefulness. Physiological parameters include heart rate, respiratory rate and pattern, oxygen saturation,

Diagnostic procedures	Arterial puncture, bronchoscopy, endoscopy, heel lancing, lumbar puncture, retinopathy of prematurity examination, suprapubic bladder tap, venipuncture
Therapeutic procedures	Bladder catheterization, central line insertion/removal, chest tube insertion/removal, chest physiotherapy, dressing change, gavage tube insertion, intramuscular injection, peripheral venous catheterization, tracheal tube insertion/removal, mechanical ventilation, tracheal suctioning, postural drainage, adhesive tape removal, ventricular tap
Surgical procedures	Circumcision
	Other surgical procedures

Table 8. Commonly performed painful procedures in the neonatal intensive care unit.

and blood pressure. These parameters are also important, but less specific, as alterations may be the result of the underlying disease process rather than pain. In the mechanically ventilated neonate with neuromuscular blocking therapy, pain must be evaluated based on changes in heart rate or blood pressure. Biological markers for pain such as emotional sweating (palm or sole, measured by skin conductance or galvanic skin response) or increased stress hormones (serum or saliva cortisol) are used in research but have limited clinical utility. Among the validated neonatal pain scales, premature infant pain profile (PIPP) assesses procedural pain, and neonatal pain, agitation, and sedation scale (N-PASS) assesses ongoing pain and sedation in both term and preterm neonates, providing an advantage over other available neonatal pain assessment tools (**Table 9**) [62–65].

5.2. Therapeutic approach

Neonatal pain is best managed using a tiered approach. Painful procedures should be avoided when possible through the use of noninvasive monitoring and bundling of laboratory blood draws. Non-pharmacological therapy, such as nonnutritive sucking, oral sucrose, breast or bottle feeding, and swaddling, can be used during mildly painful events (i.e., lab draws, line insertion, removal of adhesives, wound treatment, bladder catheterization). Topical anesthetics may be used prior to skin-breaking procedures, though caution must be exercised in the preterm neonate as the epidermis is structurally and functionally immature, increasing the risk of toxicity. Acetaminophen is effective for mild pain and as an adjuvant for moderate to severe pain. Ketamine is a potent analgesic and NMDA antagonist that can be utilized during moderate to severe painful procedures of short duration or as an adjuvant to prevent opioid tolerance. Systemic opioid analgesics are utilized to treat moderate to severe pain in conjunction with the above therapies (**Table 10**) [66, 67]. Analgesic medications are most reliable when given intravenously, as oral absorption is unpredictable in the neonate [64, 68].

Pain scale	Variables included	Type of pain assessed
Premature infant pain profile (PIPP)	Heart rate, oxygen saturation, facial actions	Procedural, postoperative
Neonatal infant pain score (NIPS)	Facial expression, crying, breathing patterns, arm/leg movement, arousal	Procedural
Neonatal facial coding system (NFCS)	Facial actions	Procedural
Neonatal pain, agitation, and sedation scale (N-PASS)	Crying, irritability, facial expression, extremity tone, vital signs	Procedural, postoperative, mechanically ventilated patients
Cry, requires oxygen, increased vital signs, expression, sleeplessness (CRIES)	Crying, facial expression, sleeplessness, requires oxygen to stay at >95% saturation, increased vital signs	Postoperative
COMFORT scale	Movement, calmness, facial tension, alertness, respiration rate, muscle tome, heart rate, blood pressure	Postoperative, critical care
Douleur Aigue du Nouveau-ne (DAN)	Facial expression, limb movements, vocal expression	Procedural

Table 9. Summary of validated neonatal pain scales.

Medication	Intermittent dose	Infusion dose	Adverse effects
Acetaminophen	10 mg/kg IV/PO	N/A	None reported*
NSAIDS	Not recommended	N/A	Unwanted ductal closure, gastropathy, nephropathy, NEC, IVH, surgical bleeding
Morphine	0.05–0.1 mg/kg IV	0.005–0.03 mg per hour	Respiratory depression, decreased gastrointestinal motility, hypotension, urinary retention
Fentanyl	1 mcg/kg IV	0.5–2 mcg/kg per hour	Respiratory depression, hypotension, muscle rigidity, hypothermia
Ketamine	0.5–2 mg/kg IV	0.5–1 mg/kg per hour	Respiratory depression, increased secretions

NSAIDS, nonsteroidal anti-inflammatory drugs; NEC: necrotizing enterocolitis; IVH: intraventricular hemorrhage
*No reported adverse effects at therapeutic doses. Known hepatotoxicity with overdosing.

Table 10. Recommended analgesic dosing for neonates.

Postsurgical pain should be anticipated and preemptively treated to mitigate the pain and stress response. In conjunction with analgesic medications, local anesthetics may be administered as a field block, as a targeted nerve block, or as an epidural block (**Table 11**) to effectively treat procedural and surgical pain. Care must be taken during the placement of

Block	Indications
Caudal epidural block	Lower abdominal surgery, inguinal herniorrhaphy, circumcision, orchidopexy, lower limb and pelvic orthopedic surgery
Caudal epidural catheter *	*Lumbar level*: lower abdominal, pelvic, and lower limb surgery *Thoracic level*: upper abdominal, renal, or thoracic surgery
Paravertebral block (via catheter)	Unilateral thoracic or renal surgery
Intercostal nerve blocks	Thoracic surgery, multiple levels typically required
Brachial plexus block (axillary or infraclavicular)	PICC line placement, ischemic limb salvage (arterial vasodilation)
Rectus sheath block	Umbilical/paraumbilical hernia, laparoscopic surgery, pyloromyotomy
Transversus abdominis plane (TAP) block	Lower abdominal surgery
Penile block	Circumcision
Femoral nerve block	PICC line placement lower limbs, muscle biopsy, skin graft, clubfoot repair

*Non-tunneled caudal epidural catheters should be removed after 72 hours or sooner when visible signs of soiling are present to minimize infectious risks.

Table 11. Neuraxial and peripheral nerve block indications.

local anesthetics, as unintended intravascular delivery can lead to systemic toxicity manifesting as altered consciousness, seizures, hemodynamic instability, and ultimately cardiovascular collapse. Safe practice includes aspiration prior to injection, slow incremental dosing, adherence to maximum dosing guidelines, and appropriate dose reductions for the neonate (**Table 12**) [69]. Local anesthetic toxicity must be promptly recognized and treated (**Table 13**) [70].

Local anesthetic	**Standard maximum dose ***	**Recommended neonatal dose**	**Comments**
Bupivacaine	2.5 mg/kg	1 mg/kg	Commonly used for field blocks and wound infiltration
Ropivacaine	3 mg/kg	1.5 mg/kg	Decreased motor block and cardiotoxicity compared with bupivacaine Vasoconstrictor effects (avoid using for digital and penile blocks)
Lidocaine	5 mg/kg	2.5 mg/kg	
Prilocaine	Not recommended	Not recommended	Concern for methemoglobinemia
Chloroprocaine	14 mg/kg	7 mg/kg	No plasma accumulation due to short half life
Topical anesthetic	**Maximum dose**		**Comments**
Eutectic mixture of local anesthetics (EMLA)	1 g/5 kg	1 g	Equal parts lidocaine and prilocaine Maximum skin contact 1 hour Risk of methemoglobinemia increased in premature neonates

*Maximum doses are additive and not independent of each other; *local anesthetic dosing should be decreased by 50% in neonates.*

Table 12. Commonly used local anesthetics.

Local anesthetic toxicity (LAST) management
• Obtain help
• Managing the airway, administering 100% oxygen
• Treat seizure activity (benzodiazepines preferred)
• Alert nearest facility capable of cardiopulmonary bypass
• Support cardiovascular function (prolonged CPR, reduced epinephrine doses)
• Institute 20% lipid emulsion therapy (lipidrescue.org)

Table 13. Treatment of local anesthetic toxicity.

Author details

Marissa Vadi*, Chelan Nour, Patrick Leiter and Harmony Carter

*Address all correspondence to: mvadi@llu.edu

Loma Linda University School of Medicine, Loma Linda, CA, USA

References

[1] Abman SH, Chatfield BA, Hall SL, McMurty IF. Role of endothelium derived relaxing factor during transition of pulmonary circulation at birth. Am J Physiol. 1990;**259**:H1921–H1927.

[2] Hagen PT, Scholz DG, Edwards WD. Incidence and size of patent foramen ovale during the first 10 decades of life: An autopsy of 965 normal hearts. Mayo Clin Proc. 1984;**59**:17–20.

[3] Robertson NRC. Perinatal physiology. In: Godfrey S, Baum JD, editors. Clinical Paediatric Physiology. London: Blackwell Scientific Publications; 1979. pp. 134–192.

[4] Rudolph AM, Heymann MA. Fetal and neonatal circulation and respiration. Annu Rev Physiol. 1974;**36**:187–207.

[5] Muller N, Volgyesi G, Bryan ME, Bryan AC. The consequences of diaphragmatic muscle fatigue in the newborn infant. J Pediatr. 1979;**95**:793–797.

[6] Keens TG, Bryan AC, Levison H, Ianuzzo CD. Developmental pattern of muscle fiber types in human ventilatory muscles. J Appl Physiol Respir Environ Exerc Physiol. 1978;**44**:909–913.

[7] Cochrane WH. Anatomy and physiology of the newborn related to anesthesia. Can Anaesth Soc J. 1961;**8**:169–176.

[8] Katz-Salamon M, Lagercrantz H. Hypoxic ventilatory defence in very preterm infants: Attenuation in long-term oxygen treatment. Arch Dis Child Fetal Neonatal Ed. 1994;**70**:F90–F95.

[9] Drukkar A, Guignard JP. Renal aspects of the term and preterm infant: A selective update. Curr Opin Pediatr. 2002;**14**:175–182.

[10] Yon JH, Daniel-Johnson J, Carter LB, Jevtovic-Todorovic V. Anesthesia induces neuronal cell death in the developing rat brain via the intrinsic and extrinsic apoptotic pathways. Neuroscience. 2005;**135**:815–827. DOI: 10.1016/j.neuroscience.2005.03.064

[11] SmartTots. Consensus Statement on the use of Anesthetic and Sedative Drugs in Infants and Toddlers [Internet]. 2015. Available from: http://smarttots.org/about/consensus-statement/ [Accessed 2016-10-17].

[12] American Society of Anesthesiologists. ASA Physical Status Classification System [Internet]. 2014. Available from: https://www.asahq.org/resources/clinical-information/asa-physical-status-classification-system [Accessed 2016-10-30].

[13] Cote CJ, Goudsouzian NG, Liu LM, Dedrick DF, Szyfelbein SK. Assessment of risk factors related to the acid aspiration syndrome in pediatric patients – gastric ph and residual volume. Anesthesiology. 1982;**56**:70–72.

[14] Apfelbaum JL, Caplan RA, Connis RT, Epstein BS, Nickinovich DG, Warner MA. Practice guidelines for preoperative fasting and the use of pharmacologic agents to reduce the risk of pulmonary aspiration: Application to healthy patients undergoing elective procedures: An updated report by the American Society of Anesthesiologists Committee on Standards and Practice Parameters. Anesthesiology. 2011;**114**:494–511. DOI: 10.1097/ALN.0b013e3181fcbfd9

[15] Warner MA, Warner ME, Warner DO, Warner LO, Warner EJ. Perioperative pulmonary aspiration in infants and children. Anesthesiology. 1999;**90**:66–71.

[16] Olsson GL, Hallen B, Hambraeus-Jonzon K. Aspiration during anaesthesia: A computer-aided study of 185,358 anaesthetics. Acta Anaesthesiol Scand. 1986;**30**:84–92.

[17] Walker RW. Pulmonary aspiration in pediatric anesthetic practice in the UK: A prospective survey of specialist pediatric centers over a one-year period. Paediatr Anaesth. 2013;**23**:702–711.

[18] Borland LM, Sereika SM, Woelfel SK, Saitz EW, Carrillo PA, Lupin JL, Motoyama EK. Pulmonary aspiration in pediatric patients during general anesthesia: Incidence and outcome. J Clin Anesth. 1998;**10**:95–102.

[19] Krane EJ, Haberkern CM, Jacobson LE. Postoperative apnea, bradycardia, and oxygen desaturation in formerly premature infants: Prospective comparison of spinal and general anesthesia. Anesth Analg. 1995;**80**:7–13.

[20] Sale SM, Read JA, Stoddart PA, Wolf AR. Prospective comparison of sevoflurane and desflurane in formerly premature infants undergoing inguinal herniotomy. Br J Anaesth. 2006;**96**:774–778. DOI: 10.1093/bja/ael100

[21] Davidson AJ, Morton NS Arnup SJ, de Graaff JC, Disma N, Withington DE, Frawley G, Hunt RW, Hardy P, Khotcholava M, von Ungern Sternberg BS, Wilton N, Tuo P, Salvo I, Ormond G, Stargatt R, Locatelli BG, McCann ME. Apnea after awake regional and general anesthesia in infants: The general anesthesia compared to spinal anesthesia study–comparing apnea and neurodevelopmental outcomes, a randomized controlled trial. Anesthesiology. 2015;**123**:38–54. DOI: 10.1097/ALN.0000000000000709

[22] Cote CJ, Zaslavsky A, Downes JJ, Kurth CD, Welborn LG, Warner LO, Malviya SV. Postoperative apnea in former preterm infants after inguinal herniorrhaphy. A combined analysis. Anesthesiology. 1995;**82**:809–822.

[23] Kelly DH, Shannon DC. Treatment of apnea and excessive periodic breathing in the full-term infant. Pediatrics. 1981;**68**:183–186.

[24] American Society of Anesthesiologists. Standards for Basic Anesthetic Monitoring [Internet]. 2015. Available from: http://www.asahq.org/~/media/sites/asahq/files/public/resources/standards-guidelines/standards-for-basic-anesthetic-monitoring.pdf [Accessed 2016-08-01].

[25] Taneja B, Srivastava V, Saxena KN. Physiological and anaesthetic considerations for the preterm neonate undergoing surgery. J Neonatal Surg. 2012;**1**:14.

[26] Hillier SC, Krishna G, Brasoveanu E. Neonatal anesthesia. Semin Pediatr Surg. 2004;**13**:142–151. DOI: 10.1053/j.sempedsurg.2004.04.002

[27] Pani N, Panda CK. Anaesthetic consideration for neonatal surgical emergencies. Indian J Anaesth. 2012;**56**:463–469. DOI: 10.4103/0019-5049.103962

[28] Schindler E, Kowald B, Suess H, Niehaus-Borquez B, Tausch B, Brecher A. Catheterization of the radial or brachial artery in neonates and infants. Paediatr Anaesth. 2005;**15**:677–682. DOI: 10.1111/j.1460-9592.2004.01522.x

[29] Freeman JJ, Gadepalli SK, Siddiqui SM, Jarboe MD, Hirschi RB. Improving central line infection rates in the neonatal intensive care unit: Effect of hospital location, site of insertion, and implementation of catheter-associated bloodstream infection protocols. J Pediatr Surg. 2015;**50**:860–863. DOI: 10.1016/j.jpedsurg.2015.02.001

[30] Lerman J, Sikich N, Kleinman S, Yentis S. The pharmacology of sevoflurane in infants and children. Anesthesiology. 1994;**80**:814–824.

[31] Taylor RH, Lerman J. Minimum alveolar concentration of desflurane and hemodynamic responses in neonates, infants, and children. Anesthesiology. 1991;**75**:975–979.

[32] Cameron CB, Robinson S, Gregory GA. The minimum anesthetic concentration of isoflurane in children. Anesth Analg. 1984;**63**:418–420.

[33] Cote CJ, Lerman J, Anderson BJ, editors. A Practice of Anesthesia for Infants and Children. 5th ed. Philadephia: Elsevier Saunders; 2013. 111 p. DOI: 10.1213/ane.0b013e3182a00428

[34] Pittaway A. Principles of anaesthesia for term neonates: An updated practical guide. Anaesth Intensive Care. 2011;**12**:95–98. DOI: 10.1016/j.mpaic.2010.11.002

[35] Davis PJ, Cladis FP, Motoyama EK, editors. Smith's Anesthesia for Infants and Children. 8th ed. Philadelphia: Elsevier Mosby; 2011. pp. 192–195. DOI: 10.1016/c2009-0-49104-9

[36] Brandom BW, Fine GF. Neuromuscular blocking drugs in pediatric anesthesia. Anesthesiol Clin North America. 2002;**20**:45–58. DOI: 10.1016/S0889-8537(03)00054-3

[37] Micromedex. Succinylcholine Chloride [Internet]. 2016. Available from: http://www.micromedexsolutions.com/micromedex2/librarian/CS/A5B83B/ND_PR/evidencexpert/ND_P/evidencexpert/DUPLICATIONSHIELDSYNC/392347/ND_PG/evidencexpert/ND_B/evidencexpert/ND_AppProduct/evidencexpert/ND_T/evidencexpert/PFActionId/evidencexpert.DoIntegratedSearch?SearchTerm=succinylcholine# [Accessed 2016-09-01].

[38] Engelhardt T. Rapid sequence induction has no use in pediatric anesthesia. Paediatr Anaesth. 2015;**25**:5–8. DOI: 10.1111/pan.12544

[39] Won YJ, Lim BG, Lee DK, Kim H, Kong MH, Lee IO. Sugammadex for reversal of rocuronium-induced neuromuscular blockade in pediatric patients: A systematic review and meta-analysis. Medicine (Baltimore). 2016;**95**:e4678. DOI: 10.1097/MD.0000000000004678

[40] Bailey AG, McNaull PP, Jooste E, Tuchman JB. Perioperative crystalloid and colloid fluid management in children: Where are we and how did we get here? Anesth Analg. 2010;**110**:375–390. DOI: 10.1213/ANE.0b013e3181b6b3b5

[41] Arya VK. Basics of fluid and blood transfusion therapy in paediatric surgical patients. Indian J Anaesth. 2012;**56**:454–462. DOI: 10.4103/0019-5049.103960

[42] Boldt J. Use of albumin: An update. Br J Anaesth. 2010;**104**:276–284. DOI: 10.1093/bja/aep393

[43] Uhing MR. The albumin controversy. Clin Perinatol. 2004;**31**:475–488.

[44] Gray R. Which colloid to choose for neonates, infants and children. South Afr J Anaesth Analg. 2015;**21**:56–58.

[45] Cote CJ, Lerman J, Anderson BJ, editors. A Practice of Anesthesia for Infants and Children. 5th ed. Philadephia: Elsevier Saunders; 2013. 198 p. DOI: 10.1213/ane.0b013e3182a00428

[46] Davies P, Robertson S, Hegde S, Greenwood R, Massey E, Davis P. Calculating the required transfusion volume in children. Transfusion. 2007;**47**:212–216.

[47] Keir AK, Stanworth SJ. Neonatal plasma transfusion: An evidence-based review. Transfus Med Rev. 2016;**30**:174–182. DOI: 10.1016/j.tmrv.2016.07.001

[48] Sloan SR, Parker RI. Current status of platelet transfusion in pediatric patients. Transfus Med Rev. 2016;**30**:230–234. DOI: 10.1016/j.tmrv.2016.07.006

[49] Goel R, Cushing MM, Tobian AA. Pediatric patient blood management programs: Not just transfusing little adults. Transfus Med Rev. 2016;**30**:235–241. DOI: 10.1016/j.tmrv.2016.07.004

[50] International Association for the Study of Pain. IASP Taxonomy [Internet]. 2012. Available from: http://www.iasp-pain.org/Taxonomy#Pain [Accessed: 2016-09-07].

[51] Anand KJ, Sippell WG, Aynsley-Green A. Randomised trial of fentanyl anaesthesia in preterm babies undergoing surgery: Effects on the stress response. Lancet. 1987;**1**:62–66. DOI: 10.1016/S0140-6736(87)90065-1

[52] Anand KJ, Hickey PR. Pain and its effects in the human neonate and fetus. N Engl J Med. 1987;**317**:1321–1329. DOI: 10.1056/NEJM198711193172105

[53] Rutter N, Doyal D. Neonatal care and management of pain: Historical and ethical issues. Semin Neonatol. 1998;**3**:297–302. DOI: 10.1016/S1084-2756(98)80084-5

[54] Anand KJ, International Evidence-Based Group for Neonatal Pain. Consensus statement for the prevention and management of pain in the newborn. Arch Pediatr Adolesc Med. 2001;**155**:173–180. DOI: 10.1001/archpedi.155.2.173

[55] Anand KJ, Scalzo FM. Can adverse neonatal experiences alter brain development and subsequent behavior? Biol Neonate. 2000; **77**:69–82. DOI: 10.1159/000014197

[56] Montirosso R, Casini E, Del Prete A, Zanini R, Bellu R, Borgatti R, NEO-ACQUA Study Group. Neonatal developmental care in infant pain management and internalizing behaviours at 18 months in prematurely born children. Eur J Pain. 2016;**20**:1010–1021. DOI: 10.1002/ejp.826

[57] Grunau RE, Holsti L, Haley DW, Oberlander T, Weinberg J, Solimano A, Whitfield MF, Fitzgerald C, Yu W. Neonatal procedural pain exposure predicts lower cortisol and behavioral reactivity in preterm infants in the NICU. Pain. 2005;**113**:293–300. DOI: 10.1016/j.pain.2004.10.020

[58] Victoria NC, Murphy AZ. Exposure to early life pain: Long term consequences and contributing mechanisms. Curr Opin Behav Sci. 2016;**7**:61–68. DOI: 10.1016/j.cobeha.2015.11.015

[59] Victoria NC, Murphy AZ. The long-term impact of early life pain on adult responses to anxiety and stress: Historical perspectives and empirical evidence. Exp Neurol. 2016;**275**:261–273. DOI: 10.1016/j.expneurol.2015.07.017

[60] Fitzgerald M. What do we really know about newborn infant pain? Exp Physiol. 2015;**100**:1451–1457. DOI: 10.1113/EP085134

[61] Maxwell LG, Malavolta CP, Fraga MV. Assessment of pain in the neonate. Clin Perinatol. 2013;**40**:457–469. DOI: 10.1016/j.clp.2013.05.001

[62] Hummel P, van Dijk M. Pain assessment: Current status and challenges. Semin Fetal Neonatal Med. 2006;**11**:237–245. DOI: 10.1016/j.siny.2006.02.004

[63] Ballantyne M, Stevens B, McAllister M, Dionne K, Jack A. Validation of the premature infant pain profile in the clinical setting. Clin J Pain. 1999;**15**:297–303.

[64] Witt N, Coynor S, Edwards C, Bradshaw H. A guide to pain assessment and management in the neonate. Curr Emerg Hosp Med Rep. 2016;**4**:1–10. DOI: 10.1007/s40138-016-0089-y

[65] Hillman BA, Tabrizi MN, Gauda EB, Carson KA, Aucott SW. The neonatal pain, agitation and sedation scale and the bedside nurse's assessment of neonates. J Perinatol. 2015;**35**:128–131. DOI: 10.1038/jp.2014.154

[66] Morton NS. Local and regional anaesthesia in infants. Contin Educ Anaesth Crit Care Pain. 2004;**4**:148–151. DOI: 10.1093/bjaceaccp/mkh041

[67] Bosenberg A, Flick RP. Regional anesthesia in neonates and infants. Clin Perinatol. 2013; **40**:525–538. DOI: 10.1016/j.clp.2013.05.011

[68] Anand KJ, Aranda JV, Berde CB, Buckman S, Capparelli EV, Carlo WA, Hummel P, Lantos J, Johnston CC, Lehr VT, Lynn AM, Maxwell LG, Oberlander TF, Raju TN, Soriano SG, Walco GA. Analgesia and anesthesia for neonates: Study design and ethical issues. Clin Ther. 2005;**27**:814–843. DOI: 10.1016/j.clinthera.2005.06.021

[69] Gunter JB. Benefit and risks of local anesthetics in infants and children. Paediatr Drugs. 2002;**4**:649–672.

[70] American Society of Regional Anesthesia and Pain Medicine. Checklist for Treatment of Local Anesthetic Systemic Toxicity [Internet]. 2016. Available from: https://www.asra.com/advisory-guidelines/article/3/checklist-for-treatment-of-local-anesthetic-systemic-toxicity [Accessed: 2016-10-30].

4

Imaging Evaluation of Liver Tumors in Pediatric Patients

Chengzhan Zhu, Bingzi Dong and Qian Dong

Abstract

Imaging plays crucial roles in the management of pediatric patients with suspected liver malignant tumors. Three-dimensional (3D) imaging could significantly improve the resection rate of pediatric tumors and increase the safety of the surgery. With the development of medical imaging, 3D reconstruction technology, the innovation of liver surgery and the proposal of precise hepatectomy, the intrahepatic vascular anatomy of the liver and liver segmentectomy based on that vascular anatomy have become well developed. With the analysis of 3D digital liver, we proposed a new type of liver classification system: Dong's digital liver classification system. And we measured the normal total liver volume from neonate to aging making a reference for surgeons all around the world. And the Human Digital Liver Database was established by the Affiliated Hospital of Qingdao University and Hisense Company, aiming to collect digital liver from neonates, children, adults, and the elderly, from normal livers, livers with cancer, and simulated livers resected using Hisense CAS. Then we showed one case report of patient with giant liver tumor. With the application of Hisense CAS and our data, we successfully removed the tumor. We believe that the new techniques in imaging will help surgeons to accomplish better operations.

Keywords: three-dimensional imaging, liver tumor, digital liver classification, total liver volume, Human Digital Liver Database

1. Introduction

Liver tumors constitute 1–4% of all solid tumors in children, of which 40% are benign. They mainly include hemangioma, liver hamartoma, and liver cell adenoma. Malignant tumors mainly include hepatoblastoma (HB), hepatocellular carcinoma (HCC), malignant liver mesothelioma, and rhabdomyosarcoma [1]. For most hepatic malignancies, hepatectomy or liver transplantation is optimal for cure. Resectability can be limited by multifocality, bilobar involvement, vascular thrombus or vascular invasion, extension to hepatic hilum, and distant metastasis [2]. If the tumor cannot be resected at initial imaging evaluation, the child is usually first treated with chemotherapy and/or radiation, and then re-imaged. For this reason, proper imaging evaluation of the liver is necessary which will shorten the surgical waiting duration and increase the success of the resection. In the cases where liver resection has high morbidity and high incidence, liver transplantation is recommended.

Imaging plays crucial roles in the management of pediatric patients with suspected liver tumors. MR imaging is recommended for children than computed tomography (CT) because of less radiation [3, 4]. However, CT could clearly show the liver anatomy and be helpful in staging, which is widely used in preoperative evaluation in the pediatric patients [3, 5]. Moreover, if the CT or MR imaging indicates a malignant mass, CT of the chest should be performed to assess the presence of lung metastasis [6].

In our experience, three-dimensional imaging can significantly improve the resection rate of pediatric tumors and increase the safety of the surgery [7]. In our center, we prefer CT scans for preoperative evaluation of pediatric liver tumors. However, it is very important to avoid non-contrast and multiphase images, and use low-dose CT scan in pediatric patients. CT phase of portal venous are very useful for evaluation of primary malignant liver tumors in children.

2. Common malignant liver tumors in pediatric patients

2.1. Hepatoblastoma (HB)

HB comprises 1% of all pediatric malignancies. HB most often occurs in infants and young children between 6 months and 4 years old. The median age of occurrence is 18 months. After 5 years of age, it becomes rare but histologically more aggressive in children over 8 years old. It occurs equally in males and females [8]. Based on radiological imaging, preoperative staging system (Pretreatment Extent of Disease or PRETEXT) which define extent of liver parenchyma involvement is an important guideline for treatment selection [9]. The new international surgical guidelines, which are being developed for the upcoming Pediatric Hepatic International Tumor Trial, will recommend primary surgical resection at diagnosis for PRETEXT I and II tumors of which the radiographic margin on the middle hepatic vein is wide [10].

As staging and treatment are mainly dependent on imaging, high-quality radiographic imaging has come to be of vital importance. For imaging assessment, both contrast-enhanced CT and MRI are recommended. Non-contrast CT typically shows a relatively well-defined, heterogeneous mass, slightly hypodense compared with liver tissue, with or without calcifications. On contrast-enhanced CT (**Figure 1**), the tumor reveals a heterogeneous enhancement, which may be hyperdense relative to liver parenchyma in the early arterial postcontrast phase and usually appears iso- or hypodense on delayed images (11). Invasion of the portal vein and its subsequent thrombosis must be evaluated in all suspected cases of hepatoblastoma. The tumor thrombus can even spread along IVC and encroach in the lumen of right atrium.

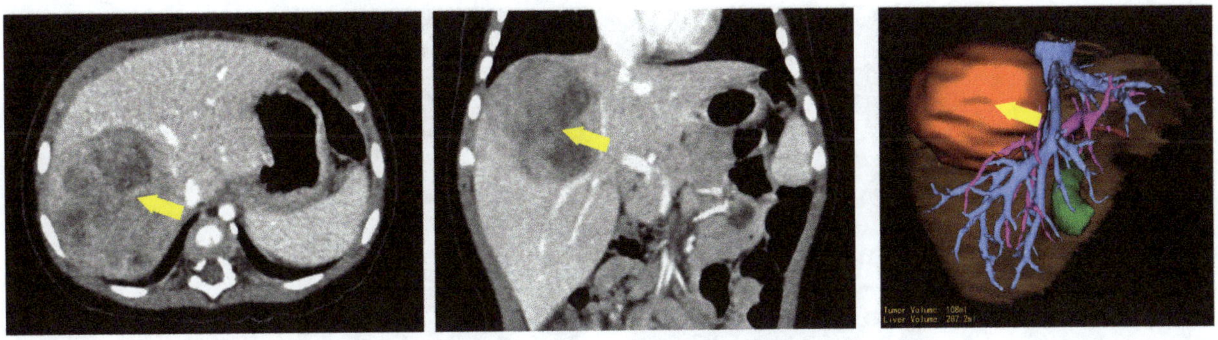

Figure 1. CT and three-dimensional reconstructed liver of PRETEXT II hepatoblastoma resectable at diagnosis (white arrow).

Metastasis may be seen in lymph nodes and lung parenchyma; it is rare in the brain and bones [11]. Twenty percent of HBs present with metastasis and most of them are in the lungs; therefore CT chest is necessary for staging.

2.2. Hepatocellular carcinoma (HCC)

The incidence of HCC in children was 0.5–1.0 cases per million children [12]. Different from HB, the median age of occurrence in children with HCC is 10 to 11.2 years [3]. The male to female ratio is 2:1 in young children, but it increases with age. Unlike adults, in whom HCC usually accompanies underlying liver disease, only 20–35% of children with HCC children have underlying liver disease [13]. HCC in children is now considered a distinct tumor family consisting of adult type HCC and variants, fibrolamellar HCC, and transitional liver cell tumor [14]. HCC is usually multifocal and may present with a variable number and distribution of tumor nodules. Recognizing HCC lesions smaller than 1.0 cm is still difficult.

In fibrolamellar HCCs, tumor cells are circumscribed by bundles of acellular collagen. This form is seen more frequently in adolescents than in adults and has better prognosis. HCCs are highly variable and show non-characteristic features on CT imaging: the tumors may be homogeneous or heterogeneous, solitary or multifocal, well- or ill-defined. On unenhanced CT images, HCCs typically appear isodense or slightly hypodense relative to liver parenchyma. On enhanced CT, they show early arterial contrast enhancement and rapid washout. HCCs are often inconspicuous on delayed scans. HCC sometimes invades the vasculature in the liver, and even the inferior vena cava may be seen [11]. The diagnosis of underlying cirrhosis may help during differential diagnosis, but it is rare in children. Three-dimensional CT image (**Figure 2**) analysis techniques are now available to estimate tumor volume and provide detailed information regarding the intrahepatic anatomy that resembles the actual intraoperative findings [15]. CT volumetry may permit calculation of resected tumor volume and anticipated size of the remnant liver in planning resection [16]. Plain CT of the chest should be performed to rule out the lung metastases. As for HB, tumor staging is an important consideration in determining the plan of treatment and prognosis. The PRETEXT staging system is recommended because it is currently the only staging system that allows surgical planning [9]. HCC is relatively chemoresistant. Complete resection or liver transplantation of localized tumor is the best option. In the SIOPEL-1 report, the overall resection rate was 36% and the 5 y OS and EFS was 28 and 17% respectively [13]. For liver transplantation, patient survival was

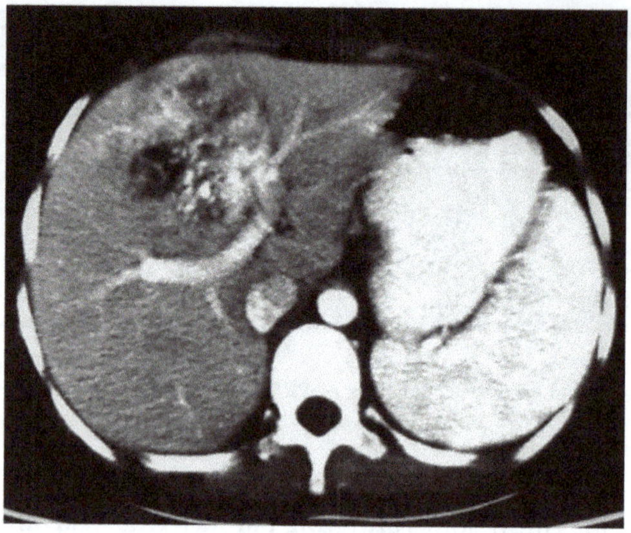

Figure 2. CT of hepatocellular carcinoma in pediatric patient.

63% at 5 years and 58% at 10 years in a study of orthotopic liver transplantation in 41 HCC children <18 years. Recurrence was the primary cause of death in 86% [17]. The outcomes of liver transplantation in HCC are not as good as that for HB.

2.3. Pediatric hepatic sarcomas

Pediatric hepatic sarcomas include undifferentiated embryonal sarcoma (UES), biliary rhabdomyosarcoma, and angiosarcoma [5]. UES is a rare malignant neoplasm, and its the incidence is higher than the other two types of sarcoma. UES was recently shown to share genetic features with mesenchymal harmatoma. Diagnosis of UES is usually between 6 and 10 years but some studies report presentation in young teenagers [18]. The tumor appears on ultrasound as a hetero-echoic mass, and a hypodense multicystic lesion on CT scan or MRI (**Figure 3**), usually exceeding 10 cm in size, with a predominance for involving the right hepatic lobe [19].

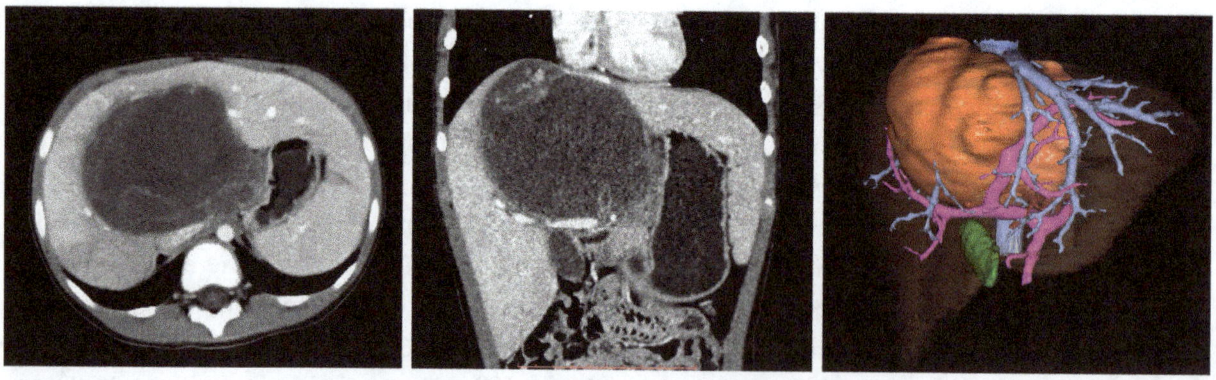

Figure 3. CT and three-dimensional reconstructed liver of undifferentiated embryonal sarcoma.

3. Value of CT scan in guiding the surgical treatment

The objective of surgery is to achieve complete resection of the tumor, both macro- and microscopically, which is paramount for cure of malignant liver cancers. The liver resection strategy is based on pre-operative understanding of liver segmentation, vascular occlusion techniques, and experience in performing different types of hepatectomy, including extensive resection (left and right trisegmentectomies). Although abdominal CT should only be considered if MR imaging is not available or contraindicated, there are some limitations of MRI in some hospitals at developing countries. In our experience, MRI is the best available technique for diagnosing liver tumors, but its value is less clear in preoperatively evaluating the resectability of liver tumors especially in pediatric patients. The development and rapid clinical acceptance of single-detector helical CT during the last decade and, more recently, the introduction of multidetector CT (MDCT) have resulted in significant improvements in the study of the liver. MDCT makes it possible to precisely image the vascular anatomy, including the anomalous branches, feeding arteries, or drainage veins. Moreover, each image phase could be independently and simultaneously extracted or combined. In addition to technical advances, such as shorter scanning times, multiplanar imaging, and improved ability to perform multiphasic contrast-enhanced studies, newer and better intravenous contrast media and advances in post-acquisition data processing techniques have renewed researchers' enthusiasm for using hepatic CT scanning [11].

Furthermore, the software program for volumetry provides a proposed remnant liver volume and an optimal cut line of the liver. Various preoperative simulations can thus be considered. This volumetric analysis positively contributes to the safety of the procedure by assisting in the selection of the optimal operations. Preoperative evaluation of the relationship between the tumor and surrounding vasculature was simulated to perform liver resection with 3D software (**Figure 4**).

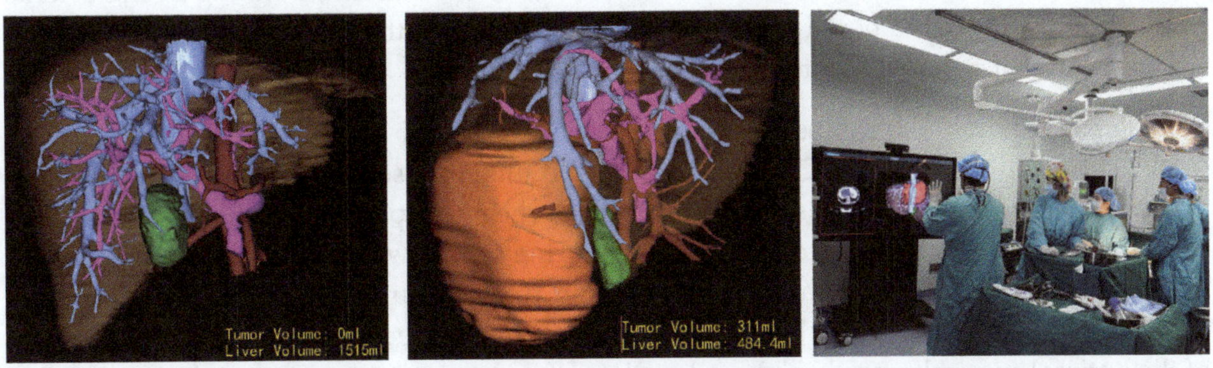

Figure 4. Three-dimensional reconstructed liver indicating total liver volume, liver tumor volume, and intraoperative navigation system.

4. 3D simulation software and Hisense Computer Assisted Surgery System (Hisense CAS)

With the development of three-dimensional simulation software, it is possible to achieve virtual hepatectomy, which can assist the surgeons planning the operation. The development of three-dimensional simulation software makes it possible to achieve virtual hepatectomy, which can assist surgeons to plan the operation, especially the complicated one. The history of 3D simulation software as it relates to hepatectomy can be divided into three stages: [1] successful 3D rendering of liver structures due to the introduction of multidetector row CT in the 1990s [20, 2] virtual hepatectomy depending on the reconstruction of the liver using 3D simulation software since 2000 [21, 3] the clinical practice and popularization of virtual hepatectomy using software packages since 2005, such as operation planning and operative navigation [22]. In some developed countries, such as Japan, virtual hepatectomy has routinely been performed in adult patients undergoing anatomic liver resection. It helps surgeons to plan the operative approach precisely, accurately position the lesion range, and be familiar with the operative route. Hisense Computer Assisted Surgery System (Hisense CAS) is a 3D simulation software package specifically developed for pediatric patients. It can provide precise and exquisite 3D visualization of pediatric liver structures using DICOM data from conventional CT. Considering that children have more refined anatomical structures, the accuracy of Hisense CAS was improved. Hepatectomy can be simulated on a personal computer, and the results can be shared with anyone in the cooperative team. Hisense CAS allows a surgeon to instantaneously manipulate the liver simulation in the operating room using a gesture-controlled display (**Figure 4**).

CT imaging can be performed using a 64-row-MDCT Scanner (Sensation64; Siemens, Erlangen, Germany) with the following parameters: kVp 120, mAs 100, slice collimation 0.625 mm, feed/rotation 12 mm, and rotation time 0.5 s. Patients received 2.0 ml/kg of an iodinated contrast agent (Ultravist; Bayer HealthCare LLC, Germany) to delineate the hepatic vasculature, which was administered intravenously using an automated injector system (CT 9000; Liebel-Flarsheim, Cincinnati, OH) at a rate of 2.0 ml/s. Automated bolus tracking with bolus detection on the level of the ascending aorta assured accurate timing of the arterial phase. For display of the portal and hepatic venous anatomy, third and fourth CT image sets were acquired at 10 and 40 s after the arterial imaging [23].

Four steps are required for transferring the CT DICOM file into 3D digital liver using Hisense CAS: [1] upload the primary CT DICOM data into the Hisense CAS; [2] auto or semi-automatically reconstruct the liver structures (liver parenchyma, portal vein, hepatic veins, and tumors) in a 3D context by extraction of neighboring voxels with a similar CT density, and automatically calculate the total liver volume and tumor volume; [3] virtual liver resection using the software (automatically calculating the remnant liver volume); and [4] assessment of the optimal surgical procedures based on the virtual hepatectomy. The surgical team could communicate and discuss the surgical liver anatomy with radiologists or pediatricians based on 3D reconstruction, such as the tumor locations, the appearance of the vessel branches, or approach of liver resection. Various virtual surgical strategies could be explored in the Hisense CAS. Finally, the surgical team could develop the optimal plan of operation [7].

5. Dong's digital liver classification

With the development of medical imaging, 3D reconstruction technology, the innovation of liver surgery and the proposal of precision hepatectomy, the intrahepatic vascular anatomy of the liver and liver segmentectomy based on that vascular anatomy have become well developed. With the analysis of 3D digital liver, we proposed a new type of liver classification system: Dong's digital liver classification system. Professor Dong Qian of the Affiliated Hospital of Qingdao University analyzed the anatomy of thousands of digital human livers from newborns to the elderly to build a new system of liver classification based on intrahepatic vascular anatomy [24].

1260 cases of normal human liver were rendered into 3D digital livers using their DICOM files. Based on the anatomical variation of the portal branches supplying liver segments, we built our Dong's digital liver classification system.

We divided the digital liver into four groups based on the type of segmentation and the variations in portal vein anatomy. Type A livers are similar to Couinaud or Cho's segmentation, containing eight segments (**Figure 5**). Type B livers have nine segments because there are three subdivisions of right-anterior portal vein (**Figure 6**). The defining characteristic of Type C is the variation in the right-posterior portal vein, which is arcuate-shaped (**Figure 7**). Type C-a livers have arcuate-shaped right-posterior portal veins and right-anterior portal veins like those in Type A livers. Type C-b livers have arcuate-shaped right-posterior portal veins and right-anterior portal veins like those in Type B livers. Type D livers have anomalous portal vein variations, which require three-dimensional simulation and individualized liver resection plan (**Figure 8**).

Type A: Similar to Couinaud [25] or Cho's segmentation [26], containing eight segments (**Figure 5**).

Segment I (3–6 P1 branches): Caudate lobe. There are 3–6 small branches (P1) originating from the back of right and left portal vein, surrounded by 5–8 tiny short hepatic veins.

Segments II and III: The left portal vein divides into the third-grade portal vein (P2 and P3) and perfuses the upper and lower outer sides of the left liver, which contains segments II and III.

Segment IV: Portal veins divided from the left portal vein perfuse the inner part of the left liver.

Segments V and VIII: The right portal vein divides into the right anterior and posterior branches, and then the anterior trunk further divides into several branches. (**Figure 5**).

Segments VI and VII: The right posterior portal vein further divides into right anterior (P6) and posterior branches (P7). The anterior branches perfuse segment VI, the lower outer area of the right liver.

Type B: Nine segments due to three subdivisions of right-anterior portal vein (**Figure 6**).

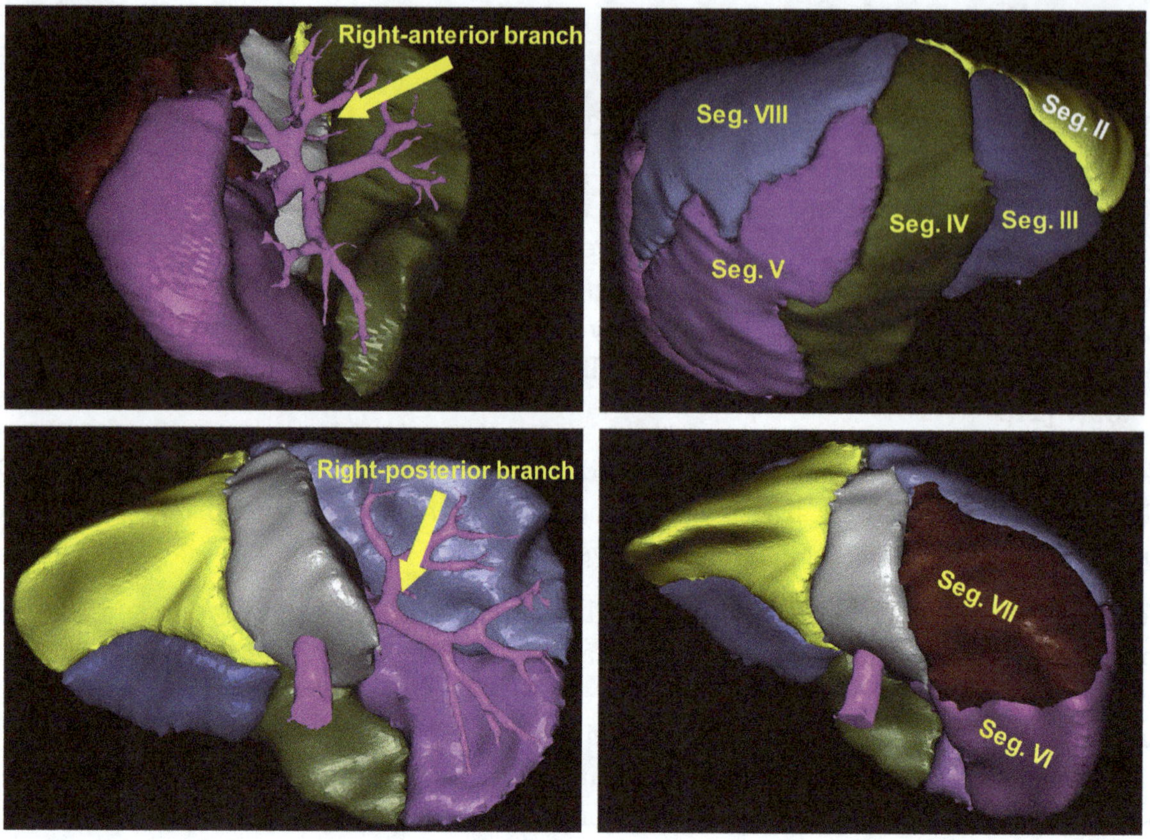

Figure 5. Right-anterior and right-posterior part of liver anatomy indicating Type A segmentation of Dong's digital liver classification system, similar to Couinaud or Cho's segmentation.

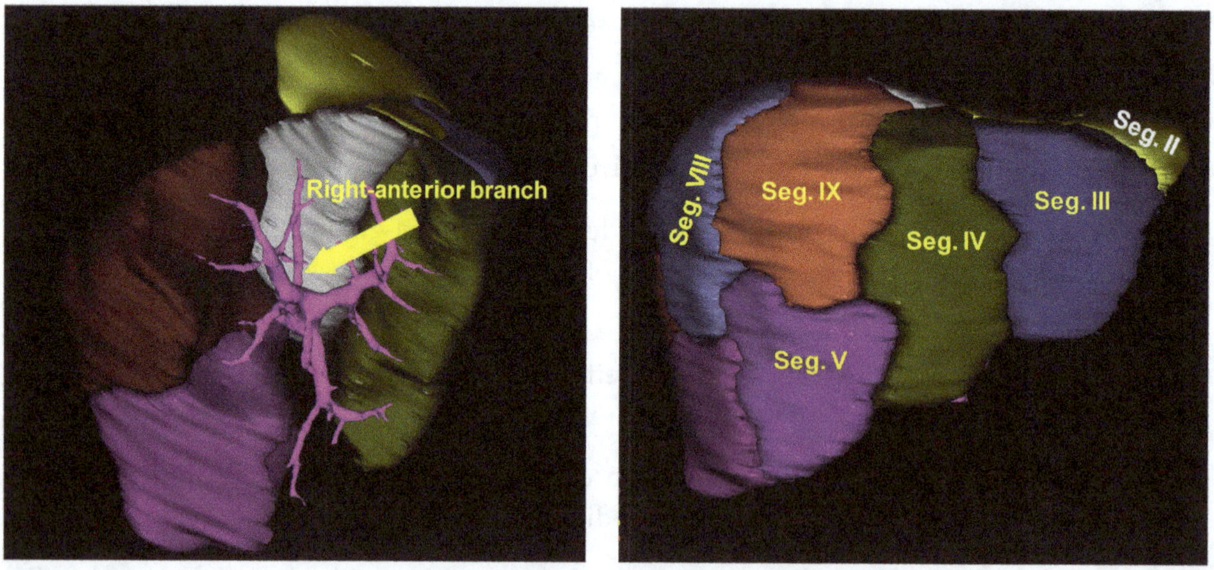

Figure 6. Right-anterior part of liver anatomy indicating Type B segmentation of Dong's digital liver classification system.

Type C: The right posterior portal vein does not divide into main branches as in Type A or B livers, whose portal veins separate into 5–11 branches from an arcuate trunk. During precise hepatectomy, it is difficult to resect only segments VI or VII as in Type A and Type B. The prevalence of Type C livers is not high, but it makes a considerable difference in precise surgery. Cases in which the right posterior portal vein is arcuate type and the right anterior portal vein separates into only P8 and P5 are defined as Type C-a (**Figure 7**). When the right posterior portal vein is arcuate type and the right anterior portal vein separate to P5, P8, and P9, we define it as Type C-b.

Type D: This is a catchall category, appearing in about 12.43% of all livers. It includes all variations that cannot be classified into any of the previous three types (**Figure 8**).

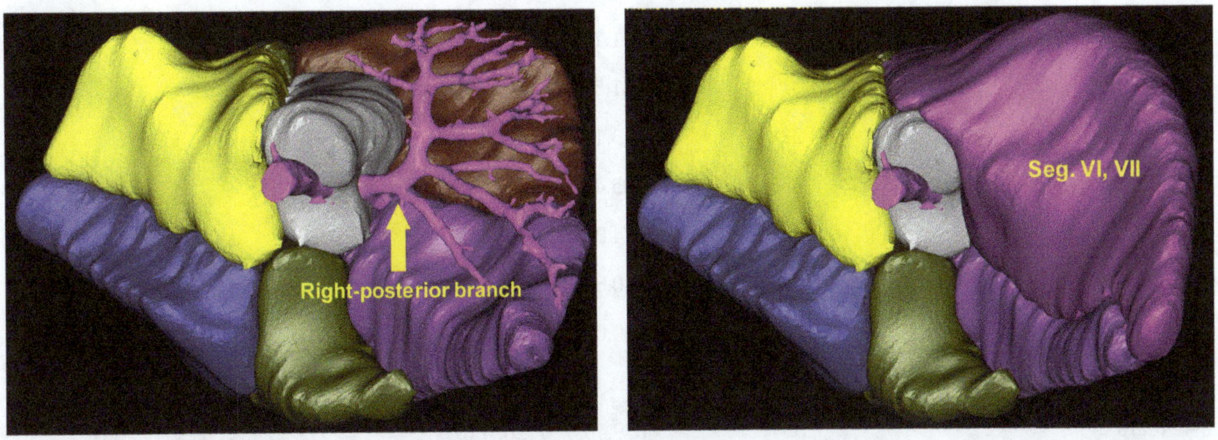

Figure 7. Type C livers have arcuate-shaped right-posterior portal veins.

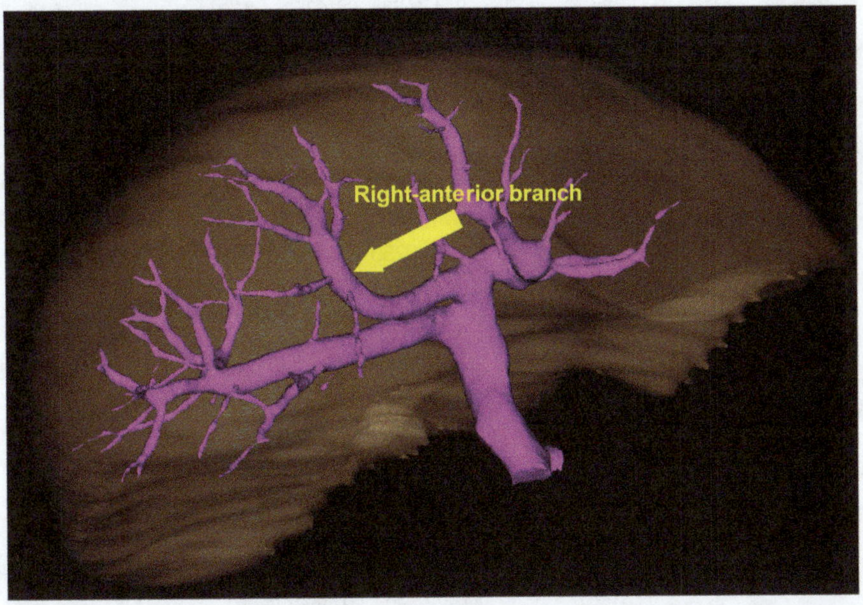

Figure 8. Rare variation of portal vein which is classified into Type D segmentation.

6. Measurement of liver volume from neonates to the elderly

Total liver volume, the basic unit of liver function, is an important factor to evaluate the resectability of liver cancer. There have been many studies of the total liver volume and necessary remnant liver volume in adult patients but only a few reports regarding liver volume in children. Because measured total liver volume has been proposed as the golden standard of liver volume for preoperative surgical plan, we tried to summarize the average total liver volume of Chinese patients of different ages, from neonates to the elderly.

Age	N	Liver volume (cm³)
<1 Month	28	140.0339 ± 50.0707
1–3 Months	26	191.1462 ± 38.9132
4–6 Months	31	261.5065 ± 70.9437
7–9 Months	22	273.1917 ± 50.0732
10–12 Months	33	305.4692 ± 36.3323
1–2 Years	56	374.3617 ± 65.8447
2–3 Years	66	440.8111 ± 71.4779
3–4 Years	58	500.0037 ± 103.2837
4–5 Years	49	549.4533 ± 84.6325
5–6 Years	33	639.4677 ± 126.7067
6–7 Years	44	722.0357 ± 140.8796
7–8 Years	44	824.6372 ± 137.9766
8–9 Years	32	844.4633 ± 93.6353
9–10 Years	37	935.8571 ± 189.1018
10–11 Years	29	985.0464 ± 121.0802
11–12 Years	27	1048.9250 ± 167.5279
12–13 Years	29	1118.4593 ± 155.2817
13–14 Years	22	1125.0250 ± 147.9899
14–18 Years	30	1323.8862 ± 226.3454
18–30 Years	42	1361.8682 ± 205.3783
30–40 Years	74	1381.1037 ± 300.3834
40–50 Years	139	1423.7647 ± 216.9305
50–60 Years	197	1343.2768 ± 246.6878
60–70 Years	181	1284.4183 ± 190.7129
70–80 Years	106	1263.1282 ± 170.2464
80–100 Years	21	1089.3429 ± 199.0259
Total	1456	

Table 1. Standard liver volume range (X ± S, cm³).

Upper abdominal CT films from 1456 children (enhanced CT 837, plain CT 619) aged 1 day to 100 years were selected. None had any history of liver disease, and CT had been performed for other clinical purposes. The patients were divided into 26 groups by age (**Table 1**).

7. Human Digital Liver Database

The Human Digital Liver Database (HDLD) was established by the Affiliated Hospital of Qingdao University and Hisense Company, aiming to collect digital liver from neonates, children, adults, and the elderly, from normal livers, livers with cancer, and simulated livers resected using Hisense CAS. The link of the HDLD is http://www.hdldb.net, which now is only available in Chinese (the English version is being translated now). The HDLD will show the digital liver in image and video form. All visitors could study the updated clinical cases at any angle of reconstructed 3D digital liver, including the vascular system, anatomical differences in the liver, and the correlation between vascular and liver tumors. The HDLD will also provide the intra-operation video comparing to the preoperative surgical plan, to help doctors and medical students better understand the anatomy and surgical procedure of pediatric liver resection, especially for patients with giant liver tumors (**Figure 9**).

7.1. Normal children and adult digital liver database

Vascular anatomical variation and total liver volume are two of the more important factors that surgeons consider when making surgical plans. We have collected thousands of CT scan data from across the nation. We would like to establish a digital liver database showing the reconstructed digital liver and separate these digital livers into different groups according to the anatomical variations in liver vasculature and liver volume (**Figure 9**). The Dong's Digital Liver Classification was established based on our collection of digital livers. We believe that a normal digital liver database may serve as an important reference for surgeons all around world.

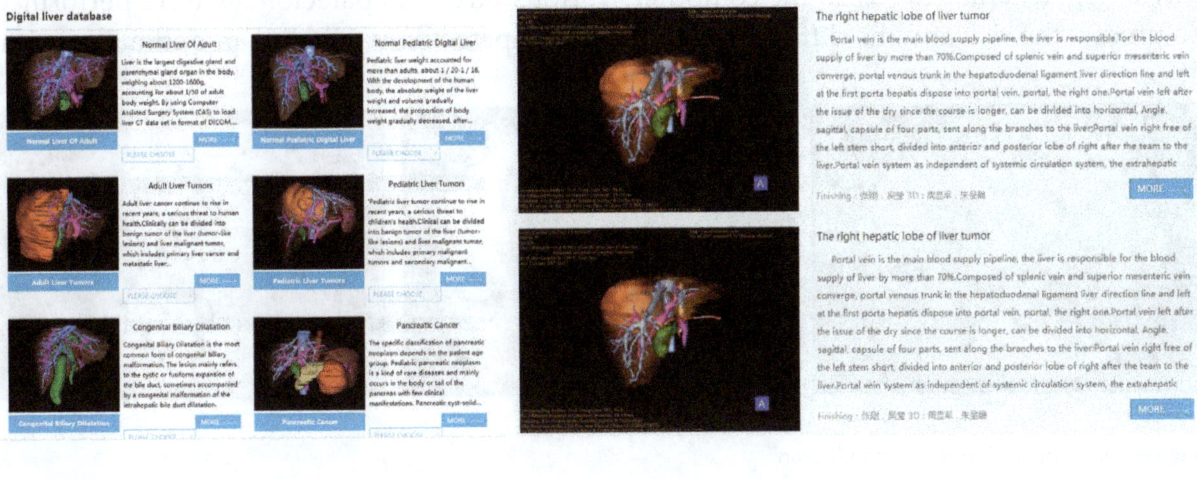

Figure 9. The Human Digital Liver Database.

7.2. Liver tumor database and simulated liver surgery

The liver tumor database shows the reconstructed digital liver image and simulated liver resection according to the surgeon's preoperative plan, and the intraoperative video of clinical cases, aiming to share the experience gained by staff at our center freely around the world. With the help of Hisense CAS, the successful surgical resection of liver tumors in pediatric patients has improved in our center. With the 3D simulation, we have found that we can clearly understand the anatomical variation in intrahepatic vasculature, the correlation of vasculature with liver tumors, and calculate the remnant liver volume of the simulated liver easily. In the database, we would like to show some difficult cases, such as those with very large liver tumors and those with vascular variation.

8. Clinical application of Hisense CAS for diagnosis and surgical plans in children with large liver tumors

An 11-month-old male infant was referred with abdominal distension and loss of appetite for the past 2 months [27]. Upon examination, a firm, non-tender mass with a smooth surface was evident arising from the right lobe of the liver, which filled the abdominal cavity. Serum ALT, AST, GGT, ALP, and Alb were normal. Both serum α-fetoprotein (AFP) and carcinoembryonic antigen (CEA) levels were within normal ranges. Ultrasound (US) revealed a well-defined, multicystic mass involving the liver. Enhanced CT images similarly showed a giant cystic mass with minimally enhanced septation and peripheral solid components (**Figure 10**).

The DICOM data obtained from the CT images were uploaded to 3D simulation software, the Hisense Computer Assisted Surgery System (Hisense, China) to simulate the liver. The relationship between HMH and the intrahepatic vasculature was revealed in a 3D context (**Figure 11**). The right hepatic vein (RHV), the middle hepatic vein (MHV), and the left hepatic vein (LHV) were confluent with a common trunk. The hepatic veins (HVs), the portal veins (PVs), and the inferior vena cava (IVC) were displaced, with no obvious infiltration or encasement. The volume of both the functional liver and the HMH was automatically calculated. The positional relationship between the vessels and HMH could be confirmed from any angle instantaneously in the computer. Various virtual hepatectomies were performed to predict the risk and the difficulty of the actual hepatectomy. Finally, an optimal surgical

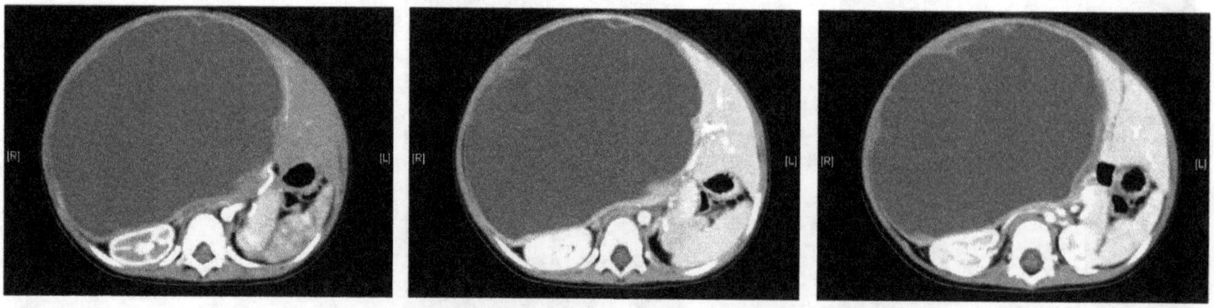

Figure 10. Preoperative enhanced CT scan.

plan was developed using 3D simulation software to safeguard RHV. The enucleation of HMH for the case was performed after adequate preoperative preparation.

After laparotomy, the fluid was aspirated using a 20 G needle from the cystic components of HMH to reduce its volume, thereby facilitating surgical resection. The resection line at the rim of HMH, which was indicated by virtual hepatectomy was made using the electrotome. The hepatic portal occlusion was used to reduce the risk of bleeding. The hepatic parenchyma was dissected using the CUSA system. The intrahepatic vessels were dissected to be safeguarded or else ligated and divided, a matter that had been assessed by the virtual hepatectomy. After 20 min, the HMH was removed with surrounding rim of normal liver tissue. The right hepatic vein was successfully safeguarded. The remnant liver volume was about 210 ml, which approximately equaled the automatically calculated remnant liver volume (230.1 ml). There was no anatomical discrepancy between the operation and the 3D simulation. The convalescence was uneventful. Histopathology confirmed the diagnosis of mesenchymal hamartoma (**Figure 12**).

In summary, three-dimensional (3D) imaging could significantly improve the resection rate of pediatric tumors and increase the safety of the surgery. Dong's digital liver classification system and human digital liver classification system will be useful for surgeons all around the world.

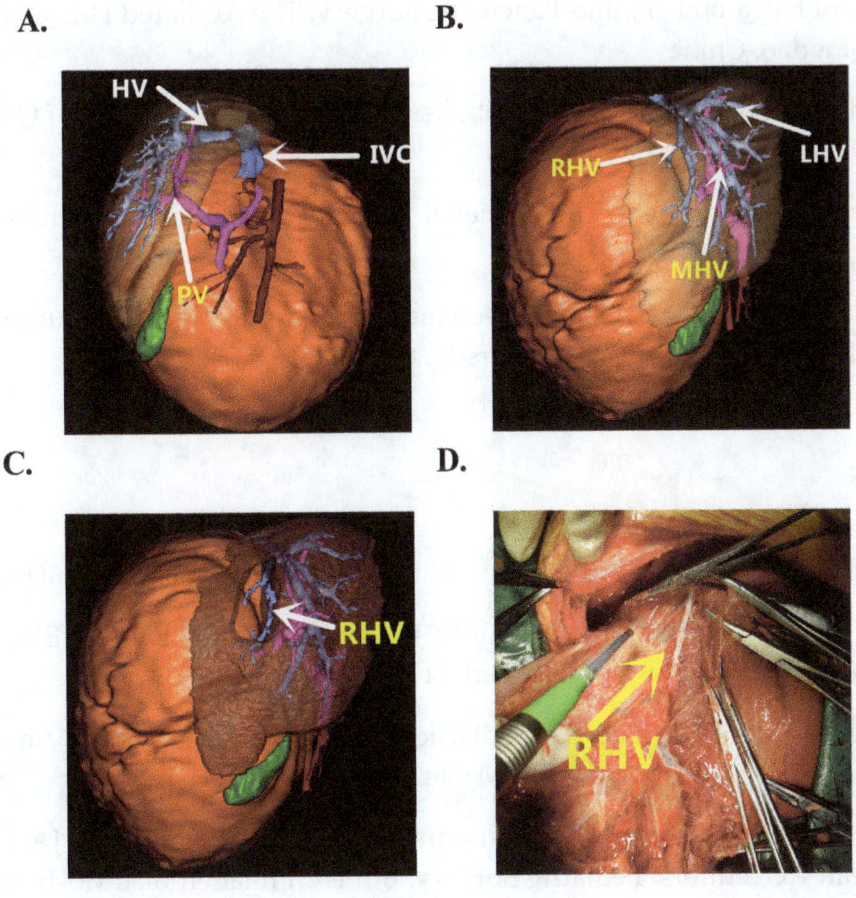

Figure 11. Comparison of 3D simulation and intraoperative liver anatomy.

A. 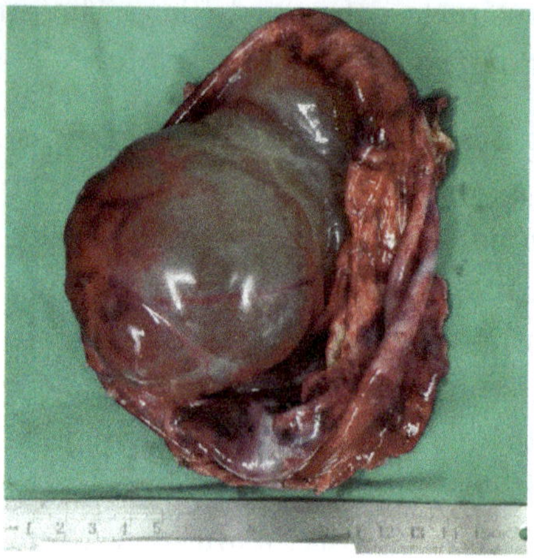 B. 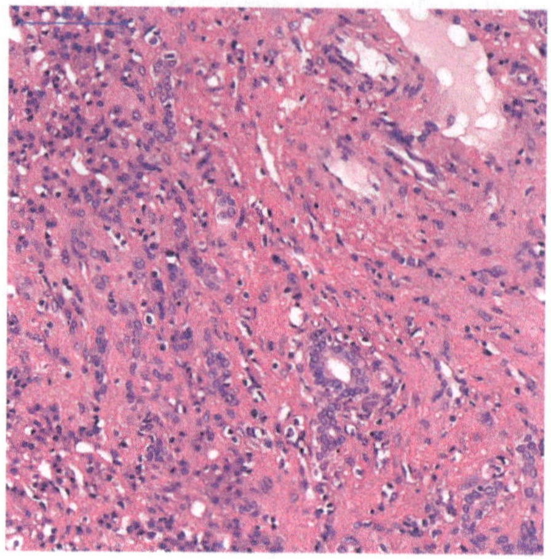

Figure 12. Resected HMH tumor and pathology.

Author details

Chengzhan Zhu[1,4], Bingzi Dong[2] and Qian Dong[3,4]*

*Address all correspondence to: 13608968352@163.com

1 Department of Hepatobiliary and Pancreatic Surgery, The Affiliated Hospital of Qingdao University, Qingdao, China

2 Department of Endocrinology and Metabolism, The Affiliated Hospital of Qingdao University, Qingdao, China

3 Pediatric Surgery Department, The Affiliated Hospital of Qingdao University, Qingdao, China

4 Shandong Key Laboratory of Digital Medicine and Computer Assisted Surgery, The Affiliated Hospital of Qingdao University, Qingdao, China

References

[1] Stocker JT. Hepatic tumors in children. Clinics in Liver Disease. 2001;**5**(1):259-281 viii-ix

[2] LaBerge JM. Liver tumors. In: O'Neill JA Jr, Grosfeld JL, Fonkalsrud EW, et al., editors. Principles of Pediatric Surgery. 2nd ed. St Louis: Mosby; 2003

[3] Yikilmaz A, George M, Lee EY. Pediatric hepatobiliary neoplasms: An overview and update. Radiologic Clinics of North America. 2017;**55**(4):741-766

[4] De Ugarte DA, Atkinson J. Liver tumors. In: Grosfeld JL, O'Neill JA Jr, Fonkalsrud AG, Coran AG, editors. Pediatric Surgery. 6th ed. Philadelphia: Mosby-Elsevier; 2006. pp. 502-505

[5] Aronson DC, Meyers RL. Malignant tumors of the liver in children. Seminars in Pediatric Surgery. 2016;**25**(5):265-275

[6] Roebuck DJ. Assessment of malignant liver tumors in children. Cancer Imaging. 2009; **9 Spec No A**:S98-S103

[7] Zhang G, Zhou XJ, Zhu CZ, Dong Q, Su L. Usefulness of three-dimensional(3D) simulation software in hepatectomy for pediatric hepatoblastoma. Surgical Oncology. 2016;**25**(3):236-243

[8] Czauderna P, Haeberle B, Hiyama E, Rangaswami A, Krailo M, Maibach R, et al. Novel global rare tumor database yields new prognostic factors in hepatoblastoma and becomes a research model. European Journal of Cancer. 2016;**52**:92-101

[9] Brown J, Perilongo G, Shafford E, Keeling J, Pritchard J, Brock P, et al. Pretreatment prognostic factors for children with hepatoblastoma-- results from the International Society of Paediatric Oncology (SIOP) study SIOPEL 1. European Journal of Cancer. 2000;**36**(11):1418-1425

[10] Czauderna P, Otte JB, Aronson DC, Gauthier F, Mackinlay G, Roebuck D, et al. Guidelines for surgical treatment of hepatoblastoma in the modern era--recommendations from the Childhood Liver Tumour Strategy Group of the International Society of Paediatric Oncology (SIOPEL). European Journal of Cancer. 2005;**41**(7):1031-1036

[11] Dong Q, Chen J. CT scan of pediatric liver tumors. In: Subburaj K, editor. CT Scanning Techniques and Applications. Intech; 2011

[12] Darbari A, Sabin KM, Shapiro CN, Schwarz KB. Epidemiology of primary hepatic malignancies in U.S. children. Hepatology. 2003;**38**(3):560-566

[13] Czauderna P, Mackinlay G, Perilongo G, Brown J, Shafford E, Aronson D, et al. Hepatocellular carcinoma in children: Results of the first prospective study of the International Society of Pediatric Oncology group. Journal of Clinical Oncology. 2002;**20**(12): 2798-2804

[14] Agarwala S. Primary malignant liver tumors in children. The Indian Journal of Pediatrics. 2012;**79**(6):793-800

[15] Su L, Dong Q, Zhang H, Zhou X, Chen Y, Hao X, et al. Clinical application of a three-dimensional imaging technique in infants and young children with complex liver tumors. Pediatric Surgery International. 2016;**32**(4):387-395

[16] Shoup M, Gonen M, D'Angelica M, Jarnagin WR, DeMatteo RP, Schwartz LH, et al. Volumetric analysis predicts hepatic dysfunction in patients undergoing major liver resection. Journal of Gastrointestinal Surgery. 2003;**7**(3):325-330

[17] Austin MT, Leys CM, Feurer ID, Lovvorn HN 3rd, O'Neill JA Jr, Pinson CW, et al. Liver transplantation for childhood hepatic malignancy: A review of the United Network for Organ Sharing (UNOS) database. Journal of Pediatric Surgery. 2006;**41**(1):182-186

[18] Plant AS, Busuttil RW, Rana A, Nelson SD, Auerbach M, Federman NC. A single-institution retrospective cases series of childhood undifferentiated embryonal liver sarcoma (UELS): Success of combined therapy and the use of orthotopic liver transplant. Journal of Pediatric Hematology/Oncology. 2013;**35**(6):451-455

[19] Cao Q, Ye Z, Chen S, Liu N, Li S, Liu F. Undifferentiated embryonal sarcoma of liver: A multi-institutional experience with 9 cases. International Journal of Clinical and Experimental Pathology. 2014;**7**(12):8647-8656

[20] Hashimoto D, Dohi T, Tsuzuki M, Horiuchi T, Ohta Y, Chinzei K, et al. Development of a computer-aided surgery system: Three-dimensional graphic reconstruction for treatment of liver cancer. Surgery. 1991;**109**(5):589-596

[21] Lamade W, Glombitza G, Fischer L, Chiu P, Cardenas CE Sr, Thorn M, et al. The impact of 3-dimensional reconstructions on operation planning in liver surgery. Archives of Surgery. 2000;**135**(11):1256-1261

[22] Souzaki R, Ieiri S, Uemura M, Ohuchida K, Tomikawa M, Kinoshita Y, et al. An augmented reality navigation system for pediatric oncologic surgery based on preoperative CT and MRI images. Journal of Pediatric Surgery. 2013;**48**(12):2479-2483

[23] Fuchs J, Warmann SW, Szavay P, Kirschner HJ, Schafer JF, Hennemuth A, et al. Three-dimensional visualization and virtual simulation of resections in pediatric solid tumors. Journal of Pediatric Surgery. 2005;**40**(2):364-370

[24] Zhou X, Dong Q, Zhu C, Chen X, Wei B, Duan Y, et al. The role and significance of digital reconstruction technique in liver segments based on portal vein structure. Chinese Journal of Surgery. 2018;**56**(1):61-67

[25] Couinaud C. The anatomy of the liver. Annali Italiani di Chirurgia. 1992;**63**(6):693-697

[26] Cho A, Okazumi S, Miyazawa Y, Makino H, Miura F, Ohira G, et al. Proposal for a reclassification of liver based anatomy on portal ramifications. American Journal of Surgery. 2005;**189**(2):195-199

[27] Zhao J, Zhou XJ, Zhu CZ, Wu Y, Wei B, Zhang G, et al. 3D simulation assisted resection of giant hepatic mesenchymal hamartoma in children. Computer Assisted Surgery (Abingdon). 2017;**22**(1):54-59

5

Neonatal Tumors

Kenneth W. Gow and Matthew Dellinger

Abstract

Neonatal tumors encompass a group of heterogeneous neoplasms that demonstrate anatomic locations, behavior patterns, histologic features, and treatment responses that are distinct from neoplasms found in older children. The majority of neonatal tumors are benign, with malignant lesions accounting for only 2% of childhood cancers. However, histologically benign tumors can lead to detrimental effects on the fetus and newborn due to their size and location in relation to vital structures. An understanding of the incidence, appearance, and typical locations of neonatal tumors can provide important diagnostic information and guide treatment decisions. Although surgical intervention is the mainstay of therapy for many neonatal tumors, it is important to recognize that some lesions will regress spontaneously, whereas others may respond to noninvasive treatment modalities. In this chapter, we explore the epidemiology of neonatal tumors and provide a location-based classification schema to aid in diagnosis. A summary of the presentation, diagnosis, and management of the most common neonatal tumors is provided as well.

Keywords: neonatal tumors, sacrococcygeal teratoma, neuroblastoma, infantile hepatic hemangioma, mesenchymal hamartoma, ovarian cyst, cervical lymphatic malformation, rhabdomyosarcoma, congenital mesoblastic nephroma

1. Introduction

Neonatal tumors encompass a group of heterogeneous neoplasms that are diagnosed prenatally or within the first 30 days of life. Neonatal tumors demonstrate anatomic locations, behavior patterns, histologic features, and treatment responses that are distinct from neoplasms found in older children [1]. The preponderance of information regarding the epidemiology of neonatal tumors is provided through the experience of single institutions. The true incidence of these lesions is unknown, as studies do not always account for pregnancies with a prenatally diagnosed mass that end in stillbirth, miscarriage, or early termination of pregnancy.

Most solid neoplasms identified in neonates are benign [2]. The incidence of a malignant tumor is 1 in every 12,500–27,500 live births, accounting for 2% of all childhood cancers [1]. Distinguishing between benign and malignant neoplasms can prove to be challenging in this group of patients. The features of a tumor that denote malignancy in adults, such as high nuclear-cytoplasmic ratio, high mitotic rate, and anaplasia, may be present in benign lesions in children and neonates [3]. Neonatal tumors are also unique in that they arise from embryonic and immature tissue as a result of intrinsic dysfunction of cellular growth and proliferation [3, 4]. As opposed to adult tumors, environmental exposures are believed to play little to no role in tumorigenesis [4]. Some malignant lesions have minimal potential for invasion or metastasis, while histologically benign lesions can be lethal due to their size and location.

Although less than 10% of childhood cancers arise in the setting of a cancer predisposition syndrome, any neonatal tumor should raise concern for this possibility [5]. The presence of associated congenital anomalies, multifocal or bilateral disease, and cancer in close relatives is suggestive of an underlying cancer predisposition syndrome [6]. Several specific types of tumors, including retinoblastoma, adrenocortical carcinoma, pleuropulmonary blastoma, hepatoblastoma, and Wilms' tumor, show a strong association with a cancer predisposition syndrome [5]. Since the presence of genetically derived lesions can have implications for these children and their family members, genetic counseling and testing should be offered.

2. Diagnosis

A thorough history and physical examination are paramount in the evaluation of a newborn. However, many anomalies can be detected prior to birth. The ability to diagnose neoplasms in utero has evolved significantly with improvement in imaging modalities. Fetal ultrasonography, magnetic resonance imaging (MRI), and echocardiography offer physicians the opportunity to diagnose a variety of congenital diseases in the prenatal period [7–9]. Ultrasonography is a critical component of the prenatal obstetric evaluation and is currently the standard of care. Prenatal ultrasound provides vital information regarding gestational age, number of fetuses, fetal health, and the presence of congenital anomalies [9]. Ultrasound and MRI are preferred because they avoid the damaging effects of ionizing radiation.

For decades, ultrasonography has been the principal imaging modality for prenatal diagnosis of fetal anomalies [10]. The benefits of ultrasound are numerous, including wide availability, low cost, noninvasiveness, and the ability, to provide real-time evaluation of the fetus. One shortcoming of ultrasound is that results are operator dependent and can vary with the experience and expertise of the examiner [11]. In a systematic review of ultrasound for fetal assessment in early pregnancy, Bricker et al. [12] determined the overall sensitivity for detection of fetal anomalies to be 44.7%. However, the sensitivities of the included studies showed great variability, ranging from 15 to 85.3%. In addition to operator experience, gestational age, anomaly type, and equipment quality impact the accuracy of screening prenatal ultrasound [12].

In the past two decades, magnetic resonance imaging (MRI) has become increasingly utilized as an adjunct to ultrasound in the evaluation of fetal and neonatal anomalies [8, 10, 13].

One driving force behind this phenomenon is the development of ultrafast MRI, which limits fetal motion artifact and does not require maternal-fetal sedation [11]. The greatest utility of MRI appears to occur in cases where sonographic findings are equivocal or further diagnostic information is desired [11, 14, 15]. MRI is also particularly useful in illustrating anatomic relationships between neoplasms and adjacent structures, characterizing intracranial and soft tissue lesions, in cases of oligohydramnios and in cases of maternal obesity [11, 14, 15].

In the most recent Guidelines for Diagnostic Imaging in Pregnancy and Lactation, the American College of Obstetricians and Gynecologists states that there is no evidence of harm from tissue heating, acoustic damage, or teratogenesis when using MRI in pregnancy [16]. However, one issue that merits discussion is the use of gadolinium contrast dye to enhance fetal imaging. In practice, gadolinium is administered as a gadolinium-chelate molecule that is water-soluble and can cross the placenta into fetal circulation. Following filtration and excretion by the fetal kidneys, these molecules can accumulate in amniotic fluid with the ability to release potentially toxic gadolinium ions [17]. Although the effect of free gadolinium ions on the fetus is unknown, the current recommendation is to abstain from the routine use of MRI contrast agents unless the benefits can be shown to clearly outweigh this theoretical risk [17].

The diagnosis of a neonatal tumor has a profound emotional impact on a family and raises questions about accuracy of diagnosis, prognosis, treatment options, and long-term outcomes [18]. While technological improvements in imaging modalities have led to better sensitivity in diagnosing congenital anomalies, the false-positive rate is far from negligible [19]. Care should be taken in making definitive statements about diagnosis and prognosis on prenatal imaging as normal anatomic variants can have the appearance of a neoplastic process and some lesions will regress spontaneously. Conversely, sonographic findings of polyhydramnios, fetal hydrops, hepatosplenomegaly, and placentomegaly should raise suspicion for an undiagnosed tumor.

Finally, having diagnostic imaging that points to anomalies will allow the care team to have prenatal discussions and do important planning. Depending on all tests done, the parents should be offered possible diagnoses, complications, and outcomes. However, one needs to be guarded with prognostication, and consideration for termination of the pregnancy must be very carefully made including all knowns and unknowns. Assuming that the plans are for delivery, early diagnosis will allow for planning around the delivery; the location of the birthing center (closer to home vs. in a maternal-neonatal center), the means of birth (vaginal vs. Cesarean section vs. ex utero intrapartum treatment (EXIT)), the personnel required for the birth aside from those needed to care for the mother (neonatologist, pediatric anesthesiologist, pediatric otolaryngologist, pediatric general surgeon, pediatric cardiothoracic surgeon), and logistics with regard to coordination of the team including diagnostic and operative services.

3. Anatomic considerations/locations

Neonatal tumors represent a varied group of neoplasms that are discovered in multiple locations throughout the body (**Figure 1**). The diversity observed is not surprising since these lesions arise

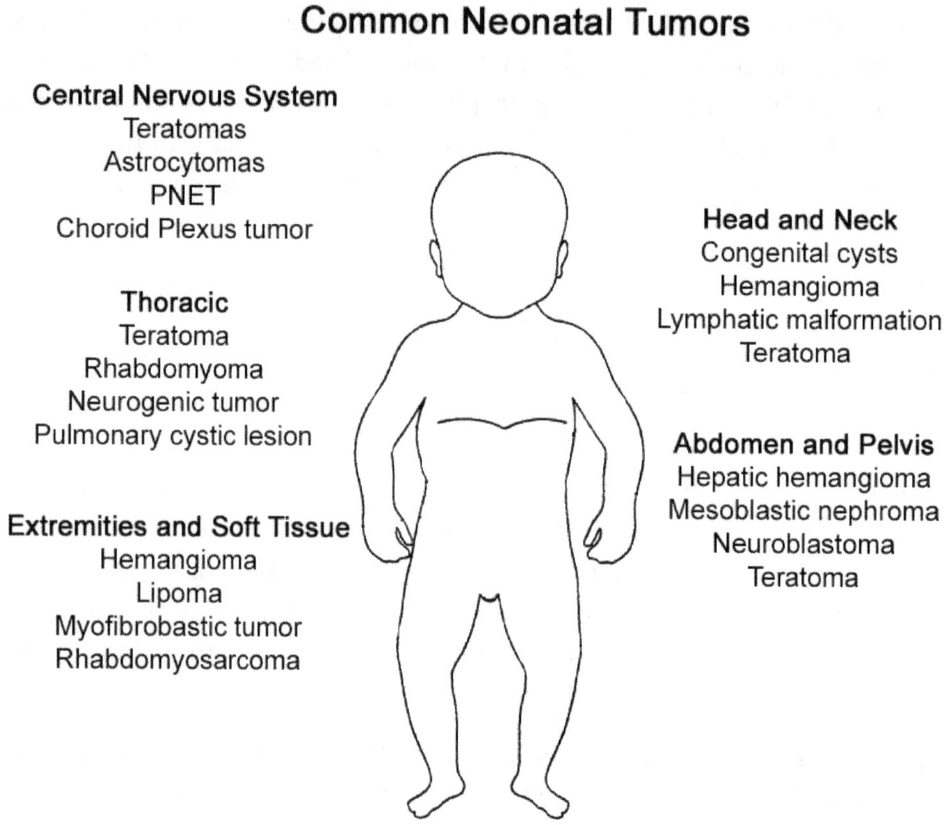

Figure 1. Common neonatal tumors based on location.

from abnormalities in fetal and neonatal development. Teratomas, particularly sacrococcygeal teratomas, are the most common neonatal tumor [1, 20, 21]. Neuroblastoma is the second most common neoplasm in neonates and the leading cause of malignancy in this group of patients. In order to decrease frequency, soft tissue tumors, central nervous system (CNS) tumors, leukemia, and renal tumors are the next most common tumor types recognized [1, 20, 21]. **Table 1** provides a brief summary of the most frequently encountered neonatal tumors. Knowledge of the incidence, appearance, and typical locations of these lesions can provide important diagnostic

Type	Percentage
Extracranial teratoma	24–30%
Neuroblastoma	23–30%
Soft tissue tumors	8–12%
Leukemia	6–12%
CNS tumors	6–10%
Renal tumors	5–7%
Hepatic tumors	5%
Cardiopulmonary tumors	<3%

Table 1. Distribution of commonly occurring neonatal tumors [1, 18, 20, 21].

information. In particular, the location of the lesion gives a wealth of information regarding the differential diagnosis. The following discussions provide a location-based review of common neonatal tumors, which is intended to provide the clinician a basis to create a differential diagnosis to plan for management. Later, specific histologic diseases will be presented to allow tailoring of therapy.

4. Central nervous system

Primary central nervous system (CNS) neoplasms are the most common solid tumor in childhood and the leading cause of cancer death in this group of patients [22]. Fortunately, this is a rare entity with an estimated incidence of 5.57 cases per 100,000 children between the ages of 0 and 19 [23]. In neonates, CNS tumors are the fifth most common solid malignancy, which occur less frequently than lesions found in older children. Brain tumors in fetuses and neonates are unique in that they are often supratentorial, while lesions in older children are typically infratentorial [24]. The rarity of neonatal brain tumors and the absence of a national pediatric CNS cancer registry make it difficult to ascertain a true incidence [25].

In a retrospective review of 250 cases of perinatal brain tumors, Isaacs [24] found that the most common tumors were teratomas (29.6%), astrocytomas (18.8%), primitive neuroectodermal tumors (13.2%), and choroid plexus tumors (13.2%). Those children presenting with choroid plexus tumors, low-grade astrocytomas, and gangliogliomas had the best survival, while intracranial teratomas and neuroectodermal tumors exhibited the worst prognosis [24]. The 5-year survival rate for neonatal brain tumors, regardless of treatment modality, is 23–36% [25]. The management of these patients includes surgical resection, chemotherapy, and irradiation, although any treatment decision should be coordinated through a multidisciplinary approach. Regardless of the histologic subtype and associated prognosis, the identification of a neonatal brain tumor is a devastating and life-altering experience for families.

5. Head and neck

Multiple conditions lead to the development of masses occurring in the head and neck of pediatric patients. The differential diagnosis is extensive and includes a variety of congenital, inflammatory, benign, and malignant lesions [26]. The vast majority of these lesions are benign. According to a comprehensive, 5-year review of 445 pediatric neck masses at Children's Hospital of Philadelphia, the most frequent lesions were congenital in origin (55%), followed by inflammatory masses (27%), malignant neoplasms (11%), and benign neoplasms (3%) [27]. Inflammatory lesions likely account for the most common pediatric neck masses but often resolve with conservative therapy, obviating the need for biopsy or excision [26]. The incidence and distribution of head and neck masses in the neonatal period are not as well defined.

The most common congenital head and neck lesions are branchial cleft, thyroglossal duct, and dermoid cysts. Although less common, vascular masses, lymphatic malformations, and teratomas deserve special consideration secondary to the potential to cause detrimental effects on the developing fetus and newborn. Highly vascular lesions can lead to high-output cardiac failure and hydrops fetalis. Fluid accumulation in lymphatic malformations and the nearby tissues can also lead to fetal hydrops. Mass effect and extrinsic compression from certain lesions have the potential to cause life-threatening airway obstruction as well as atypical development of adjacent structures. Cervical lymphatic malformations and cervical teratomas, two lesions responsible for these physiologic disturbances, will be discussed in greater detail later in this chapter.

Cervical vascular masses include congenital and infantile hemangiomas. An important distinction to make is that vascular malformations and congenital hemangiomas are present at birth, grow concurrently with the child, and do not involute. Vascular tumors develop in the neonatal period and demonstrate a proliferative phase followed by involution [28]. Infantile hemangiomas occur in up to 4–5% of newborns [29]. Infantile hemangiomas arise following birth, proliferate for a variable amount of time, and ultimately involute. In contrast, congenital hemangiomas proliferate in utero and are fully developed at birth. These masses can be subdivided into rapidly involuting and noninvoluting types. Congenital hemangiomas are rare, accounting for only 3% of all hemangiomas [30].

Malignant head and neck lesions are rarely diagnosed in neonates. Lymphomas are the most common head and neck malignancy in children, with 60% of these tumors being classified as non-Hodgkin's lymphoma and the remaining 40% classified as Hodgkin's lymphoma [31]. Excisional biopsy is usually necessary to provide adequate tissue to confirm the diagnosis. Following diagnosis, a multidisciplinary approach is recommended for appropriate staging and treatment [31]. Neuroblastoma is another malignancy that can be found in the head and neck of neonates. Typically, these are metastatic lesions as primary cervical neuroblastoma accounts for only 5% of neonatal neuroblastoma [32]. Some children may have a concomitant Horner's syndrome secondary to compression of the cervical sympathetic chain. Treatment of neuroblastoma is also conducted via a multidisciplinary approach, with lesions diagnosed prenatally having a better prognosis than those identified following birth [32]. Other neonatal head and neck cancers include salivary gland malignancies, thyroid cancer, and nasopharyngeal carcinoma, each of which is exceedingly rare in this population.

6. Thoracic

The differential diagnosis of fetal and neonatal thoracic tumors can be narrowed significantly with an understanding of their incidence and common locations. One useful method for organizing these tumors is to differentiate between mediastinal, pleural, and pulmonary neoplasms.

The anterior mediastinum includes the region between the sternum and pericardium below the thoracic inlet. The thymus, portions of the thyroid gland, and nodal tissue serve as potential sites for tumorigenesis. In a retrospective review of 534 fetuses and neonates diagnosed with teratomas, Isaacs [33] found that 2.6% of these masses occurred in the mediastinum. Teratomas that do occur in this region are usually located in the anterior mediastinum [34]. Sonographic identification of calcifications can help differentiate mediastinal teratomas from congenital pulmonary airway malformations and pulmonary sequestration [35]. Large mediastinal teratomas have the potential to cause lethal sequelae for the fetus and newborn. Polyhydramnios and preterm labor may develop from esophageal obstruction. High-output cardiac failure secondary to solid lesions with high vascularity can lead to fetal hydrops and intrauterine death. Perinatal decompensation and death are risks associated with intrathoracic airway obstruction. Although the thymus is included in the anterior mediastinum, thymomas are exceptionally rare in children, with most of the published cases being limited to case reports and retrospective reviews. Thyroid neoplasms and lymphoma are also extremely rare in this group of patients.

The middle mediastinum encompasses the heart and pericardium, great vessels, tracheal bifurcation, and phrenic nerves. Primary cardiac tumors are very uncommon in the fetus and neonate [36]. Of the primary cardiac tumors that occur in these patients, nearly all of them are histologically benign [37, 38]. Rhabdomyomas account for the majority of these lesions [36–38]. Fibromas, myxomas, and teratomas represent additional benign cardiac lesions with rare occurrence. Pericardial-based teratomas are also exceedingly rare. Based on their size and location, middle mediastinal tumors can have a number of detrimental physiologic effects. Dysrhythmias, impairment of cardiac function, and great vessel compression may result in fetal or neonatal demise without timely intervention.

The posterior mediastinum is bound by the pericardium and thoracic vertebrae and extends from the sternal notch inferiorly to the diaphragm. The esophagus, descending thoracic aorta, azygos veins, thoracic duct, and neural tissue are the key components of this region. Nearly all of the tumors arising in the posterior mediastinum in children are neurogenic in origin. Neurogenic tumors are named according to the type of neural tissue from which they originate. Neoplasms that arise from the sympathetic chain reflect a continuum of cellular differentiation and maturation [39]. Ganglioneuromas are benign, fully differentiated, and arise from mature Schwann and ganglion cells. These are the most common posterior mediastinal masses in children [39]. Ganglioneuroblastomas are malignant tumors of intermediate differentiation and contain both mature and immature elements of ganglion cells [39]. Neuroblastomas are also malignant tumors that are derived from immature, undifferentiated ganglion cells [39]. Neuroblastoma is the most common malignancy and second most common tumor in neonates, with approximately 5% arising in the posterior mediastinum [32]. Additional tumors include neurofibroma, neurilemoma, neurosarcoma, and paraganglioma, all of which are uncommon in neonates.

Pulmonary lesions diagnosed prenatally or in the newborn are rarely true neoplasms. The most commonly identified abnormalities are congenital pulmonary malformations, intra- and extralobar pulmonary sequestrations, and congenital lobar emphysema. Pleuropulmonary blastoma is a very rare, aggressive pulmonary malignancy. Although uncommon, it is the primary pulmonary malignancy presenting in childhood with up to 94% of cases being diagnosed in children 6 years of age and younger [40]. Type I and II pleuropulmonary blastomas possess cystic components, which can lead to misdiagnosis as benign lesions. Since pleuropulmonary blastoma is rare and over 90% of pulmonary cystic lesions in children are benign, surveillance may be an appropriate strategy with the knowledge that the emergence of solid components in the lesion warrants surgical resection [40].

7. Abdominal/retroperitoneal/pelvic

Masses discovered in the neonatal abdominal cavity, retroperitoneum, and pelvis represent a very diverse group of pathologies as would be expected based on the tissue types and organs in this region. These lesions range from small incidentally discovered masses to those occupying an entire body cavity, from benign to malignant and from purely cystic to solid neoplasms [41]. Hepatic lesions are the most common intra-abdominal neonatal tumors, while neuroblastoma and teratoma are the most common retroperitoneal and pelvic masses, respectively.

Hepatic tumors encompass a variety of benign and malignant lesions, representing only 5% of neonatal tumors. Most neonatal liver tumors are benign and discovered as an asymptomatic abdominal mass or identified on prenatal imaging [5]. In a retrospective review of 194 cases of fetal and neonatal hepatic tumors, Isaacs [42] identified hemangioma (60.3%), mesenchymal hamartoma (23.2%), and hepatoblastoma (16.5%) as the three primary tumor types. Hepatoblastoma represents the most common primary hepatic malignancy in this patient population. Serum alpha-fetoprotein is elevated in nearly half of neonates with hepatoblastoma; however, serum levels may remain elevated for several months following birth in children with benign hepatic masses or in the absence of hepatic masses [43]. Surgical resection is the primary treatment modality for hepatoblastoma with chemotherapy typically reserved for children with unresectable lesions or metastatic disease. Newborns presenting with congenital hepatoblastoma appear to have similar survival when compared to older children with similar stages of disease [43].

Renal tumors account for approximately 5–7% of neonatal tumors. Non-neoplastic pathologies, such as hydronephrosis and renal cystic disease, are far more prevalent than true neoplasms, accounting for up to 40% of neonatal abdominal masses [44]. The most common neonatal renal neoplasm is congenital mesoblastic nephroma (CMN), followed in frequency by Wilms' tumor, rhabdoid tumor, and clear cell sarcoma [44]. Juxtarenal masses are also part of the differential diagnosis with neuroblastoma being the most common of these lesions.

Although prenatal ultrasound is widely used, it is estimated that only 15% of renal masses are diagnosed prenatally [45]. Of those lesions not diagnosed via fetal ultrasound, nearly 50% are identified during routine physical examination [45]. Mesoblastic nephroma is rarely diagnosed following the first 3 months of life, while it is uncommon for Wilms' tumor to be diagnosed prior to 6 months of age [41]. Mesoblastic nephroma may be differentiated from other masses by the presence of a "ring sign" or anechoic circle surrounding the mass on sonography [46]. The optimal treatment for neonatal renal masses is surgical resection. Similar to hepatic lesions, chemotherapy is reserved for malignant lesions that are unresectable or metastatic at the time of diagnosis.

Teratomas are the most common neonatal tumors and the most prevalent pelvic neoplasms. In contrast, neonatal testicular tumors are rarely encountered in clinical practice. The tumors that do occur are usually testicular germ cell tumors such as teratomas and yolk sac tumors [47]. Diagnosis typically occurs after parents or clinicians palpate a testicular mass. Ultrasound examination distinguishes between intra- and extratesticular pathology. Yolk sac tumors are the most common testicular malignancy in children, although most masses are benign. Serum alpha-fetoprotein (AFP) is a useful adjunct in the diagnosis of testicular tumors as it is elaborated by nearly 90% of yolk sac tumors in childhood [48]. However, measuring AFP levels is less reliable in newborns as they can physiologically remain elevated for up to 1 year after birth in the absence of underlying pathology. Since most of these lesions are benign, some tumors can be excised with a testicle-sparing approach [49]. In the event that a malignancy is identified on intraoperative frozen section, radical orchiectomy is required.

Ovarian enlargement can result from a variety of pathologies including ovarian cysts, ovarian torsion, and benign and malignant neoplasms [50]. Fortunately, true neonatal ovarian masses are infrequently seen in practice. Many lesions are identified on prenatal imaging, although some children present with palpable abdominal or groin masses, endocrine abnormalities, or ambiguous genitalia and congenital anomalies [50]. The majority of fetal and neonatal ovarian masses are cystic in nature. Management of ovarian cysts includes observation for simple lesions and surgical excision for larger, more complex lesions [41]. Preservation of functional ovarian parenchyma is the foundation of management.

8. Extremities and soft tissue

Soft tissue tumors comprise a heterogeneous group of benign and malignant neoplasms that represent 8–12% of neonatal tumors [1, 20, 21]. Soft tissue tumors are a rare entity in neonates, and the true incidence is unknown. There are a wide variety of benign tumors, including vascular malformations, lipomas, lipoblastomas, and fibroblastic tumors.

Head and neck hemangiomas are the most common benign soft tissue tumors in neonates. Lipomas consist of a group of widely distributed fatty tumors that are composed of mature adipocytes with a histologic appearance identical to normal fat [51]. Lipomas are classified based on their depth, with superficial lesions being much more common than deep lesions, which are located beneath the superficial fascia [51]. Lipoblastomas are rare, benign, rapidly growing tumors that arise from embryonic white fat and typically occur on the trunk and limbs [52]. The treatment of lipomas and lipoblastomas is usually complete excision, although the extent of resection should take functional and cosmetic outcomes into consideration. Fibroblastic and myofibroblastic tumors of intermediate prognosis represent benign lesions that display locally aggressive behavior with little to no propensity to metastasize [53]. Surgical resection remains the mainstay of treatment, yet a multidisciplinary approach is often necessary as radical resection of large, invasive lesions can lead to significant disfigurement and disability [53].

In infants, rhabdomyosarcoma (32.8%) is the most common malignant soft tissue tumor, followed in frequency by infantile fibrosarcoma (24.5%) and rhabdoid tumors (14.2%) [53]. Overall, malignant soft tissue tumors are rare in neonates. Rhabdoid tumors represent rare, aggressive malignancies that typically occur not only in the kidney and brain but can also be found in various soft tissue locations [54]. These tumors are relatively chemoresistant, demonstrate early tumor recurrence following surgical resection, and portend an overall poor prognosis [54].

9. Birth considerations

Certain neonatal tumors warrant special consideration regarding fetal delivery and perinatal management. Neoplasms that compromise the fetal airway represent an immediate threat to the neonatal airway, with the potential for hypoxia, ischemic brain injury, and death [55]. Cervical teratomas, cervical lymphatic malformations, and cervical hemangiomas are the most common neoplasms with the propensity to cause extrinsic airway compression in the neck. Mediastinal tumors that compress the great vessels or intrathoracic trachea also demand specialized pre- and postnatal care. Large tumors, particularly sacrococcygeal teratomas, merit consideration for Cesarean or early delivery as a method to avoid intrauterine or perinatal complications.

Prior to the development of the ex utero intrapartum treatment (EXIT) procedure, case reports described managing obstructing cervical masses with bronchoscopy and intubation prior to division of the umbilical cord [56]. The operation on placental support (OOPS) procedure involved Cesarean delivery of the head and thorax in order to perform endotracheal intubation [57]. Inhaled isoflurane anesthesia was administered in hopes of minimizing uterine contractions in an effort to preserve fetoplacental circulation and prevent placental abruption [57]. These early procedures were felt to provide inadequate tocolysis and/or reduce the uterine volume through fetal delivery, both of which result in uterine contraction and interruption of uteroplacental gas exchange [58].

Currently, the EXIT procedure offers a more comprehensive management approach to fetal and neonatal airway obstruction. The procedure also has application in the treatment of pulmonary and mediastinal masses leading to airway obstruction or other physiologic derangements. The EXIT procedure [59] entails intubating the mother and administering deep inhalational anesthesia with high-dose (2–3%) isoflurane. Anesthetic alone provides adequate uterine relaxation in many cases, but bolus doses of terbutaline or nitroglycerin can be given when necessary. Prior to performing hysterotomy, ultrasound is used to identify the location of the fetus and placenta. Following hysterotomy, the head and thorax of the fetus are delivered, allowing for multiple procedures to be performed, including bronchoscopy, orotracheal intubation, tracheostomy, mass excision, and ECMO cannulation. Fetoplacental circulation is preserved during the procedure and mitigates the possibility of hypoxia and brain ischemia. Once the airway is secured, the umbilical cord is divided, and Pitocin is administered, while the concentration of inhalational anesthetic is decreased to low levels or discontinued. The remainder of the procedure proceeds as would be expected from a routine Cesarean section.

Mediastinal tumors of appropriate size and location have the potential to cause fetal and neonatal demise through several mechanisms. One potential presentation is fetal airway and esophageal obstruction leading to polyhydramnios and preterm labor [60]. A second presentation is great vessel compression with resulting nonimmune fetal hydrops and fetal demise [60]. Several successful management strategies have been reported. One strategy involves aspiration of the cystic component of mediastinal teratomas for size reduction and alleviation of fetal hydrops until delivery and definitive management [61]. Serial amniocenteses to reduce uterine volume followed by neonatal resection have also been reported [60, 62–64].

The EXIT procedure also serves as a useful adjunct in transitioning these children from intrauterine life to definitive airway control, ECMO cannulation, or surgical resection.

10. Common specific lesions

10.1. Teratomas

Teratomas are the most common neonatal tumors, accounting for up to 30% of these lesions in some series [1, 20, 21]. Teratomas typically occur in the midline, spanning a variety of locations from the pineal gland to the coccyx [34]. The distribution of these tumors is explained by the fact that they arise from pluripotent germ cells that arrest in abnormal locations during embryologic migration [30]. Persistent division by these aberrant nests of cells results in tumors of varying size in diverse locations.

These neoplasms include all three germ cell layers, endoderm, mesoderm, and ectoderm. Most tumors are benign and can be classified as mature or immature based on their histologic appearance. Elements of the ectoderm, particularly neural tissue, are a dominant feature of immature fetal and neonatal teratomas [65, 66]. Mature and immature teratomas also contain mesenchymal components, including smooth muscle, cartilage, fat, and bone. Endodermal features such as respiratory and gastrointestinal epithelium are much less common [33, 65, 66]. Sacrococcygeal teratomas are the most common type of these tumors, followed in frequency by intracranial, cervical, palatal and nasopharyngeal, cardiac, gastric, and mediastinal teratomas [33]. Survival rates vary considerably by location, with intracranial teratomas (11%) having the lowest survival and gastric teratomas (100%) demonstrating the best prognosis [33].

Sacrococcygeal teratomas represent 40–60% of teratomas and demonstrate a 3 to 1 female to male distribution [33, 67]. The estimated incidence is 1 in every 35,000 live births [68]. In countries where prenatal ultrasound is ubiquitous, many lesions are diagnosed in utero. In the absence of prenatal diagnosis, the classic presentation is that of a newborn with an evident mass on physical examination. Diagnosis of purely pelvic teratomas is frequently delayed [69]. Children in this category may develop urinary retention, constipation, a palpable abdominal mass, or failure to thrive. MRI serves as a useful adjunct to ultrasound in determining the degree of intrapelvic extension. In 1973, Altman et al. [69] developed a location-based classification system for sacrococcygeal teratoma. Type I tumors are mainly external (sacrococcygeal) with minimal presacral component. Type II tumors exhibit an external component on presentation but have a substantial intrapelvic component. Type III tumor indicates a tumor with minimal external component with the majority of the mass located intrapelvic and extending into the abdomen. Type IV tumors are found entirely in the presacral space without any external component. Accurate classification is critical to parental counseling and appropriate operative planning.

Large sacrococcygeal teratomas represent a challenging diagnosis due to their potential to cause perinatal complications as well as unpredictable growth patterns [70]. Potential complications associated with these tumors are numerous, consisting of premature labor from polyhydramnios or increased intrauterine volume, tumor rupture, labor dystocia, hemorrhage, maternal mirror syndrome, and fetal hydrops secondary to high-output cardiac failure in highly vascular lesions [70]. Prenatally diagnosed sacrococcygeal teratomas should undergo frequent surveillance to monitor for rapidity of growth and development of the aforementioned complications [63]. For tumors that demonstrate a predominantly solid component with high vascularity, open fetal surgery may be necessary for tumor debulking to prevent high-output cardiac failure and fetal hydrops [71]. Similar to the management options for mediastinal teratomas, cyst aspiration and serial amniocenteses are beneficial interventions in appropriately selected patients [63, 64]. Cesarean delivery should be considered in larger lesions to prevent labor dystocia, tumor rupture, and hemorrhage.

En bloc resection of the tumor and coccyx is the primary treatment modality for sacrococcygeal teratoma. Failure to remove the coccyx and gross tumor spillage appear to have the highest association with recurrence [72]. The presence of microscopically positive margins necessitates routine surveillance in the absence of yolk sac tumor elements on final pathology, while histologic confirmation of yolk sac tumor components warrants adjuvant chemotherapy [72]. The age at diagnosis correlates with the presence of underlying malignancy and overall survival. Approximately 10% of neonatal sacrococcygeal teratomas contain a yolk sac tumor with the incidence of a concurrent malignancy increasing with age [33]. The outcome of fetuses diagnosed with sacrococcygeal teratoma is worse than those diagnosed in neonates. The estimated mortality for prenatally diagnosed lesions ranges from 33 to 50% and approaches 100% when fetal hydrops is present [33, 63, 73]. Conversely, the survival for a newborn diagnosed with this disease approaches 90% following complete surgical excision [33, 63, 73].

10.2. Neuroblastoma

Neuroblastoma represents the second most common neonatal tumor, accounting for 22.5–30% of these neoplasms, and the most common congenital malignancy [1, 20, 21]. Neuroblastomas are derived from primitive neural crest cells, or neuroblasts, and can be identified in any location where sympathetic tissue exists [74, 75]. Nearly 90% of fetal and neonatal cases of neuroblastoma occur in the adrenal gland compared to 35% in infants and older children [75, 76]. The next most common sites, in order to decrease frequency, are the retroperitoneum, posterior mediastinum, and neck [32]. The incidence of neuroblastoma is approximately 1 in 100,000 children, with a mean age of diagnosis of 18 months [77]. The incidence of neuroblastoma in neonates is not as well defined as tumors occur less commonly in this age group compared to older children.

Neuroblastoma is being diagnosed with increased frequency on prenatal ultrasound due to widespread use of fetal sonography and continued technological improvement [78]. In fact, there was once an interest in screening for neuroblastoma with prenatal ultrasound, but in general this practice has been abandoned as it only succeeded in identifying lesions that could otherwise be observed and did not identify the more aggressive lesions that most are interested in identifying early. The differential diagnosis of an adrenal lesion includes adrenal hemorrhage, adrenal abscess, adrenal cyst, and renal anomalies. Nearly all cases are diagnosed during the third trimester. Identification of a solid or cystic adrenal mass should raise suspicion for the presence of an underlying neuroblastoma [78]. Postnatal MRI serves as useful to clarify the extent of disease and guide treatment options. Most mothers with a prenatal diagnosis of neuroblastoma are asymptomatic, although maternal hypertension and preeclampsia may occur due to elevated levels of catecholamines in maternal circulation [76]. In the absence of a prenatal diagnosis of neuroblastoma, presentation is variable and includes detection of a palpable abdominal mass, hepatomegaly, respiratory distress, and the presence of cutaneous nodules. Neuroblastomas are hormonally active tumors that secrete high levels of catecholamines and their by-products. The diagnosis can be further solidified by detection of these chemicals in a urine sample, although serum levels are not predictive of prognosis and do not dictate treatment.

Staging of neuroblastoma follows the International Neuroblastoma Staging System, which considers tumor location, nodal involvement, and the presence of metastases in assessing the burden of disease [79]. The majority of fetal and neonatal cases of neuroblastoma are stage I, stage II, and stage IV-S at the time of diagnosis [32, 76, 77]. Most tumors also demonstrate favorable histology including N-myc non-amplification, stroma-rich appearance, and aneuploid DNA content [32, 76, 77]. Surgical resection is the principal treatment for localized cases of neuroblastoma. In cases of unresectable disease, open or core needle biopsy provides valuable histologic information to help guide treatment decisions. Neonates with stage IV-S represent a particularly unique group of patients who have a localized tumor with metastases isolated to the liver, bone, and skin [79]. Despite the presence of metastatic disease, these children have a favorable prognosis, and many tumors undergo spontaneous regression without specific treatment. Treatment options for stage IV-S include observation, surgical resection, and chemotherapy. Chemotherapy is also employed in the neoadjuvant setting for tumors that are initially deemed to be unresectable. Overall, the prognosis for fetal and neonatal neuroblastoma is excellent, with survival ranging from 70 to 100% [32, 76, 77]. There have been favorable studies that have demonstrated success with observation with small lesions that likely represent neuroblastoma [80]. Moving forward, current staging is changing from a surgery-based staging toward image-defined risk categories with the majority of neonatal lesions falling into the low-risk categories. Therefore, we would recommend that these patients should be enrolled in current observation studies to document outcomes of this patient population.

10.3. Infantile hepatic hemangioma and mesenchymal hamartoma

Infantile hepatic hemangiomas are the most common primary liver tumors in newborns. Hemangiomas display a wide range of behavior, spanning from asymptomatic masses to those causing significant physiologic distress and potential demise [41]. Most lesions are diagnosed on prenatal imaging or found incidentally on physical examination. In some cases, the presence of cutaneous hemangiomas prompts evaluation for a concomitant hepatic mass [41]. Infantile hepatic hemangiomas are benign, vascular masses characterized by rapid postnatal growth followed by involution in childhood [42]. For this reason, asymptomatic and smaller lesions can be observed for involution through serial ultrasonography. Conversely, some lesions develop severe arteriovenous shunting, which can lead to high-output cardiac failure, fetal hydrops, and death. Other masses lead to Kasabach-Merritt syndrome, which can cause consumptive coagulopathy, thrombocytopenia, and hemolytic anemia [81]. Surgical excision is an effective management for localized lesions in children without severe physiologic derangement. Selective hepatic arterial embolization can be used to induce preoperative tumor shrinkage and in cases of refractory coagulopathy [82].

Mesenchymal hamartomas are the second most common hepatic tumor in newborns. These lesions are congenital malformations that contain elements of normal hepatic parenchyma including mesenchyme, portal venous branches, bile ducts, hepatocytes, and cysts of varying size [41]. Hamartomas are benign masses that display several chromosomal abnormalities [83]. Similar to hemangiomas, hamartomas are typically identified on prenatal imaging or found as an asymptomatic mass on physical examination. Approximately 75% are found in the right hepatic lobe with the rest involving the left lobe or both lobes [84]. Although these are histologically benign tumors, some lesions demonstrate rapid growth and result in significant physiologic disturbance. Tumors abutting the diaphragm can cause significant respiratory compromise. Compression of intra-abdominal vascular structures may lead to nonimmune fetal hydrops and fetal demise. Complete surgical excision is the optimal management for children with hepatic mesenchymal hamartomas. In tumors with large cystic components, fetal aspiration has been reported to mitigate detrimental fetal and obstetric sequelae [85].

10.4. Ovarian cysts

Ovarian cysts are the most common masses identified in neonatal girls and are nearly always benign. The etiology of ovarian cysts is not completely understood, but hormonal stimulation is felt to be responsible for this disease process [86]. In 1975, Valenti et al. [87] reported the first case of a prenatally diagnosed ovarian cyst. With improvement in ultrasonography, ovarian cysts are being identified with increasing frequency on prenatal imaging. Ultrasound provides vital information about size, location, wall characteristics, and vascularity [41]. However, many lesions are asymptomatic and would not be identified if not for routine fetal ultrasound [88].

Treatment of ovarian cysts hinges upon the risk of complications and the ability to differentiate between truly benign cysts and other ovarian neoplasms [89]. The most common complication encountered is ovarian torsion with subsequent loss of the affected ovary [86, 89]. Many cases of ovarian torsion occur prenatally, precluding the ability to intervene in an effort for ovarian preservation. Doppler evaluation is an unreliable measure of torsion in this patient population secondary to vessel size and the fact that normal flow does not exclude the diagnosis [86]. Fetal cyst aspiration is one management strategy used to mitigate the risk of in utero torsion, but there is no agreed upon size cutoff to determine when this measure should be employed.

Simple cysts less than 4–5 cm in size can be observed for spontaneous regression with serial ultrasonography [41, 86, 88, 89]. Cysts larger than 4–5 cm are candidates for cyst aspiration or surgical intervention given a higher potential for ovarian torsion [41, 86, 88, 89]. Complex ovarian cysts, cysts that fail to regress spontaneously, cysts that recur following aspiration, and those that are symptomatic should be removed surgically [89]. Preservation of ovarian parenchyma is the hallmark of surgery for ovarian cysts. Options for surgical management include cyst unroofing, partial or total cystectomy, and oophorectomy. In cases of ovarian torsion, the macroscopic appearance of the ovary does not necessarily correlate with the degree of parenchymal damage [88]. Pathologic evaluation of a portion of the cyst wall is recommended; however, the presence of an underlying malignancy is exceedingly rare.

10.5. Cervical lymphatic malformations

Lymphatic malformations are characterized by localized collections of malformed lymphatic channels that occur most commonly in the head and neck [90]. Lymphatic malformations typically occur in the posterior neck and are often associated with karyotypic abnormalities [91]. Other common locations are the trunk and extremities, the thoracic cavity, and the abdominal cavity. Traditionally, lymphatic malformations have been assigned to different categories based on histologic appearance: cavernous lymphangiomas, capillary lymphangiomas, and cystic hygroma [90]. However, the histologic classification does not seem to correlate with clinical behavior or response to therapy [90]. These masses follow a variable clinical course, with prenatally diagnosed lesions having a worse prognosis than those identified following birth [91].

Lymphatic malformations typically grow proportionally with the growth of the child, with rapid enlargement occurring as the result of trauma, hemorrhage, or infection [91]. Spontaneous infection occurs in approximately 7–30% of these masses [92]. The size and location of a given lymphatic malformation are predictive of potential adverse consequences to the developing child. Head and neck lesions can lead to fetal esophageal obstruction, resulting in polyhydramnios and preterm labor. A more serious complication is the potential for neonatal airway obstruction and rapid demise following birth. The EXIT procedure [56] offers a comprehensive management strategy to establish a definitive airway while maintaining fetoplacental circulation. However, if the lesion is soft and away from the midline, such fetuses may not require EXIT as obtaining an airway may not be difficult. Intrathoracic lymphatic malformations also have the potential to cause airway obstruction. Compression of the great vessels in the thorax and abdomen can cause high-output cardiac failure, hydrops fetalis, and fetal demise.

Many treatment modalities exist for the management of lymphatic malformations. In general, asymptomatic lesions can be observed for some time as many of these lesions will resolve without intervention. In those lesions that are large, growing, or symptomatic, therapeutic maneuvers include sclerotherapy and surgery. Prior to pursuing these therapies, the extent of the tumor and association with surrounding structures must be determined [91]. Nerves and major vessels should be preserved [90]. More complex and invasive lesions may require multiple, staged operations to achieve complete resection [90, 91]. Tumors that undergo complete macroscopic excision show the lowest recurrence rates but still return in 17% of cases [93]. Recurrences occur in up to 100% of cases following aspiration and in 40% of masses that are incompletely excised [93]. The estimated recurrence rate following injection of sclerosing agents, such as sodium tetradecanol, bleomycin, and OK-432, ranges from 50 to 100% [91, 93]. Aspiration does play a role in emergent cases to decrease the mass effect of the tumor and establish an airway [90]. In small, asymptomatic lesions, a period of surveillance to monitor for spontaneous regression may also be pursued [90].

10.6. Rhabdomyosarcoma

Soft tissue tumors account for 8–12% of neonatal tumors [1, 20, 21]. Rhabdomyosarcoma is the most common malignant soft tissue tumor in children, representing one third of these masses in infants and nearly half of soft tissue tumors found in older children [53]. Rhabdomyosarcoma is an aggressive, embryonal tumor of childhood marked by high-grade histology, local invasiveness, and a propensity to metastasize [53]. There are two main histologic subtypes: embryonal rhabdomyosarcoma accounts for nearly 70% of all cases and portends a better prognosis and alveolar rhabdomyosarcoma which is characterized by numerous chromosomal translocations and has a worse overall outcome [94]. As mesenchymal tumors that arise from skeletal muscle, rhabdomyosarcoma can occur in many locations throughout the body. The most common sites of occurrence are the head and neck followed by the genitourinary system and extremities [53]. Neonatal cases of rhabdomyosarcoma are rare. Male gender, Caucasian race, embryonal subtype, and undifferentiated histology are the predominant characteristics in neonates [95].

Rhabdomyosarcoma may be identified on prenatal imaging but more commonly presents as an identifiable mass following birth. The differential diagnosis is broad and includes many benign and malignant soft tissue tumors. Lymphatic involvement and metastatic disease are present in nearly 20% of cases at presentation [53]. The most common sites of metastasis are the lung, bone marrow, and bone. Neonatal cases of alveolar rhabdomyosarcoma may present with brain metastases and subcutaneous nodules [96]. Biopsy of the primary lesion is recommended for diagnostic purposes and to determine tumor biology to guide treatment. However, one should proceed with complete excision of smaller lesions (<5 cm) if this can be performed with clear margins and without injury to surrounding structures. Larger or difficult to excise lesions should have an incisional biopsy with a sufficient tissue sample to allow for all necessary studies (1 cm^3). Following diagnosis, tumors require staging with CT or MRI of the primary lesion, imaging of the chest, bone marrow aspiration, and bone marrow biopsy.

Treatment of neonatal rhabdomyosarcomas should be undertaken in a multidisciplinary fashion. Therapy is multimodal and includes systemic chemotherapy for metastatic disease and surgical resection and radiation for local disease. Complete surgical resection may not always be feasible, and age at diagnosis dictates the ability to give chemotherapy and radiation. Age is an independent prognostic factor with children less than 1 year of age having a worse overall prognosis than children between the ages of 1 and 10 [97, 98]. In the Intergroup Rhabdomyosarcoma Study, Lobe et al. [95] found that only 49% of 14 newborns diagnosed with rhabdomyosarcoma were alive at 3 years.

10.7. Congenital mesoblastic nephroma

Congenital mesoblastic nephroma is the most common renal tumor occurring in neonates and during the first 3 months of life [45]. In a retrospective review of 210 renal tumors in fetuses and infants less than 2 months of age, Isaacs [44] found that the four most common renal neoplasms were congenital mesoblastic nephroma (66%), Wilms' tumor (20%), rhabdoid tumor of the kidney (11%), and clear cell sarcoma of the kidney (3%). Congenital mesoblastic nephroma demonstrates a slight male predominance with a male to female ratio of 1.5 to 1 [45]. The most common presentations of mesoblastic nephroma are prenatal identification on fetal ultrasound, polyhydramnios, and palpation of an abdominal mass following birth. Sonographically, the presence of an anechoic circle or "ring sign" surrounding the mass may help differentiate congenital mesoblastic nephroma from other renal neoplasms [46]. These tumors typically demonstrate benign behavior; however, in addition to polyhydramnios, some masses may be complicated by hypertension; respiratory compromise; circulatory compromise from large, space-occupying lesions; and fetal hydrops [44].

Congenital mesoblastic nephroma (CMN) is a benign neoplasm that is characterized by leiomyomatous histology with bundles of spindle cells, rare mitoses, and lack of necrosis [99]. The tumor can be further subdivided into classic and cellular subtypes based on histological appearance. Patients with the cellular subtype of CMN tend to have larger tumor burdens and older age of presentation [99]. Additionally, many cellular mesoblastic nephromas are cystic in nature, which may lead to increased risk of rupture and higher rates of recurrence [99]. Radical nephrectomy is the mainstay of treatment for a neonate diagnosed with CMN. Patients with the classic subtype of CMN are typically cured with surgical excision alone, while aggressive tumors, which are often of the cellular subtype, may require adjuvant chemotherapy. Recurrence occurs in 5% of patients, while metastases are present in 2% of cases [44]. The overall survival for a patient diagnosed with congenital mesoblastic nephroma is 95–98% [99, 100].

11. Chemotherapy and irradiation

One of the greatest challenges in pediatric oncology is determining the appropriate dosing regimen for chemotherapeutic agents in young children [101]. Multiple factors influence the pharmacology of chemotherapeutic drugs in the newborn, including changes in blood flow, hepatic and renal development, and alterations in the amount of body composition attributed to fat and water [101]. Body surface area dosing is the most commonly employed dosing method in the pediatric setting, but there are inconsistencies in the cutoffs and magnitude for dose reductions [101]. Administration of chemotherapy in newborns should always take place under the guidance of a pediatric oncologist.

Radiation therapy is also very challenging in the pediatric patient population. Although radiation therapy has been successful in the treatment of many pediatric cancers, concerns remain about long-term side effects [102]. Growth and development failure is a primary concern for children who receive radiation therapy [102]. Other late sequelae include neurocognitive defects, infertility, cardiac and pulmonary abnormalities, gastrointestinal dysfunction, and secondary cancer development [102]. Over the last 35 years, the use of radiation therapy has declined in the treatment of many pediatric cancers, including Wilms' tumor, neuroblastoma, ALL, and non-Hodgkin's lymphoma [102]. The decision to use radiation therapy in the treatment of neonatal tumors should always include a discussion of the risks and benefits of therapy with a radiation oncologist. Of note for this patient population is the need to perform radiation under sedation as the drugs used in this treatment modality are under investigation as to potential long-term side effects.

12. Conclusion

Neonatal tumors encompass an extremely diverse, heterogeneous group of neoplasms. Neonatal tumors demonstrate a broad spectrum of behaviors and outcomes with some lesions spontaneously regressing without treatment, while others are resistant to aggressive, multimodal therapy. The majority of lesions are benign, but histologic classification is not always predictive of clinical behavior or overall outcome. Treatment of neonatal tumors requires a clear understanding of the natural history of disease and the limitations of each treatment modality. The optimal management strategy incorporates the expertise of pediatricians, pediatric surgeons, pediatric medical oncologists, and pediatric radiation oncologists.

Author details

Kenneth W. Gow* and Matthew Dellinger

*Address all correspondence to: kenneth.gow@seattlechildrens.org

Seattle Children's Hospital and the University of Washington, USA

References

[1] Moore SW, Satge D, Sasco AJ, et al. The epidemiology of neonatal tumours. Report of an international working group. Pediatric Surgery International. 2003;**19**:509–519

[2] Weitzman S, Grant R. Neonatal oncology: Diagnostic and therapeutic dilemmas. Seminars in Perinatology. 1997;**21**(1):102–111

[3] Batcup G. Cancer in the very young child—pitfalls and problems for the pathologist. British Journal of Cancer. Supplement. 1992;**18**:S5-S7

[4] Halperin E. Neonatal neoplasms. International Journal of Radiation Oncology Biology Physics. 2000;**47**(1):171–178

[5] Orbach D, Sarnacki S, Brisse HJ, et al. Neonatal cancer. Lancet Oncology. 2013;**14**:e609-e620

[6] Merks JHM, Caron HN, Hennekam RCM. High incidence of malformation syndromes in a series of 1073 children with cancer. American Journal of Medical Genetics. 2005;**134**:132–143

[7] Santos XM, Papanna R, Johnson A, et al. The use of combined ultrasound and magnetic resonance imaging in the detection of fetal anomalies. Prenatal Diagnosis. 2010;**30**:402–407

[8] Nemec SF, Horcher E, Kasprian G, et al. Tumor disease and associated congenital abnormalities on prenatal MRI. European Journal of Radiology. 2012;**81**:e115-e122

[9] Lee TC, Olutoye OO. Evaluation of the prenatally diagnosed mass. Seminars in Fetal & Neonatal Medicine. 2012;**17**:185–191

[10] Pugash D, Brugger PC, Bettelheim D, et al. Prenatal ultrasound and fetal MRI: The comparative value of each modality in prenatal diagnosis. European Journal of Radiology. 2008;**68**:214–226

[11] Chung R, Kasprian G, Brugger PC, et al. The current state and future of fetal imaging. Clinics in Perinatology. 2009;**36**:685–699

[12] Bricker L, Garcia J, Henderson J, et al. Ultrasound screening in pregnancy: A systematic review of the clinical effectiveness, cost-effectiveness, and women's views. Health Technology Assessment. 2000;**4**(16):1–193

[13] Chen MM, Coakley FV, Kaimal A, et al. Guideline for computed tomography and magnetic resonance imaging use during pregnancy and lactation. Obstetrics & Gynecology. 2008;**112**:333–340

[14] Breysem L, Bosmans H, Dymarkowski S, et al. The value of fast MR imaging as an adjunct to ultrasound in prenatal diagnosis. European Radiology. 2003;**13**:1538–1548

[15] Wagenvoort AM, Bekker MN, Go ATJI, et al. Ultrafast scan magnetic resonance in prenatal diagnosis. Fetal Diagnosis and Therapy. 2000;**15**:364–372

[16] American College of Obstetricians and Gynecologists' Committee on Obstetric Practice. Guidelines for diagnostic imaging during pregnancy and lactation. Obstetrics & Gynecology. 2016;**127**(2):e75-e80

[17] Kanal E, Barkovich AJ, Bell C, et al. ACR guidance document on MR safe practices: 2013. Expert Panel on MR Safety. Journal of Magnetic Resonance Imaging. 2013;**37**:501–530

[18] Alamo L, Beck-Popovic M, Gudinchet F, et al. Congenital tumors: Imaging when life just begins. Insights into Imaging. 2011;**2**:297–308

[19] Borsellino A, Zaccara A, Nahom A, et al. False-positive rate in prenatal diagnosis of surgical anomalies. Journal of Pediatric Surgery. 2006;**41**:826–829

[20] Isaacs H Jr. Congenital and neonatal malignant tumors. A 28-year experience at Children's Hospital of Los Angeles. The American Journal of Pediatric Hematology/Oncology. 1987;**9**(2):121–129

[21] Parkes SE, Muir KR, Southern L, et al. Neonatal tumours: A thirty-year population-based study. Medical and Pediatric Oncology. 1994;**22**:309–317

[22] Bauchet L, Rigau V, Mathieu-Daudé H, et al. Clinical epidemiology for childhood primary central nervous system tumors. Journal of Neuro-Oncology. 2009;**92**:87–98

[23] Ostrom QT, Gittleman H, Fulop J, et al. CBTRUS statistical report: Primary brain and central nervous system tumors diagnosed in the United States in 2008–2012. Neuro-Oncology. 2015;**17**:iv1-iv62

[24] Isaacs H Jr. Perinatal brain tumors: A review of 250 cases. Pediatric Neurology. 2002;**27**:333–342

[25] Magdum SA. Neonatal brain tumours—a review. Early Human Development. 2010;**86**:627–631

[26] Goins MR, Beasley MS. Pediatric neck masses. Oral & Maxillofacial Surgery Clinics of North America. 2012;**24**:457–468

[27] Torsiglieri AJ Jr, Tom LWC, Ross AJ III, et al. Pediatric neck masses: Guidelines for evaluation. International Journal of Pediatric Otorhinolaryngology. 1988;**16**:199

[28] Krol A, MacArthur CJ. Congenital hemangiomas: Rapidly involuting and noninvoluting congenital hemangiomas. Archives of Facial Plastic Surgery. 2005:**7**:307–311

[29] Kanada KN, Merin MR, Munden A, et al. A prospective study of cutaneous findings in newborns in the United States: Correlation with race, ethnicity, and gestational status using updated classification and nomenclature. Journal of Pediatrics. 2012;**161**:240–245

[30] Tranvinh E, Yeom KW, Iv M. Imaging neck masses in the neonate and young infant. Seminars in Ultrasound, CT, and MRI. 2015;**36**:120–137

[31] Dickson PV, Davidoff AM. Malignant neoplasms of the head and neck. Seminars in Pediatric Surgery. 2006;**15**(2):92–98

[32] Isaacs H Jr. Fetal and neonatal neuroblastoma: Retrospective review of 271 cases. Fetal and Pediatric Pathology. 2007;**26**:177–184

[33] Isaacs H Jr. Perinatal (fetal and neonatal) germ cell tumors. Journal of Pediatric Surgery. 2004;**39**(7):1003–1013

[34] Woodward PJ, Sohaey R, Kennedy A, Koeller KK. From the archives of the AFIP: A comprehensive review of fetal tumors with pathologic correlation. Radiographics. 2005;**25**(1):215–242

[35] Wienk MA, Van Geijn HP, Copray FJ, Brons JT. Prenatal diagnosis of fetal tumors by ultrasonography. Obstetrical & Gynecological Survey. 1990;**45**:639–653

[36] Isaacs H Jr. Fetal and neonatal cardiac tumors. Pediatric Cardiology. 2004;**25**:252–273

[37] Chan HS, Sonley MJ, Moes CA, Daneman A, Smith CR, Martin DJ. Primary and secondary tumors of childhood involving the heart, pericardium, and great vessels. A report of 75 cases and review of the literature. Cancer. 1985;**56**:825–836

[38] Van der Hauwaert LG. Cardiac tumours in infancy and childhood. British Heart Journal. 1971;**33**:125–132

[39] Jaggers J, Balsara K. Mediastinal masses in children. Seminars in Thoracic and Cardiovascular Surgery. 2004;**16**:201–208

[40] Priest JR, Williams MG, Hill DA, et al. Pulmonary cysts in early childhood and the risk of malignancy. Pediatric Pulmonology. 2009;**44**:14–30

[41] Chandler JC, Gauderer MWL. The neonate with an abdominal mass. Pediatric Clinics of North America. 2004;**51**:979–997

[42] Isaacs H Jr. Fetal and neonatal hepatic tumors. Journal of Pediatric Surgery. 2007; **42**:1797–1803

[43] Trobaugh-Lotrario AD, Chaiyachati BH, Meyers RL, et al. Outcomes for patients with congenital hepatoblastoma. Pediatric Blood & Cancer. 2013;**60**:1817–1825

[44] Isaacs H Jr. Fetal and neonatal renal tumors. Journal of Pediatric Surgery. 2008;**43**: 1587–1595

[45] Powis M. Neonatal renal tumors. Early Human Development. 2010;**86**:607–612

[46] Kelner M, Droullé P, Didier F, et al. The vascular "ring" sign in mesoblastic nephroma: Report of two cases. Pediatric Radiology. 2003;**33**:123–128

[47] Manivel JC. Testicular germ cell tumors (TGCTs) in neonates and infants. Seminars in Diagnostic Pathology. 2016;**33**(6):410–148

[48] Ross JH. Prepubertal testicular tumors. Urology. 2008;**74**:94–99

[49] Ross J, Rybicki L, Kay R. Clinical behavior and a contemporary management algorithm for prepubertal testis tumors: A summary of the Prepubertal Testis Tumor Registry. Journal of Urology. 2002;**168**:1675–1679

[50] Quint EH, Smith YR. Ovarian surgery in premenarchal girls. Journal of Pediatric & Adolescent Gynecology. 1999;**12**:27–30

[51] Navarro OM, Laffan EE, Ngan BY. Pediatric soft-tissue tumors and pseudotumors: MRI imaging features with pathologic correlation. Radiographics. 2009;**29**:887–906

[52] Bruyeer E, Lemmerling M, Poorten VV, et al. Paediatric lipoblastoma in the head and neck: Three cases and review of literature. Cancer Imaging. 2012;**12**:484–487

[53] Ferrari A, Orbach D, Sultan I, et al. Neonatal soft tissue sarcomas. Seminars in Fetal & Neonatal Medicine. 2012;**17**:231–238

[54] Bourdeaut F, Fréneaux P, Thuille B, et al. Extra-renal non-cerebral rhabdoid tumours. Pediatric Blood & Cancer. 2008;**51**:363–368

[55] Marwan A, Crombleholme TM. The EXIT procedure: Principles, pitfalls, and progress. Seminars in Pediatric Surgery. 2006;**15**:107–115

[56] Langer JC, Tabb T, Thompson P, et al. Management of prenatally diagnosed tracheal obstruction: Access to the airway in utero prior to delivery. Fetal Diagnosis and Therapy. 1992;**7**:12–16

[57] Skarsgard ED, Chitkara U, Krane EJ, et al. The OOPS procedure (operation on placental support): In utero airway management of the fetus with prenatally diagnosed tracheal obstruction. Journal of Pediatric Surgery. 1996;**31**:826–828

[58] McNamara H, Johnson N. The effect of uterine contractions on fetal oxygen saturation. British Journal of Obstetrics and Gynaecology. 1995;**102**:644–647

[59] Mychaliska GB, Bealer JF, Graf JL, et al. Operating on placental support: The ex utero intrapartum treatment procedure. Journal of Pediatric Surgery. 1997;**32**:227–231

[60] Merchant AM, Hedrick HL, Johnson MP, et al. Management of fetal mediastinal teratoma. Journal of Pediatric Surgery. 2005;**40**:228–231

[61] Takayasu H, Kitano Y, Kuroda T, et al. Successful management of a large fetal mediastinal teratoma complicated by hydrops fetalis. Journal of Pediatric Surgery. 2010;**45**: e21-e24

[62] Dumbell HR, Coleman AC, Pudifin JM, et al. Prenatal ultrasonographic diagnosis and successful management of mediastinal teratoma. A case report. South African Medical Journal. 1990;**20**:481–483

[63] Hedrick HL, Flake AW, Crombleholme TM, et al. Sacrococcygeal teratoma; Prenatal assessment, fetal intervention, and outcome. Journal of Pediatric Surgery. 2004;**39**:430–438

[64] Makin EC, Hyett J, Ade-Ajayi N, et al. Outcome of antenatally diagnosed sacrococcygeal teratomas: Single-center experience (1993–2004). Journal of Pediatric Surgery. 2006;**41**:388–393

[65] Isaacs H Jr. Perinatal (congenital and neonatal) neoplasms: A report of 110 cases. Pediatric Pathology. 1985;**3**:165–216

[66] Werb P, Scurry J, Ostor A, et al. Survey of congenital tumors in perinatal necropsies. Pathology. 1992;**24**:247–253

[67] Billmire DF, Grosfeld JL. Teratomas of childhood: Analysis of 142 cases. Journal of Pediatric Surgery. 1986;**21**:548–551

[68] Pantoja E, Liobet R, Gonsales-Flores B. Retroperitoneal teratoma: Historic review. Journal of Urology. 1976;**115**:520–523

[69] Altmann RP, Randolph JG, Lilly JR. Sacrococcygeal teratoma: American Academy of Pediatrics Surgical Section Survey 1973. Journal of Pediatric Surgery. 1974;**9**:389–398

[70] Roybal JL, Moldenhauer JS, Khalek N, et al. Early delivery as an alternative management strategy for selected high-risk fetal sacrococcygeal teratomas. Journal of Pediatric Surgery. 2011;**46**: 1325–1332

[71] Adzick NS. Open fetal surgery for life-threatening fetal anomalies. Seminars in Fetal & Neonatal Medicine. 2010;**15**(1):1–8

[72] De Backer A, Madern GC, Hakvoort-Cammel FGAJ, et al. Study of the factors associated with recurrence in children with sacrococcygeal teratoma. Journal of Pediatric Surgery. 2006;**41**:173–181

[73] Holterman AX, Filiatrault D, Lallier M, et al. The natural history of sacrococcygeal teratomas diagnosed through routine obstetric sonogram: A single institution experience. Journal of Pediatric Surgery. 1998;**33**:899–903

[74] Fisher JPH, Tweddle DA. Neonatal neuroblastoma. Seminars in Fetal & Neonatal Medicine. 2012;**17**:207–215

[75] Lonergan GJ, Schwab CM, Suarez ES, et al. Neuroblastoma, ganglioneuroblastoma, and ganglioneuroma: Radiologic-pathologic correlation. Radiographics. 2002;**22**:911–934

[76] Acharya S, Jayabose S, Kogan SJ, et al. Prenatally diagnosed neuroblastoma. Cancer. 1997;**80**:304–310

[77] Kostyrka B, Li J, Soundappan SV, et al. Features and outcomes of neonatal neuroblastoma. Pediatric Surgery International. 2011;**27**:937–941

[78] Ho PTC, Estroff JA, Kozakewich M, et al. Prenatal detection of neuroblastoma. A ten year experience from the Dana Farber Cancer Institute and Children's Hospital. Pediatrics. 1993;**92**(3):358–364

[79] Brodeur GM, Pritchard J, Berthold F, et al. Revisions of the international criteria for neuroblastoma diagnosis, staging, and response to treatment. Journal of Clinical Oncology. 1993;**11**:1466–1467

[80] Nuchtern JG, London, WB, Barnewolt CE, et al. A prospective study of expectant observation as primary therapy for neuroblastoma in young infants: A Children's Oncology Group study. Annals of Surgery. 2012;**256**(4):573–580

[81] Haisley-Royster C, Enjolras O, Frieden IJ, et al. Kasabach-Merritt phenomenon: A retrospective study of treatment with vincristine. Journal of Pediatric Hematology/Oncology. 2002;**24**(6):459–462

[82] Kullendorff CM, Cwikiel W, Sandstrom S. Embolization of hepatic hemangiomas in infants. European Journal of Pediatric Surgery. 2002;**12**(5):348–352

[83] Murthi GV, Paterson L, Azmy A. Chromosomal translocation in mesenchymal hamartoma of liver: What is its significance? Journal of Pediatric Surgery. 2003;**38**(10):1543–1545

[84] Stringer MD, Alizai NK. Mesenchymal hamartoma of the liver: A systematic review. Journal of Pediatric Surgery. 2005;**40**:1681–1690

[85] Tsao K, Hirose S, Sydorak R, et al. Fetal therapy for giant hepatic cysts. Journal of Pediatric Surgery. 2002;**37**(10):e31

[86] Bagolan P, Giorlandino C, Nahom A, et al. The management of fetal ovarian cysts. Journal of Pediatric Surgery. 2002;**37**(1):25–30

[87] Valenti C, Kassner EG, Yermakov V, et al. Antenatal diagnosis of a fetal ovarian cyst. American Journal of Obstetrics and Gynecology. 1975;**123**:216–219

[88] Galinier P, Carfagna L, Juricic M, et al. Fetal ovarian cysts management and ovarian prognosis: A report of 82 cases. Journal of Pediatric Surgery. 2008;**43**:2004–2009

[89] Brandt ML, Luks FI, Filiatrault D, et al. Surgical indications in antenatally diagnosed ovarian cysts. Journal of Pediatric Surgery. 1991;**26**(3):276–282

[90] Bloom DC, Perkins JA, Manning SC. Management of lymphatic malformations. Current Opinion in Otolaryngology & Head and Neck Surgery. 2004;**12**:500–504

[91] Gallagher PG, Mahoney MJ, Gosche JR. Cystic hygroma in the fetus and newborn. Seminars in Perinatology. 1999;**23**(4):341–356

[92] Wiswell TE, Miller JA. Infections of congenital cervical neck masses associated with bacteremia. Journal of Pediatric Surgery. 1986;**21**:173–174

[93] Alqahtani A, Nguyen LT, Flageole H, et al. 25 years' experience with lymphangiomas in children. Journal of Pediatric Surgery. 1999;**34**(7):1164–1168

[94] De Giovanni C, Landuzzi L, Nicoletti G, et al. Molecular and cellular biology of rhabdomyosarcoma. Future Oncology. 2009;**5**:1449–1475

[95] Lobe TE, Wiener ES, Hays DM, et al. Neonatal rhabdomyosarcoma: The IRS experience. Journal of Pediatric Surgery. 1994;**29**:1167–1170

[96] Rodriguez-Galindo C, Hill DA, Onyekwere O, et al. Neonatal alveolar rhabdomyosarcoma with skin and brain metastases. Cancer. 2001;**92**:1613–1620

[97] Sultan I, Casanova M, Al-Jumaily U, et al. Soft tissue sarcomas in the first year of life. European Journal of Cancer. 2010;**46**:2449–2456

[98] Joshi D, Anderson JR, Paidas C, et al. Age is an independent prognostic factor in rhabdomyosarcoma: A report from the Soft Tissue Sarcoma Committee of the Children's Oncology Group. Pediatric Blood & Cancer. 2004;**42**(1):64–73

[99] Furtwaengler R, Reinhard H, Leuschner I, et al. Mesoblastic nephroma—a report from the Gesellschaft fur Pädiatrische Onkologie und Hämatologie (GPOH). Cancer. 2006;**106**:2275–2283

[100] Howell CG, Othersen HB, Kiviat NE, et al. Therapy and outcome in 51 children with mesoblastic nephroma: A report of the National Wilms' Tumor Study. Journal of Pediatric Surgery. 1982;**17**:826–831

[101] Veal GJ, Boddy AV. Chemotherapy in newborns and preterm babies. Seminars in Fetal and Neonatal Medicine. 2012;**17**(4):243–248

[102] Jairam V, Roberts KB, Yu JB. Historical trends in the use of radiation therapy for pediatric cancers: 1973–2008. International Journal of Radiation Oncology Biology Physics. 2013;**85**(3):e151-e155

6

Perioperative Care of the Neonate

Shelly Haug, Sara Farooqi, Anamika Banerji and Andrew Hopper

Abstract

Care of the perioperative neonate requires careful consideration of many aspects including the impact of anesthesia and surgery on multiple organ systems. Neonatal care should include close attention to achieving homeostasis and stability in the perioperative period. This chapter will address the critical elements in the management of the surgical neonate.

Keywords: neonate, surgical care, Neonatal Intensive Care Unit (NICU)

1. Preoperative care of the neonate

Care of the preoperative surgical neonate starts with a comprehensive history and physical examination on admission. It is important to focus on airway, respiratory, cardiac, and renal abnormalities which may impact surgery. Preoperative lab studies should include a complete blood count with differential, basic metabolic panel, coagulation studies and cross match blood screening [1, 2].

Preoperative airway management includes consideration of need for intubation and mechanical ventilation and chest radiography to confirm endotracheal tube position, to assess lung volumes and to evaluate cardiomegaly. Endotracheal intubation is often completed by the neonatal intensive care physician though at times pediatric anesthesia may prefer this responsibility; therefore, communication is important.

Additional preoperative goals include optimizing ventilation and oxygenation, correcting abnormal electrolytes and pH and ensuring adequate perfusion. Lab work should forewarn clinicians of anemia and thrombocytopenia which should be corrected with goal neonatal hematocrit of 30–35% and platelet count greater than 100,000 preoperatively. Coagulation studies should be normalized with fresh frozen plasma and cryoprecipitate as needed prior to surgery. In cases of liver dysfunction, consider vitamin K administration. Disseminated intravascular coagulation should be considered and treated if sepsis is suspected. Ideally, surgery should be deferred if sepsis is suspected.

Adequate intravenous access is necessary prior to surgery. The need for central venous line placement should be determined and discussed with the anesthesiologist and pediatric surgeon in advance. If percutaneous central venous line placement is unsuccessful, central venous line may need to be placed by surgery. Factors that should be weighed in determining the need for central line placement include type of surgery, anticipated recovery time and anticipated length of time to regain bowel function. If the neonate is expected not to tolerate adequate enteral volumes for appropriate nutrition or to be nil per os (NPO) for greater than 2 – 5 days, then central line access should be considered [3].

Length of NPO status should be discussed with the surgeon. For elective procedures requiring anesthesia or sedation, the American Society of Anesthesiologists recommends neonates be NPO for at least 4 hours if fed breast milk and 6 hours if fed formula prior to surgery [4]. NPO status is at times outweighed by the need for emergency surgery in cases of critical illness.

Choice of intravenous fluid replacement is in large part dictated by the disease process, surgery and type of therapy anticipated [5]. Intravenous fluids should include provision for maintenance fluids and, if indicated, fluid and electrolyte replacement to correct deficits and for surgical conditions with anticipated fluid loss (see **Table 1**). Neonates are born with excess total body water in comparison with muscle mass and fat. The more preterm neonates have increased extracellular fluid. After birth, there is a shift of fluid from the extracellular compartment that results in salt and water diuresis by 48 to 72 hours and physiological weight loss in the first week of life. Failure to have adequate diuresis is associated with increased morbidities including pulmonary edema, tissue edema, symptomatic patent ductus arteriosus, necrotizing enterocolitis (NEC) and chronic lung disease [5–8]. Neonates are more sensitive to hypovolemia due to relatively low cardiac contractility. Maintenance fluid replacement should allow for the initial loss of extracellular fluid diuresis over the first week of life while maintaining normal intravascular volume and tonicity reflected by heart rate, urine output, electrolytes and acid/base status [5].

Birth weight (g)	Insensible water loss (mL/kg/day)	Total water requirement by age (mL/kg/day)		
		Day 1–2	Day 3–7	Day 8–30
<750	100+	100–200	120–200	120–180
750–1000	60–70	80–150	100–150	120–180
1001–1500	30–65	60–100	80–150	120–180
>1500	15–30	60–80	100–150	120–180

Adapted from Ref. [45].

Table 1. Maintenance fluid requirements during the first month of life [5].

Careful estimation of ongoing pathogenic fluid losses is important to determine the best volume and composition of fluid replacement. Estimation of fluid and electrolyte losses can be difficult especially in conditions that predispose to third spacing such as sepsis, hypoalbuminemia, intra-abdominal infection, postoperative abdominal surgery or cardiac surgery. Calculating daily gross intake and output along with serial weight can help to estimate fluid loss. Electrolyte losses can be estimated by multiplying the volume of fluid loss by the electrolyte content of the type of body fluid (see **Table 2**) [5].

Fluid source	Sodium (mmol/L)	Potassium (mmol/L)	Chloride (mmol/L)
Stomach	20–80	5–20	100–150
Small intestine	100–140	5–15	90–120
Bile	120–140	5–15	90–120
Ileostomy	45–135	3–15	20–120
Diarrheal stool	10–90	10–80	10–110

Adapted from Ref. [45].

Table 2. Electrolyte content of body fluids [5].

Normal saline boluses of 10–20 mL/kg should be given to maintain adequate renal perfusion to ensure normal urine output (2–3 mL/kg/hour). Fluid should also be given to maintain normal blood pressure based on gestational age. Caution should be used when administering greater than 40 mL/kg of fluid boluses to support blood pressure as this should prompt evaluation regarding the cause of hypotension. Fluid boluses must be balanced by the risk of patent ductus arteriosus in at-risk preterm neonates. Need to increase total fluid intake may be better tolerated by gradually increasing overall total daily fluid rate rather than by giving fluid boluses. Metabolic acidosis can be buffered by the administration of sodium acetate in fluids given to maintain central line patency. Hypoproteinemia should be corrected slowly if possible preoperatively to ensure better postoperative wound healing. An early assessment of serum albumin should be considered, as this may be reflective of prognosis for severity of gastroschisis. In most instances, administration of albumin for fluid replacement and to correct hypoalbuminemia should be discouraged as the albumin leaks into the tissues and contributes to tissue edema. Consideration should be given to placement of a Foley catheter for very long procedures or very unstable or chemically paralyzed neonates. Perfusion should be monitored and normalized. Assessment of tissue perfusion includes measuring blood pressure by peripheral cuff or by arterial line placement. Monitoring arterial blood pressure by indwelling arterial line is indicated for critically ill neonates if a period of postoperative instability is expected, if the neonate is requiring vasopressors or for frequent blood sampling.

Significant morbidity and mortality of perioperative neonates are related to hypoxic/ischemic events. Most intensive care units monitor perfusion index as part of skin surface oxygen saturation monitoring [9, 10]. More institutions are using near infrared spectroscopy (NIRS) to assess tissue perfusion. While pulse oximetry provides a measure of arterial oxygen saturation, it may not be particularly useful for determining oxygen delivery to the tissues. NIRS regional oximetry measures the balance between local oxygen delivery and consumption beneath the sensor. NIRS provides an end-organ measure of not only oxygenation, but also perfusion. NIRS can be used as a continuous, real-time, noninvasive bedside monitor using infrared light sensors of regional tissue oxygenation and hemodynamics [11]. It is United States Food and Drug Administration (FDA) approved for use in neonates, including those less than 2.5 kg. Regional tissue oxygen saturation reflects a ratio of arterial and venous blood (25:75%) and the balance between oxygen delivery and tissue consumption. NIRS monitoring usually includes measuring cerebral and somatic, either renal or mesenteric, regional oxygen saturation. There are norms of average NIRS values for cerebral, renal and mesenteric areas of monitoring, providing a noninvasive measure of end-organ oxygenation and perfusion [12]. These norms vary between term and preterm neonates (see **Table 3**).

rSO2	Term	Preterm
Cerebral (%)	66–89	66–83
Renal (%)	75–97	64–87
Mesenteric (%)	63–87	32–66

Values differ by sensor type with neonatal sensors reading 10% higher. Adapted from Refs. [13, 14].

Table 3. Normal ranges of regional oxygen saturation (rSO2) in term [13] and preterm [14] neonates.

Gastric decompression by Replogle sump tube should be discussed with surgeon and must be considered for neonates with intestinal obstruction. Cases to strongly consider gastric decompression include surgical necrotizing enterocolitis, Hirschsprung's disease, intestinal atresias, gastroschisis and omphalocele.

Preoperative labs should be obtained within 24 hours of planned surgery to ensure infection is ruled out. Prophylactic antibiotics should be given within 1 hour of skin entry [1]. At some hospitals, this timing is best achieved if antibiotic such as cefazolin is given in the preoperative surgical area as part of a preoperative checklist. Antibiotic choice should be dependent on disease process. Suspected perforation should be treated with broad-spectrum antibiotics that specifically include Gram-negative and anaerobic coverage. Length of therapy and choice of antibiotics may change depending on the intraoperative findings and culture results.

2. Common conditions of the surgical neonate

Although various conditions require specific management, the initial management of the surgical neonate consists of gastric decompression with placement of a Replogle tube, imaging including abdominal radiographs, and fluid and electrolyte management. The use of antibiotics is dependent upon the suspected pathology. Specialized management considerations are reviewed for the following conditions.

2.1. Gastroschisis

Gastroschisis is a congenital anterior abdominal wall defect that occurs to the right of the umbilical cord insertion that results in herniation of abdominal contents and thereby permitting bowel exposure to amniotic fluid in utero [15]. Abdominal contents generally contain the small intestine; however, larger defects may contain the stomach and colon [16]. Compared to an omphalocele defect, there is no transparent sac to protect the intestine and gastroschisis is not usually associated with other congenital syndromes. However, it may be associated with other gastrointestinal abnormalities such as malrotation, atresia or stenosis. A neonate with a prenatal diagnosis of gastroschisis should preferably be delivered at an institution with multidisciplinary care, influx into maternal-fetal medicine service, neonatal intensive care team and pediatric surgery. At the time of delivery, the neonate should be placed in a bowel bag enclosed to the neonate's axilla. This bag protects the bowel and also helps to retain body heat. Given the location of the defect, the neonate should be placed right side down to avoid tension on the mesenteric vasculature. A Replogle tube should be placed at the time of delivery to allow for abdominal decompression. All neonates should receive empiric broad-spectrum antibiotics, preferably ampicillin and gentamicin. Immediate intubation is not required if the neonate's respiratory status is stable. Some medical experts recommend a controlled, elective intubation to avoid unnecessary airway trauma. Surgical management is dependent on the defect. Surgical options include primary closure, staged reduction with a silo or sutureless umbilical closure [17]. In order to prepare the neonate for surgery, a secure airway should be established as well as adequate intravenous access. Due to the nature of the defect, umbilical lines are contraindicated in gastroschisis. Chemical paralysis is generally dependent on the preference of the surgeon and may be required in neonates with a large defect. When defect size or abdominal pressure issues prevent primary closure, placement of a silo allows for gradual reduction in the intestine into the abdominal cavity. With a silo, abdominal contents are gently "squeezed" into the abdomen daily. Once the contents are reduced, the neonate is taken to the operating room for closure. After the defect is closed, nasogastric decompression is continued until return of bowel function.

Special consideration must be taken in regard to fluid management in gastroschisis due to insensible fluid loss and postoperative third-space fluid shifts. Amount of postoperative fluid administration should generally be less than prior to gastroschisis closure and be balanced with perfusion and urine output [18]. See discussion of preoperative fluid management. Potential complications associated with gastroschisis include ileus, sepsis, intestinal atresias, malabsorption, wound infection and necrotizing enterocolitis [16].

2.2. Omphalocele

An omphalocele is a congenital ventral abdominal wall defect of the umbilical ring that results in abdominal viscera herniation and is associated with chromosomal, cardiac and/or genitourinary abnormalities [19]. Immediate postnatal management should include protection of the herniated viscera with sterile saline-soaked gauze, and stabilization of viscera to ensure blood supply to the bowel is not kinked by the weight of the bowel. The neonate may be placed right side down or with towels placed under the bowel to help support the externalized intestine.

Gastric decompression should be initiated with placement of a Replogle tube on continuous low suction to prevent bowel distention. If volume of gastric drainage exceeds approximately 10 mL/kg per 12 hour shift, gastric fluid should be replaced with 0.9% sodium chloride.

Potential problems with omphalocele include risk of hypothermia due to high heat loss from the exposed bowel as well as risk of vasoconstriction, decreased tissue perfusion and metabolic acidosis [19]. Fluids and electrolyte replacement will need to anticipate additional fluid losses due to the specific disease pathology. Maintenance of intravascular fluid volume is necessary to ensure adequate tissue perfusion and preservation of bowel wall perfusion [19, 20].

Other factors to consider include prevention of sepsis by administering broad-spectrum antibiotic therapy. Due to the association with other anomalies, neonates with omphalocele should be evaluated with chest and abdominal radiography, renal and abdominal ultrasound as well as echocardiogram prior to operation [19]. Repair of the defect will be a primary or a staged closure depending on the size of the defect. Potential postoperative complications include significant increase in intra-abdominal pressures that may compromise venous blood return and hemodynamic and/or respiratory stability due to diaphragmatic elevation [19].

Another important consideration in neonates with omphalocele is the risk of pulmonary hypertension [21]. All neonates with omphalocele should be monitored for evidence of pulmonary hypertension between the second and seventh day after birth as they may not initially present with signs of pulmonary hypertension. Diagnosis should be suspected based on increased oxygen requirement and increased pre- and postductal gradient and confirmed by increased right ventricular pressures (greater than 40 mmHg) on echocardiogram [21].

Short-term postoperative complications include necrotizing enterocolitis, prolonged ileus and respiratory distress. If primary closure is done, the neonate will require assisted ventilation and may require muscle relaxants for a time. It is important to ensure adequate ventilation and oxygenation by adjusting inspiratory and end expiratory pressures to maintain adequate lung volumes as the abdominal distention postoperatively may be aggravated by fluid third spacing due to capillary leak syndrome. Postoperative pain management usually requires continuous infusion of morphine and should be titrated according to appropriate neonatal pain scales (see pain section later in chapter) [22]. Long-term complications include prolonged dependence on parenteral nutrition, gastroesophageal reflux, parenteral nutrition-related liver disease, feeding intolerance and neurodevelopmental delay [19]. When bowel function returns postoperatively, initiation of enteral feeds should be done with breast milk or an elemental formula such as Elecare or Neocate, starting with small volumes and advancing slowly [23, 24]. Neonates with giant omphalocele usually require prolonged time to achieve full enteral feeds, especially if complicated by respiratory insufficiency requiring intubation shortly after delivery or symptoms of gastroesophageal reflux postoperatively [24].

2.3. Obstruction

See further detail (**Table 4**).

Type	Presentation	Diagnosis	Preoperative care	Treatment	Postoperative care
Duodenal atresia	Few hours after birth; bilious vomiting, no distention	Abdominal film; "double-bubble" sign	Gastric decompression, IV fluids	Diamond-shaped duodenoduodenostomy	Feeding dependent upon bowel function
Malrotation with volvulus	At 3–7 days; bilious vomiting, rapid deterioration with volvulus	Ultrasound and contrast studies; "upper GI spiral" sign, abnormal location of the superior mesenteric vessels	Gastric decompression, IV fluids, STAT surgery for symptomatic patients	Ladd's procedure	Feeding dependent upon bowel function
Jejunoileal atresia	Within 1 day of birth; vomiting, abdominal distention	Abdominal film; air-fluid levels	Gastric decompression, IV fluids	Resection and anastomosis	Feeding dependent upon bowel function
Meconium ileus	Immediately after birth; abdominal distention, bilious vomiting	Abdominal film; distention, air-fluid levels, "ground-glass" sign	Gastric decompression, IV fluids	Enterostomy if complicated; gastrografin enema	Acetylcysteine (Mucomyst), pancreatic enzymes
Necrotizing ileus	Varied timing; feeding intolerance, abdominal distention, vomiting, bloody stools	Serial abdominal films; distention, ileus, pneumatosis intestinalis, portal venous gas	Gastric decompression, IV fluids, antibiotics for 7 to14 days, serial imaging, STAT surgery if perforated	Resection of necrotic bowel and enterostomy	Feeding reinitiation with slow advancement after antibiotic course completion and normal imaging

Adapted from Ref. [25].

Table 4. Neonatal obstruction [25].

2.4. Necrotizing enterocolitis

Necrotizing enterocolitis (NEC) is the most common emergent neonatal gastrointestinal diseases among premature neonates [26]. The mortality rate of NEC may range from 20 to 30% with the highest mortality in those neonates who require surgery [27]. Often, an inverse relationship between gestational age and frequency of NEC exists. Therefore, the smaller the neonate, the higher the clinical suspicion for this disease.

Typically, NEC presents with feeding intolerance, hematochezia and abdominal distention. Clinical progression of the disease may ensue rapidly from abdominal discoloration, worsening distention with intestinal perforation leading to clinical deterioration with hypotension, metabolic acidosis and thrombocytopenia requiring intensive medical and surgical support. At the moment of suspicion for NEC, the neonate should be placed NPO and gastric decompression initiated. Intravenous fluid hydration must be provided, along with an urgent surgical consultation. Intravenous antibiotics should be started once NEC is suspected that often include "triple therapy" consisting of Gram-positive, Gram-negative and anaerobic bacteria coverage. Immediate and serial abdominal radiographs should be obtained to assess the presence of pneumatosis intestinalis, one of the hallmarks to diagnose NEC. Laboratory testing should include blood cultures, complete blood count (CBC) to assess for leukocytosis and thrombocytopenia, and C-reactive protein. Serial two-view abdominal radiographs should be obtained to assess for progression. While there are no universally accepted criteria for NEC, Bell's staging system is often used to describe the stages and severity of this disease. The staging is described as follows (see **Table 5**).

Stage/classification	Systemic signs	Abdominal signs	Radiographic signs
IA; suspected	Temperature instability, apnea, bradycardia, lethargy	Gastric residuals, abdominal distention, emesis, heme-positive stool	Normal or intestinal dilation, mild ileus
IB; suspected	Same as above	Gross hematochezia	Same as above
IIA; definite, mildly ill	Same as above	Same as above with absent bowel sounds with or without abdominal distention	Intestinal dilation, ileus, pneumatosis intestinalis
IIB definite, moderately ill	Same as above plus mild metabolic acidosis and thrombocytopenia	Same as above, plus absent bowel sounds, definite tenderness, with or without abdominal cellulitis or right lower quadrant mass	Same as IIA plus ascites
IIIA advanced, severely ill, intact bowel	Same as IIB plus hypotension, bradycardia, severe apnea, combined respiratory and metabolic acidosis, DIC and neutropenia	Same as above, plus signs of peritonitis, marked tenderness and abdominal distention	Same as IIA plus ascites
IIIB advanced, severely ill, perforated bowel	Same as IIIA	Same as IIIA	Same as above plus pneumoperitoneum

Adapted from Ref. [28].

Table 5. Modified Bell's staging criteria for necrotizing enterocolitis [28].

3. Comparison between acute and elective surgical management

Operative intervention of the acutely ill neonate is less desirable but often unavoidable. In situations of intestinal perforation or a hemodynamically compromised neonate, all efforts should be made to ensure a near stable status of the neonate [1, 2, 5]. If a neonate requires emergent surgical intervention, communication with the surgical team, anesthesiology and neonatology team to discuss diagnosis and planned intervention must be made as soon as possible. Most important in management is establishing a stable airway and adequate intravenous or central line access. Pertinent imaging including radiographs and ultrasound should be readily available for evaluation by the surgical team. The neonatal team should ideally be at bedside to intervene in case of clinical deterioration per Pediatric Advance Life Support

(PALS) guidelines. Informed consent for surgery must be obtained with the parents or guardian either in person or via telephone.

One common routine elective operation in neonates is gastrostomy tube placement. A gastrostomy tube or "g-tube" is a small feeding tube that is surgically or percutaneously placed in the stomach for feeding or decompression of air or drainage. Surgical placement is either laparoscopic or open and may be done in association with other procedures [29]. Gastrostomy tubes may be needed for preterm neonates with continued inadequate oral feeding once corrected to term if gastrostomy tube feeding is expected to be needed for greater than 4 weeks. Prior to gastrostomy tube placement, the surgeon may request radiographs to evaluate anatomy of the upper gastrointestinal tract. After gastrostomy tube placement, the neonate may have minor pain at the incision site. Intravenous fluids may be required for the first 24 hour to provide parenteral nutrition to allow the site to heal. Generally, the neonate may be restarted on previous feeds at 25% of the total expected volume, and advanced gradually to full enteral feeds via the g-tube within 24–36 hours as tolerated.. A frequent complication of gastrostomy tubes includes dislodgment, usually within the first 2 weeks after its placement [29]. When this occurs, a physician should replace the tube as soon as possible, so the hole in the stomach does not close. A small amount of leaking is normal and may require protective cream application to the skin. A gastrostomy tube may be left in place permanently or temporarily dependent on the neonate's needs [29].

Another common elective surgical procedure includes inguinal hernia repair. An inguinal hernia repair is an internal opening in the inguinal canal through which fluids and/or intestines may pass through [30]. The neonate may have minor pain at the incision site postoperatively that should be controlled with acetaminophen or small doses of morphine. Neonates should be monitored for postoperative respiratory complications such as apnea and oxygen desaturation. Neonates at risk include those with a history of prematurity, especially if still less than 45 weeks corrected gestational age, and neonates with comorbidities including chronic lung disease, history of necrotizing enterocolitis, anemia, low birth weight or former apnea episodes [31, 32]. Healthy, older neonates may generally be repaired as an outpatient [31].

4. Postoperative care of the neonate

Postoperative management should begin with face-to-face communication between the senior clinician caring for the neonate after surgery and the surgeon as well as the anesthesiologist. The neonatologist should be informed of major events that may have occurred during the surgery, the surgery that was performed, the anesthesia the neonate received during the surgery and postoperatively in recovery (especially if paralytic agents were used), as well as the volume and type of fluids or blood products given during the operation.

Temperature homeostasis is important in the postoperative period. Neonates undergoing operative procedures in the operating room are at increased risk of thermal instability. Hypothermia of postoperative neonates leads to an increased risk of adverse respiratory events including increased need for respiratory and cardiac interventions compared to normothermic neonates [33]. Furthermore, hypothermia may cause protein catabolism, hypokalemia and changes in glucose metabolism. Postoperative interventions include applying warm temperature regulating blankets, decreasing skin exposure and warming operative rooms [34].

If the neonate remains intubated postoperatively, obtain a blood gas and chest radiography immediately following return to the ICU to assess oxygenation, ventilation, chest expansion and endotracheal tube position. It is important for clinicians to understand postoperative neonates are prone to apnea and periodic breathing while recovering from anesthesia and in response to pain and pain medications. Neonates are also prone to hypoxemia due to transient decrease in functional residual capacity of the lungs and ventilation/perfusion mismatch. Adequate lung tidal volumes of 6–8 mL/kg expiratory lung volumes should be maintained to prevent atelectasis. Blood gas pH should be maintained at 7.35–7.45 with pCO2 of 40–55 for most neonates. Once the neonate is awake and consistently breathing spontaneously, the clinician should rapidly wean the ventilator and extubate per blood gases if possible. Weaning off mechanical ventilation should be weighed against the need for additional pain control. Surgery should be made aware of neonates requiring nasal continuous positive airway pressure (CPAP) or nasal intermittent mandatory ventilation (IMV) postextubation. Ideally, continuous narcotic infusion for pain control should be at a minimum or discontinued prior to extubation. The clinician should also monitor for the development of pulmonary hypertension by clinical symptoms, pre- and postductal oxygen gradient and confirm by echocardiography [1].

Immediate postoperative labs should include evaluation of hemoglobin/hematocrit. If blood loss is over 15% and not already replaced during the operative period, clinicians should consider replacing with packed red blood cells [35, 36]. Electrolytes should be evaluated in the immediate postoperative period and also monitored every 6 hours for invasive procedures or every 8–12 hours for less intensive procedures for the first 24-hours postoperatively [1].

Surgical neonates may have significant third-space losses depending on the magnitude of the procedure. Phases of fluid resuscitation change with time postoperatively. In the immediate postoperative time period, fluid and blood replacement is often required. Postoperative days 2–4 are often phases of third spacing and vascular leak during which some element of fluid replacement is required in conjunction with diuretics to help mobilize fluids. Avoidance of massive anasarca is important. Abdominal compartment syndrome is especially important to consider in the context of abdominal closures with decreased perfusion and the potential for decreased urine output. Gastroschisis patients are especially prone to large fluid losses. If total parenteral nutrition is not immediately available, D5 lactated ringers should be given. Initial fluids should be given at 150–175 mL/kg/day. Total parenteral nutrition should be optimized to include protein of 3–4 g/kg/day to minimize catabolic state and promote wound healing. Dextrose may need to be adjusted postoperatively due to hyperglycemia secondary to stress and increased fluid administration. Therefore, Accuchecks should be monitored frequently, and glucose infusion rate (GIR) should be adjusted. GIR should be maintained 4–8 μg/kg/min to maintain blood glucose levels of 100–160 mg/dL. Electrolytes should be normalized as much as possible [5]. Consideration of starting enteral nutrition should be discussed when the neonate shows intestinal readiness, presence of bowel sounds and passing gas. Clinicians should monitor for postoperative ileus from the surgery and/or ileus due to pain medications. Antireflux medications should be avoided in the neonate unless for specific surgical cases such as tracheoesophageal fistula where such medications have proven to be necessary. Reflux medications lead to abnormalities of intestinal flora and have been shown to increase neonatal mortality [37].

Special fluid consideration must be made for those neonates with gastroschisis that have undergone repair. Once they are repaired, their fluid losses significantly decrease, and thus, parenteral nutrition must be adjusted shortly after surgical closure. Total fluid administration should be decreased to approximately 140–150 mL/kg/day [38], based on the assessment of the neonate's fluid losses. Clinicians should be cautious of fluid volumes as overhydration may lengthen hospital stay and delay enteral feeding [38].

Hypotension secondary to hypovolemia may be treated with 10–20 mL/kg boluses of normal saline or if hypotension is persistent and severe, the clinician should consider fresh frozen plasma. If anemic, packed red blood cells may be used. Albumin should rarely be used and only with great caution as it may worsen third-space fluid losses in neonates. Low albumin is often partially dilutional and when not exacerbated by dilutional effects, is best addressed through maximizing protein delivery through nutrition. Replacement of any gastric output should be considered with 0.45 normal saline with 10 mEq of potassium chloride per liter. If output is large, consider replacing more frequently (i.e., every 4 hours to run over 4 hours versus once a shift over 1 hour if lower output). Replacement of gastric fluid is important to maintain fluid balance but must be balanced with urine output and overall body edema. Vasopressor therapy may be considered for the critically ill postoperative neonate if fluid replacement is already optimized and neonate remains hypotensive with signs of decreased end-organ perfusion. Steroid therapy to aid adrenal stress response may also improve hemodynamic stability; however, it should be used cautiously as steroids may decrease immune response if there is concern for infection.

Fluid status must be monitored closely, and urine output should be maintained at a minimum of 1 mL/kg/hour. The clinician must balance the neonate's overall fluid status as measured by weight, urine output, body wall edema, blood pressure, heart rate and overall clinical status. Edematous neonates may still have low intravascular volumes, and thus, diuretics would possibly exacerbate hypotension.

Blood pressure should be monitored closely, at least hourly if there is no arterial line access. Hypotension in the postoperative period is considered a sign of hypovolemia until proven otherwise. Skin perfusion should be monitored which can be done by NIRS or perfusion index of pulse oximetry monitoring. All tubes and drains should be monitored closely postoperatively for patency, function and how secure they are attached to the patient. Output of sumps, chest tubes, wound drains and Foley catheters should be followed. Pending resolution of ileus and improvement in outputs each should be removed at the earliest time point to prevent infection with persistent foreign bodies.

Prevention of infection is important. White blood cell count, C-reactive protein trend and bandemia should be monitored and blood cultures obtained if concern for infection rises [1]. Be especially cautious of hygienic precautions when handling tubes, drains and any wound dressing changes. The need for postoperative antibiotic coverage should be discussed between the neonatal clinician and surgeon.

5. Pain management, sedation and paralysis review

Pain control should be titrated based on the type of surgery. More invasive surgeries will likely require immediate postoperative pain management including a narcotic drip for the first 24 – 48 hours [39]. Consider morphine 20-50 micrograms/kg/hour or Fentanyl 3 micrograms/kg/hour with as needed (PRN) dosing for breakthrough pain. Pain management should be transitioned to PRN dosing when able. Titration of pain medication should be assessed through reliable and accurate neonatal pain assessment scoring tools such as the "Neonatal Pain, Agitation and Sedation Scale" (N-PASS) [40] or "Crying, Requires increased oxygen administration, Increased vital signs, Expression and Sleeplessness" (CRIES) [41]. A combination of behavioral observations such as facial expression, body posture and tone and physiologic symptoms such as heart rate, blood pressure and oxygen saturation should be taken into consideration by the neonatal pain score used [22].

Nonnarcotic pain management methods should be used such as Sweet-Ease and intravenous Tylenol 20 mg/kg/dose every 6 hours for a 24-48 hour period, unless contraindicated or if there is concern for liver dysfunction. The neonate should be monitored closely for urinary retention if Foley catheter is not in place. The stomach should be decompressed. Nonpharmacological pain management includes protective neonatal positioning if possible with the neonate supported in the flex position. Environmental stimulation should be minimized with decreased lighting, noise and touch.

Use of chemical paralytic agents postoperatively should only be used in cases where there is concern for wound dehiscence, large irreducible gastroschisis or patient instability. Paralytics should be used for shortest time possible, as the use will increase the likelihood of third-spacing fluids, urinary retention and anasarca [39].

6. Follow-up of the surgical neonate

The care of a neonate following discharge from the ICU is one that requires a multidisciplinary approach. The patient's pediatrician, neonatologist in the High Risk Follow Clinic (when appropriate), various therapists and the primary surgeon will need to see the neonate after discharge [42]. Follow-up visits include neurodevelopment assessment scales using Bayley III and WPPSI-II scores. While there are certain risk factors innate to sick neonates that make them prone to developmental delay such as prematurity and/or congenital defects, there are data to suggest that neonates who require surgical intervention experience initial developmental delays as compared with their healthy counterparts [43]. While there is ample evidence of suboptimal developmental outcomes in neonates requiring cardiac surgery, the data for those undergoing repair of conditions such as gastroschisis suggest that outcomes are similar to those of their healthy cohorts [44]. Those neonates who have had significant surgical intervention and those with severe outcomes such as short gut syndrome require a lifelong close follow-up with the surgical team.

Author details

Shelly Haug*, Sara Farooqi, Anamika Banerji and Andrew Hopper

*Address all correspondence to: shaug@llu.edu

Loma Linda University Children's Hospital, Loma Linda, CA, USA

References

[1] Philadelphia TCH of Perioperative Care Newborns/Infants—Clinical Pathway: ICU and Inpatient. http://www.chop.edu/clinical-pathway/perioperative-care-newborns-infants-clinical-pathway. Published August 12, 2014. Accessed October 23, 2016.

[2] Rowe MI, Rowe SA. The last fifty years of neonatal surgical management. *Am J Surg*. 2000;180(5):345–352.

[3] Percutaneous Placement of Central Venous Catheters. University of Iowa Children's Hospital. https://uichildrens.org/health-library/percutaneous-placement-central-venous-catheters. Published September 12, 2012. Accessed November 27, 2016.

[4] American Society of Anesthesiologists Committee. Practice guidelines for preoperative fasting and the use of pharmacologic agents to reduce the risk of pulmonary aspiration: application to healthy patients undergoing elective procedures: an updated report by the American Society of Anesthesiologists Committee on Standards and Practice Parameters. *Anesthesiology*. 2011;114(3):495–511. doi:10.1097/ALN.0b013e3181fcbfd9

[5] Dell KM. Fluid, Electrolytes, and Acid-Base Homeostasis. In R. J. Martin, A. A. Fanaroff, & M. C. Walsh (Authors), Fanaroff and Martin's neonatal-perinatal medicine: diseases of the fetus and infant. Philadelphia, PA: Elsevier/Saunders. 2015;613–627.

[6] Bell EF, Warburton D, Stonestreet BS, Oh W. High-volume fluid intake predisposes premature infants to necrotising enterocolitis. *Lancet Lond Engl*. 1979;2(8133):90.

[7] Bell EF, Warburton D, Stonestreet BS, Oh W. Effect of fluid administration on the development of symptomatic patent ductus arteriosus and congestive heart failure in premature infants. *N Engl J Med*. 1980;302(11):598–604. doi:10.1056/NEJM198003133021103

[8] Marshall DD, Kotelchuck M, Young TE, et al. Risk factors for chronic lung disease in the surfactant era: a North Carolina population-based study of very low birth weight infants. *Pediatrics*. 1999;104(6):1345–1350. doi:10.1542/peds.104.6.1345

[9] Piasek CZ, Van Bel F, Sola A. Perfusion index in newborn infants: a noninvasive tool for neonatal monitoring. *Acta Paediatr Oslo Nor 1992*. 2014;103(5):468–473. doi:10.1111/apa.12574

[10] Terek D, Altun Koroglu O, Ulger Z, Yalaz M, Kultursay N. The serial changes of perfusion index in preterm infants with patent ductus arteriosus: is perfusion index clinically significant? *Minerva Pediatr*. 2016;68(4):250–255.

[11] Koch HW, Hansen TG. Perioperative use of cerebral and renal near-infrared spectroscopy in neonates: a 24-h observational study. *Pediatr Anesth*. 2016;26(2):190–198. doi:10.1111/pan.12831

[12] Alderliesten T, Dix L, Baerts W, et al. Reference values of regional cerebral oxygen saturation during the first 3 days of life in preterm neonates. *Pediatr Res*. 2016;79(1–1):55–64. doi:10.1038/pr.2015.186

[13] Chock V. NIRS Educational Module. November 2016. http://neonatology.stanford.edu/content/dam/sm/neonatology/documents/NIRS%20Educational%20Module.pdf.

[14] McNeill S, Gatenby JC, McElroy S, Engelhardt B. Normal cerebral, renal and abdominal regional oxygen saturations using near-infrared spectroscopy in preterm infants. *J Perinatol*. 2011;31(1):51–57. doi:10.1038/jp.2010.71

[15] Wilson RD, Johnson MP. Congenital abdominal wall defects: an update. *Fetal Diagn Ther*. 2004;19(5):385–398. doi:10.1159/000078990

[16] Lund CH, Bauer K, Berrios M. Gastroschisis: incidence, complications, and clinical management in the neonatal intensive care unit. *J Perinat Neonatal Nurs*. 2007;21(1):63–68.

[17] O'Connell RV, Dotters-Katz SK, Kuller JA, Strauss RA. Gastroschisis: a review of management and outcomes. *Obstet Gynecol Surv*. 2016;71(9):537–544. doi:10.1097/OGX.0000000000000344

[18] Bonasso PC, Lucke-Wold B, Hobbs GR, Vaughan RA, Shorter NA, Nakayama DK. Excessive postoperative fluid administration in infants with gastroschisis. *Am Surg*. 2016;82(8):704–706.

[19] McNair C, Hawes J, Urquhart H. Caring for the newborn with an omphalocele. *Neonatal Netw NN*. 2006;25(5):319–327. doi:10.1891/0730-0832.25.5.319

[20] Philippart AI, Canty TG, Filler RM. Acute fluid volume requirements in infants with anterior abdominal wall defects. *J Pediatr Surg*. 1972;7(5):553–558. doi:10.1016/0022-3468(72)90212-6

[21] Baerg JE, Thorpe DL, Sharp NE, et al. Pulmonary hypertension predicts mortality in infants with omphalocele. *J Neonatal-Perinat Med*. 2015;8(4):333–338. doi:10.3233/NPM-15915011

[22] Bhalla T, Shepherd E, Tobias JD. Neonatal pain management. *Saudi J Anaesth*. 2014;8(Suppl 1):S89–S97. doi:10.4103/1658-354X.144085

[23] Spatz DL, Schmidt KJ. Breastfeeding success in infants with giant omphalocele. *Adv Neonatal Care Off J Natl Assoc Neonatal Nurses*. 2012;12(6):329–335. doi:10.1097/ANC.0b013e31826150c5

[24] Haug S, St Peter S, Ramlogan S, et al. The impact of breast milk, respiratory insufficiency and GERD on enteral feeding in infants with omphalocele. *J Pediatr Gastroenterol Nutr*. November 2016. doi:10.1097/MPG.0000000000001463

[25] Kimura K, Loening-Baucke V. Bilious vomiting in the newborn: rapid diagnosis of intestinal obstruction. *Am Fam Physician*. 2000;61(9):2791–2798.

[26] Neu J, Walker WA. Necrotizing Enterocolitis. *N Engl J Med*. 2011;364(3):255–264. doi:10.1056/NEJMra1005408

[27] Fitzgibbons SC, Ching Y, Yu D, et al. Mortality of necrotizing enterocolitis expressed by birth weight categories. *J Pediatr Surg*. 2009;44(6):1072–1076. doi:10.1016/j.jpedsurg.2009.02.013

[28] Neu J. Necrotizing enterocolitis: the search for a unifying pathogenic theory leading to prevention. *Pediatr Clin North Am*. 1996;43(2):409–432.

[29] Gastrostomy (G-Tube) Surgery | Children's Hospital Pittsburgh. Children's Hospital of Pittsburgh. http://www.chp.edu/our-services/transplant/intestine/education/patient-procedures/gastrostomy. Accessed November 23, 2016.

[30] Inguinal Hernia Repair Surgery | Children's Hospital Pittsburgh. Children's Hospital of Pittsburgh. http://www.chp.edu/our-services/urology/patient-procedures/hernia. Accessed November 23, 2016.

[31] Özdemir T, Arıkan A. Postoperative apnea after inguinal hernia repair in formerly premature infants: impacts of gestational age, postconceptional age and comorbidities. *Pediatr Surg Int*. 2013;29(8):801–804. doi:10.1007/s00383-013-3330-8

[32] Murphy JJ, Swanson T, Ansermino M, Milner R. The frequency of apneas in premature infants after inguinal hernia repair: do they need overnight monitoring in the intensive care unit? *J Pediatr Surg*. 2008;43(5):865–868. doi:10.1016/j.jpedsurg.2007.12.028

[33] Morehouse D, Williams L, Lloyd C, et al. Perioperative hypothermia in NICU infants: its occurrence and impact on infant outcomes. *Adv Neonatal Care Off J Natl Assoc Neonatal Nurses*. 2014;14(3):154–164. doi:10.1097/ANC.0000000000000045

[34] Dennison D. Thermal regulation of patients during the perioperative period. *AORN J*. 1995;61(5):827–828, 831–832.

[35] Fasano R, Luban NLC. Blood component therapy. *Pediatr Clin North Am*. 2008;55(2):421–445. doi:10.1016/j.pcl.2008.01.006

[36] Roseff SD, Luban NLC, Manno CS. Guidelines for assessing appropriateness of pediatric transfusion. *Transfusion (Paris)*. 2002;42(11):1398–1413. doi:10.1046/j.1537-2995.2002.00208.x

[37] Terrin G, Passariello A, Curtis MD, et al. Ranitidine is associated with infections, necrotizing enterocolitis, and fatal outcome in newborns. *Pediatrics*. 2012;129(1):e40–e45. doi:10.1542/peds.2011-0796

[38] Waldhausen JHT. Surgical management of gastroschisis. *NeoReviews*. 2005;6(11):e500–e507. doi:10.1542/neo.6-11-e500

[39] Committee on Fetus And Newborn and Section on Anesthesiology and Pain Medicine. Prevention and management of procedural pain in the neonate: an update. *Pediatrics*. 2016;137(2):e20154271. doi:10.1542/peds.2015-4271

[40] Hillman BA, Tabrizi MN, Gauda EB, Carson KA, Aucott SW. The Neonatal Pain, Agitation and Sedation Scale and the bedside nurse's assessment of neonates. *J Perinatol Off J Calif Perinat Assoc.* 2015;35(2):128–131. doi:10.1038/jp.2014.154

[41] Krechel SW, Bildner J. CRIES: a new neonatal postoperative pain measurement score. Initial testing of validity and reliability. *Paediatr Anaesth.* 1995;5(1):53–61.

[42] Panel SA. Referral to pediatric surgical specialists. *Pediatrics.* 2014;133(2):350–356. doi:10.1542/peds.2013-3820

[43] Ludman L, Spitz L, Landsdown R. Developmental progress of newborns undergoing neonatal surgery. *J Pediatr Surg.* 1990;25(5):469–471. doi:10.1016/0022-3468(90)90552-K

[44] Harris EL, Hart SJ, Minutillo C, et al. The long-term neurodevelopmental and psychological outcomes of gastroschisis: A cohort study. *J Pediatr Surg.* 2016;51(4):549–553. doi:10.1016/j.jpedsurg.2015.08.062

[45] Fanaroff AA, Martin FJ (eds). Neonatal and Perinatal Medicine: Diseases of the Fetus and Newborn (10th edition). St. Louis: Mosby; 1997, p 672.

7

Anesthetic Neurotoxicity in Pediatric Patients

Ayse B. Ozer and Sibel Ozcan

Abstract

In recent years, an increasing number of publications have shown the negative effects of anesthetics on the developing brain and have made inquiries about anesthesia for pediatric patients in practice. Anesthesia is applied to millions of children for surgery, imaging, and other invasive procedures; the issue is very serious and concerns. In this chapter, experimental and clinical studies about the issue have been summarized. As a result, anesthetic drugs except alpha-2 adrenergic agonist anesthetic (NMDA antagonist or a GABA agonist) used in pediatric patients (especially if there is no painful situation) have potential neurotoxicity. Particularly, if anesthesia exposure was applied in the fragile period (the first 4 years) and if used at higher concentrations or repeated anesthesia application, adverse effects of anesthesia exposure on the developing brain have been claimed. But, the issue is not fully clarified yet.

Keywords: anesthesia, neurotoxicity, neonatal, developing brain

1. Introduction

Since the beginning of the modern anesthesia (nearly 170 years), millions of people have received inhalation anesthetics, intravenous anesthetics, or a combination in order to create general anesthesia. These drugs have been applied in all age groups, from newborns who may be only a few hours old to geriatric patients. In fact, pediatric patients comprise a significant proportion of the total number of patients treated with general anesthesia, a trend that will continue well into the future.

Pediatric patients are not miniature versions of adult physiology. Pediatric patients differ significantly from adults and among other pediatric patients in anatomical, physiological, and pharmacological characteristics. Many centers have established a separate pediatric anesthesia subspecialty in order to meet the appropriate anesthetic requirements of newborns, premature infants, infants, children, and adolescents. In particular, neonates carry 10 times more mortality and morbidity risk compared to other pediatric age groups. The most common complications in this age group involve the cardiovascular and respiratory system [1]. Holzman [2] noted that the practitioner's experience and the presence of existing respiratory, cardiac, or muscular disease are the key factors that determine the risk of mortality and morbidity. Hemodynamic disturbances due to hypotension, hypertension, tachycardia, bradycardia, asystole, or other arrhythmias arising in the cardiovascular system and respiratory system issues such as hypopnea, apnea, hypoxia, hypocapnia, or hypercapnia can lead to disturbances in microcirculation to the central nervous system (CNS). Although the rate of complications has been reduced through improved understanding of the anatomical, physiological, and pharmacological characteristics of pediatric patients, advances in monitoring methods, and practitioner specialization, the risks are never completely eliminated.

Despite recent advances in the field of pediatric anesthesia, an increasing number of recent reports point to the adverse effects of anesthetics on the developing brain, raising concerns about the application of anesthesia in pediatric patients. As early as 1965, Sir Austin Bradford Hill recognized this issue at a meeting of the Royal Society of Medicine, stating: "How do we determine what are physical, chemical and psychologic hazards of occupation and in particular those that are rare and not easily recognized?" and "… the available human studies … cannot exclude the possibility that the anesthesia- induced neurotoxicity observed in many animal studies may also occur in children" [3]. Although it has been nearly 50 years from that meeting of the Royal Society of Medicine, the short- and long-term effects of anesthesia applications in pediatric patients remain poorly understood. In this chapter, the acute and long-term effects of anesthesia and anesthetics on the developing brain are summarized.

2. Definitions

Neurotoxicity of anesthetic substances on the developing brain is determined by a reduction in neural density and apoptosis in experimental studies and by disturbances in memory, attention, learning, and motor activity in clinical studies [4–6]. Although anesthetic agents used in neonates have known neurotoxic effects, there are valid reasons for using these agents even in vulnerable patients. Because pain itself has a neurotoxic effect, anesthesia-analgesia application in painful conditions may have a net neuroprotective effect [7, 8]. It should also be noted that in cases of hypoxia-ischemia or trauma, administration of anesthetics reduces the infarct volume by reducing the metabolic rate, decreasing intracranial pressure, eliminating free oxygen radicals, and reducing secondary injury [9–11]. Another positive effect is neuroplasticities. These are described as the neurophysical and neurochemical ability to improve compliance against environmental changes and damage when used in depressive disorders and diseases. Neuroplasticity refers to the increase in intercellular connections. Agents that enhance neuroplasticity have raised new hope for the treatment of neurodegenerative diseases [12–14].

3. Other factors that may cause neurotoxicity

Anesthetics are just one of many potential sources of perioperative neurotoxicities. Patient-related factors, such as genetic anomalies, prematurity, sepsis, infection, and vascular diseases, can cause perioperative toxicity. Additionally, hormonal, metabolic, inflammatory, or cardiovascular changes caused by trauma or surgery, hemodynamic disturbances, hypoxia, hypo-/hypercapnia, hypo-/hyperglycemia, electrolyte imbalances, and temperature variations that occur due to anesthesia can also contribute to the development of perioperative neurotoxicity [15–18].

4. Experimental studies

4.1. Inhalation anesthetics

In an experimental study by Shen et al. [4], sevoflurane was applied to neonatal (PND3, PND7, and PND14) and adult rats (PNW7) at concentrations ranging from 1% to 4%. Spatial memory was then assessed in adulthood using the Morris water maze (MWM) test. The PNW7 rats were less sensitive to sevoflurane than neonatal rats. Memory defects were apparent in groups treated with repeated low doses or a single high-dose anesthetic. The authors concluded that neonatal exposure to sevoflurane can result in memory defects in adulthood, with greater deficits seen in animals treated with multiple doses in a short period of time. As a result, the authors recommend that exposure to anesthesia during the neonatal period should be limited in dose and duration. Another study has shown that 4-hour sevoflurane exposure (2.5%) resulted in reduced hippocampal postsynaptic density protein-95 expression without causing any neuronal loss and was associated with learning and memory disturbances [19].

Another experimental study reported that 0.5% minimum alveolar concentration (MAC) sevoflurane applied for 6 hours had no significant effect on apoptosis and S100β levels. Conversely, isoflurane, which is given in the same circumstances, was shown to increase the level of apoptosis and S100β levels [20]. In another study, which evaluated the effects of inhalation anesthetics in neonatal rats, it was demonstrated that sevoflurane, isoflurane, and desflurane increased caspase-3 levels. Interestingly, nitrous oxide application (up to 150% concentration) for 6 hours did not cause neuroapoptosis; however, apoptosis was increased when nitrous oxide was applied with isoflurane [21]. Halothane administered during the prenatal period was associated with neurodegeneration and behavioral changes [22, 23]. Xenon, the currently preferred anesthetic, does not cause neuroapoptosis when used alone; on the contrary, xenon reduced the effects of other inhalation anesthetics when administered first [24].

4.2. Intravenous anesthetics

Zou et al. [5] have examined the effect of ketamine anesthesia duration in newborn rhesus monkeys (PND5, PND6) through silver and Fluoro-Jade C stains and caspase-3 immunostain. Three hours exposure to ketamine did not produce any significant histochemical change, whereas profound brain cell death was observed in the frontal cortex among subjects that were under the effect of ketamine for 9 or 24 hours. In cell culture study of Bosnjak et al. [25], they demonstrated that ketamine decreases neuronal viability time and dose dependently, leads to neuronal ultrastructural abnormalities, causes depolarization of mitochondrial membrane potential, induces apoptotic pathway, causes cytochrome c release from mitochondria into cytosol, and induces free oxygen radical production.

Yu et al. examined neuroapoptosis and long-term behavioral changes in PND7 rats that were given single and repetitive doses of propofol. Their findings included reduction in neuron density, morphological changes in pyramidal cells, apoptosis, and suppressed release of excitatory neurotransmitters. Additionally, these effects were more pronounced among the group that was subject to repeated doses of propofol [26].

Benzodiazepines (clonazepam, diazepam, and midazolam), which are intravenous anesthetics, have controversial effects on apoptosis; however, barbiturates (pentobarbital, phenobarbital) clearly increase apoptosis. The few studies that have examined the effects of sodium thiopental reported that exposure did not result in increased apoptosis [27–33]. Thompson [34] has suggested high-dose narcotic anesthetic for neonatal and infant. But, fetal and neonatal chronic exposure to opioids has been associated with neuronal changes. Although opioid-based anesthesia and opioids coadministered with inhalation anesthetics have been shown to reduce apoptosis, safety has not been demonstrated with these preparations [35, 36]. However, these studies are controversial and their safety has been in question. Another study has demonstrated that dexmedetomidine, the current intravenous anesthetic, reduces prenatal toxicity caused by propofol [37].

5. Pathogenesis

The molecular pathogenesis of anesthesia-induced neurotoxicity has also been investigated in experimental studies.

Neonates are born with approximately 100 billion neurons, and the number of neurons does not increase over time. The neonatal brains weigh approximately 300–400 g. Increased myelination, synapse formation, neuron maturation, and proliferation of glial cells increase the weight of the brain to 1100 g at 3 years of age and 1300–1400 g at adulthood. A newborn infant has approximately 50 trillion synapses, increasing to 1000 trillion within the first year of life and decreasing to 500 trillion in adulthood. Critical periods for brain development are the intrauterine period, the first 3 years of life and puberty [38–40].

Thus, brain maturation is not complete at birth, and there is a heterogeneous maturation process in the brain following birth. Maturation is particularly slow in the cortex and in the limbic system [38–40]. Alteration of neurotransmission in the immature brain due to anesthesia exposure may lead to future impairments.

Synaptogenesis has been defined as the most important period of brain development, also described as the "fragile period" or "critical period." Synaptogenesis consists of five phases. The greatest leap in synapse formation occurs in phase 3, which is sometimes referred to as the "big bang." Phase 3 corresponds to the neonatal period. Following phase 3, synaptogenesis continues with the same speed during phase 4. This phase is referred to as the plateau phase, corresponding to infancy and adolescence. During phase 5, which occurs during adulthood, synaptogenesis continues, but it is limited and localized [41]. The initiation, duration, and end of these critical periods (phase 3 and phase 4) are controlled by multiple genetic and epigenetic mechanisms. The brain's sensitivity to environmental stimuli is at maximum during the neonatal and infancy period when synaptogenesis is also maximized [41].

Anesthetics elicit their effects by enhancing the activity of major inhibitory neurotransmitters gamma-aminobutyric acid (GABA) and glycine or antagonizing the N-methyl-D-aspartate (NMDA) receptors of the major excitatory neurotransmitter glutamate. During brain development, GABA facilitates cell proliferation, neuroblast migration, and dendritic maturation, and unlike in adults, it acts as an excitatory neurotransmitter during infancy rather than an inhibitory neurotransmitter [42, 43]. This is because these two mediators increase the permeability of the cell membrane to chloride ions through intrinsic chloride-conducting ion pores. After the permeability of the GABA, ligand-gated ion channel to chloride is increased, KCC2 K+/Cl-2 cotransporter aids in influx of chloride ion. Thus, the neuron is hyperpolarized and its activity is suppressed. However, because KCC2 expression is low during the early period of development, the chloride action potential is reversed by $GABA_A$ and glycine receptor activity, leading to neuronal depolarization and increased permeability to chloride. Clinical studies have shown that sevoflurane, isoflurane, and propofol cause excitability in electroencephalogram in neonates [44–46]. The major excitatory neurotransmitters glutamate and aspartate are present in the brain at very high concentrations (glutamate 10 mmol/L and aspartate 4 mmol/L). Glutamate and aspartate direct synaptic signaling at nerve terminals and control ion intake to neurons. They have been found to influence synaptogenesis, neuronal plasticity, learning, and memory [47–49]. Although the excitatory neurotransmitters are normally responsible for nerve conduction, they are also potential sources of neurotoxicity. An abnormal decrease in glutamate may disturb normal excitation, and abnormal increases may cause excitotoxicity and cell death by disturbing calcium homeostasis. Glutamate and similar amino acids have been shown to cause acute swelling in the neuron body, dendrites, and glia and also promote neuronal degeneration over extended periods of time. For this reason, there is a delicate mechanism acting in normal conditions to regulate glutamate levels in the synaptic gap involving reuptake of excess glutamate from the synaptic gap through receptors present in presynaptic end of nerve terminal and glial cells. Although glutamate is a strong and rapid-acting toxin under physiological conditions, this mechanism ensures that even direct application to the brain does not cause damage [47]. Nevertheless, pathological conditions that result in insufficiency of this system or cause release of large amounts of glutamate would lead to neuronal loss. For these reasons, anesthesia applications are believed to disrupt the balance between excitatory and inhibitory neurotransmission and thus cause neuronal injury [47–49].

Regarding neuronal viability and development, one of the most studied neurotropins in neonatal subjects is brain-derived neurotrophic factor (BDNF). Mature BDNF is formed by destruction of proBDNF in the synaptic gap by the action of plasmin. Mature BDNF binds to the TrkB receptors present on the postsynaptic membrane and enhances viability of the target cell. However, in conditions where plasmin release is reduced or blocked, such as when anesthesia is applied, proBDNF cannot be converted to the mature form, and it stimulates p75NTR instead of the TrkB receptor. Activation of p75NTR receptor, also called the "death receptor," leads to actin depolymerization and apoptosis. Head et al. [50] demonstrated that isoflurane causes apoptosis in the neonatal mice brain through this pathway.

Apoptosis is a programmed cell death that can occur in both physiological and pathological conditions. Apoptosis is physiologically present in the developing brain, occurring at a rate of approximately 1%. However, apoptosis that occurs following pathological processes like hypoxia and ischemia is typically problematic. Several experimental studies have shown that apoptosis is increased following anesthesia exposure. However, it is not possible to conduct such studies in humans. Therefore, it is difficult to estimate the rate of apoptosis following anesthesia exposure in humans to what extent this apoptosis affects maturation of the developing brain. Experimental studies have shown that anesthesia induces apoptosis via intrinsic and extrinsic pathways. Anesthesia application causes leakage of cytochrome c and translocation of Bax protein to the mitochondria, leading to activation of the apaf-1 and caspase pathways, respectively. This in turn results in lipid peroxidation via release of free oxygen radicals. Apoptosis occurs not only in intrinsic pathway but also in extrinsic pathway which activates Fas protein [51–53].

There are three publications that demonstrate the relationship between microRNA and anesthetic-induced developmental neurotoxicity; according to these publications, while propofol downregulates microRNA-21, ketamine upregulates microRNA-34a, microRNA-34c, and microRNA-124 and downregulates microRNA-137 [54–56].

In cell culture models, it has been demonstrated that neuron development is highly dependent on the actin cytoskeleton, and anesthetics are dangerous for actin regulation [57–59].

Tau protein hyperphosphorylation at serine 404 demonstrates neurodegeneration and is induced by ketamine. Therefore, microtubules are disrupted and damaged [60].

Translocator protein (TSPO, 18 kDa) is a biomarker that could be used for evaluation of reactive gliosis and microglia activity and has the potential for use in noninvasive imaging using positron emission tomography and single photon emission computed tomography [61]. The relationship between anesthesia-associated neurotoxicity and DNA methylation and gene expression has been investigated [62].

Treatment strategies to reduce neurodegeneration induced by anesthetics have also been widely investigated. Lithium, melatonin, estradiol, pilocarpine, dexmedetomidine, xenon, erythropoietin, L-carnitine, hydrogen gas, and pramipexole are among the leading candidates for this emerging therapy [63, 64].

6. Clinical studies

Although many experimental studies have been conducted, this alone is not sufficient evidence to conclude that general anesthetics have a neurotoxic effect on the developing human brain. Even within mammals, species vary widely in the rate and timing of brain development. Total maturation of the brain takes only a few weeks in the rat, while maturation of the human brain occurs over many years. In addition, the dose and duration of anesthetics used in experimental models is not directly proportional to the procedures used in patients. In some cases, experimental doses may be as much as 20 times the standard clinical dose. Adjusted for the life span of a rat, 6 hours of anesthesia may correspond to 1 month of a human life span. Again, some observations from these studies, such as lactic acidosis, hypercarbia, and hypoglycemia, have mostly been ignored. Learning ability is also disturbed in subjects that are fasted for the duration of the anesthesia treatment [43, 65, 66].

In one retrospective birth cohort study that used New York State Medicaid data collected between the years 1999 and 2002, 383 children who underwent inguinal hernia repair with anesthesia before the age of 3 were evaluated along with 5050 children who did not undergo an operation. Hazard ratios regarding behavioral and developmental disorders were reported to be 2.3 with exposure to anesthesia, 1.0 for age, 2.7 for gender, 1.2 for race, and 1.6 for birth complications [6]. Considering that elective surgeries can be postponed, exposure to anesthesia is an avoidable risk for most infants.

In another report, patients that had been overexposed to anesthesia had more learning difficulties than those who were treated with appropriate doses. The risk of learning difficulties was progressively increased with repeated exposure to anesthesia [67, 68]. The effects of anesthesia used during cesarean procedures were examined in children. Infants born under regional anesthesia exhibited fewer learning difficulties in the later stages of their life [69, 70].

One retrospective study examined 10,450 siblings born between the years 1999 and 2005 and evaluated developmental and behavioral disorders among those who did and did not receive anesthesia prior to the age of 3. The incidence of developmental and behavioral disorder was 128.2/1000/year among those who were exposed to anesthesia and 56.3/1000/year among those who were not exposed to anesthesia. Therefore, behavioral disorders were 60% more frequent among those who received anesthesia in comparison to those who did not. The estimated hazard ratio for developmental and behavioral disorders was 1:1 for those who received anesthesia once before the age of 3, 2:9 for those exposed twice, and 4 for those who had been exposed to anesthesia three or more times [71].

Meyer et al. observed development of convulsion with similar clinical characteristics in three infants under the age of 2 months, occurring after 23–30 hours of anesthesia induced and maintained using propofol. They reported that the seizures did not recur; however, two infants had progressive microcephaly and cognitive and behavioral disorder. Magnetic resonance imaging also showed white matter abnormalities [72]. The manufacturer of propofol does not recommend the use of propofol as a general anesthetic agent for children under the age of 3 [73].

Clinical studies in the literature are often retrospective, and even strong correlations are not evidence of causality. Therefore, the Mayo Anesthesia Safety in Kids (MASK) study was launched by Mayo Clinic at the suggestion of the FDA to evaluate neurotoxicity in children exposed to anesthesia. The study included children born in Olmsted County between 1997 and 2007 and who still lived there when they reached 8 years old. Those who received general anesthesia before the age of 3 were excluded from the study. Children classified as having single, multiple, or no anesthesia exposure were evaluated between the years 2007 and 2016, when they were at the age of 8–12 or 15–19 with a single session that lasted for 4 hours using the National Center for Toxicological Research-Operant Test Battery (NCTR-OTB). The NCTR-OTB test evaluates processing speed; cognitive/intellectual memory; attention, language, motor and visual-spatial, and cognitive processing; and executive functions [74].

The Pediatric Anesthesia and Neurodevelopmental Assessment (PANDA), which was conducted by the University of Columbia and followed sibling pairs under the age of 3 who underwent inguinal operation up to the age of 8–15, published four symposiums in 2-year interval. The first meeting in 2008 established the goals of the study. The second meeting in 2010 was interdisciplinary. The third meeting in 2012 was attended by different disciplines, parents, clinicians, FDA workers, and patient's rights advocates. In this meeting, attendees agreed to collaborate on advanced preclinical, clinical, and translational studies [75, 76]. Additionally in 2012, pediatric anesthesiologists and pediatric surgeons met to discuss the neurotoxicity risk of some elective procedures and anesthesia applications performed in children and specifically to discuss questions and concerns of parents. Meeting attendees, including pediatric general surgeons, urologists, plastic surgeons, and ophthalmologists, reviewed inguinal hernia, hypospadias-undescended testis, cleft lip, craniosynostosis, cataracts, and strabismus applications in early childhood. They emphasized that the amount of volatile anesthetics and sedation levels could be reduced by using balanced anesthesia methods, regional anesthesia methods, and the use of opioid and non-opioid analgesics, but the group was unable to reach a consensus on best practices [77]. At the 2014 meeting, the existing clinical studies, General Anesthesia Study (GAS), MASK, and PANDA, were evaluated, and Strategies for Mitigating Anesthesia-Related neuroToxicity in Tots (SmartTots) was presented along with the future targets of this organization. SmartTots is a public-private partnership that investigates the effects of anesthetic agents on neural development in infants and children. All panelists evaluated their anesthesia and clinical practices with the following questions [78, 79]:

- What does anesthesia mean to my patients?
- What does anesthesia mean to my practice now?

Ordering imaging studies with sedation/anesthesia.

A child requiring multiple procedures under GA overtime.

A child requiring multiple procedures from different subspecialties at the same time.

- If anesthesia affects neurodevelopment:

How will I discuss this with the parents?

Will I change my practice and how?

The 2014 report indicated that the collected data was insufficient to draw any conclusions. However, it stated 2 years later that the results would be considered as a public health problem, leading to greater awareness [78]. On the other hand, the General Anesthesia Study

(GAS), which is currently ongoing and only investigates causality, investigated cases that were less than 60 weeks from conception and greater than 26 weeks gestational age and had undergone inguinal hernia operations with sevoflurane-based general anesthesia or awake-regional anesthesia. This study was conducted in 28 hospitals from Australia, Italy, the USA, the UK, and Canada. No opioids or nitrous oxide was used. Regional techniques and intravenous acetaminophen were used for postoperative analgesia. Protocols were applied in order to prevent development of adverse states that would contribute in neurotoxicity, such as hypoglycemia, hypotension, and hypoxia. Children were assessed using the composite cognitive score of the Bayley Scales of Infant and Toddler Development III test at the age of 2 and with the Wechsler Preschool and Primary Scale of Intelligence Third Edition (WPPSI-III) Full Scale Intelligence Quotient score at the age of 5. During 2007–2013, 363 infants were enrolled in the awake-regional group, and 359 infants were enrolled in the general anesthesia group. According to the study results, the median general anesthesia duration was 54 minutes. No significant difference was found between the groups regarding cognitive composite score at 2 years of age. This study provides strong evidence that sevoflurane anesthesia lasting <1 hour in infants does not produce more severe neurotoxicity at the second year of age than awake-regional treatment. Nonetheless, the primary outcome of this study is the evaluation of neurodevelopmental state at 5 years of age, and this result has not been published yet. It was also reported in this study that early-period apnea development (<30 minutes) was less frequent in the regional anesthesia group [80].

Other discussed topics are applied anesthesia techniques to mothers during childbirth. Flick et al. determined that neuraxial labor analgesia for vaginal delivery did not cause learning disabilities in childhood [69, 70].

Another topic of discussion was how parents should be informed and the need to establish a protocol. However, since it was not possible to reach a consensus based on the current data, it was concluded that it would not be appropriate to inform parents and establish a protocol yet [81].

Author details

Ayse B. Ozer* and Sibel Ozcan

*Address all correspondence to: abelinozer@gmail.com

Faculty of Medicine, Department of Anesthesiology Intensive Care, Firat University, Elazig, Turkey

References

[1] Cohen MM, Cameron CB, Duncan PG: Pediatric anesthesia morbidity and mortality in the perioperative period. Anesth Analg 1990; **70**:160–167.

[2] Holzman RS:. Morbidity and mortality in pediatric anesthesia. Pediatr Clin North Am. 1994;**41**:239–256.

[3] Flick RP, Warner DO: a users' guide to interpreting observational studies of pediatric anesthetic neurotoxicity. The lessons of sir Bradford Hill. Anesthesiology 2012; **117**:459–462

[4] Shen X, Liu Y, Xu S, Zhao Q, Guo X, Shen R, Wang F: Early life exposure to sevoflurane impairs adulthood spatial memory in the rat. NeuroToxicology 2013;**39**:45–56

[5] Zou X, Patterson TA, Divine RL, Sadovova N, Zhang X, Hanig JP, et al: Prolonged exposure to ketamine increases neurodegeneration in the developing monkey brain. Int J Dev Neurosci 2009;**27**:727–731

[6] DiMaggio, Sun LS, Kakavouli A, Byrne MW, Li G: A retrospective cohort study of the association of anesthesia and hernia repair surgery with behavioral and developmental disorders in young children. J Neurosurg Anesthesiol 2009;**21**:286–291

[7] Sanders RD, Ma D, Brooks P, Maze M: Balancing paediatric anaesthesia: preclinical insights into analgesia, hypnosis, neuroprotection, and neurotoxicity. Br J Anaesth 2008;**101**:597–609.

[8] Hays SR, Deshpande JK. Neurotoxicity of anesthesia on developing brain. In: Baheti DK, Dhayagude SH, Deshpande JK, Menon R, editors. World clinics, anesthesia, critical care, pain, pediatric anesthesia-II. 2nd ed. New Delhi: Jaypee Brothers Medical Publishers Ltd;. 2015. p. 117–143

[9] Tawfeeq NA, Halawani MM, Al-Faridi K, Aal-Shaya WA, Taha WS: Traumatic brain injury: neuroprotective anaesthetic techniques, an update. Injury 2009;**40**:S75–S81.

[10] Burchell SR, Dixon BJ, Tang J, Zhang JH: Isoflurane provides neuroprotection in neonatal hypoxic ischemic brain injury. J Investig Med. 2013;**61**:1078–1083.

[11] Stocchetti N, Taccone FS, Citerio G, Pepe PE, Le Roux PD, Oddo M, et al: Neuroprotection in acute brain injury: an up-to-date review. Crit Care 2015;**19**:186.

[12] Kays JL, Hurley RA, Taber KH: The dynamic brain: neuroplasticity and mental health. J Neuropsychiatry Clin Neurosci. 2012;**24**:118–124.

[13] Zheng Z, Xu F: Neuroplasticity may play a role in inter-individual difference among neuropsychiatric disease treatment efficacy. Dev Psychobiol. 2012;**54**:369–371.

[14] Cramer SC, Sur M, Dobkin BH, O'Brien C, Sanger TD, Trojanowski JQ, et al: Harnessing neuroplasticity for clinical applications. Brain. 2011;**134**:1591–1609.

[15] Soriano SG, Anand KJ: Anesthetics and brain toxicity. Curr Opin Anaesthesiol 2005;**18**:293–297.

[16] Taylor J: Anaesthesia-induced developmental neurotoxicity. South Afr J Anaesth Analg 2012;**18**:242–247.

[17] Davidson AJ: Anesthesia and neurotoxicity to the developing brain: the clinical relevance. Pediatr Anesth 2011;**21**:716–721

[18] Wise-Faberowski L, Loepke A: Anesthesia during surgical repair for congenital heart disease and the developing brain: neurotoxic or neuroprotective? Pediatr Anesth 2011;**21**:554–559

[19] Wang SQ, Fang F, Xue ZG, Cang J, Zhang XG: Neonatal sevoflurane anesthesia induces long-term memory impairment and decreases hippocampal PSD-95 expression without neuronal loss. Eur Rev Med Pharmacol Sci 2013;**17**:941–950

[20] Liang G, Ward C, Peng J, Zhao Y, Huang B, Wei H: Isoflurane causes greater neurodegeneration than an equivalent exposure of sevoflurane in the developing brain of neonatal mice. Anesthesiology. 2010;**112**:1325–1334

[21] Istaphanous GK, Howard J, Nan X, Hughes EA, McCann JC, McAuliffe JJ, et al: Comparison of the neuroapoptotic properties of equipotent anesthetic concentrations of desflurane, isoflurane, or sevoflurane in neonatal mice. Anesthesiology. 2011;**114**:578–587

[22] Chalon J, Tang CK, Ramanathan S, Eisner M, Katz R, Turndorf H. Exposure to halothane and enflurane affects learning function of murine progeny. Anesth Analg 1981;**60**:794–797

[23] Quimby KL, Aschkenase LJ, Bowman RE, Katz J, Chang LW: Enduring learning deficits and cerebral synaptic malformation from exposure to 10 parts of halothane per million. Science 1974;**185**:625–627

[24] Cattano D, Williamson P, Fukui K, Avidan M, Evers AS, Olney JW, et al: Potential of xenon to induce or to protect against neuroapoptosis in the developing Mouse brain. Can J Anaesth 2008;**55**:429–436.

[25] Bosnjak ZJ, Yan Y, Canfield S, Muravyeva MY, Kikuchi C, Wells CW, et al: Ketamine induces toxicity in human neurons differentiated from embryonic stem cells via mitochondrial apoptosis pathway. Curr Drug Saf. 2012;7:106–119.

[26] Yu D, Jiang Y, Gao J, Liu B, Chen P: Repeated exposure to propofol potentiates neuroapoptosis and long-term behavioral deficits in neonatal rats. Neurosci Lett. 2013;**534**:41–46.

[27] Ikonomidou C, Bittigau P, Ishimaru MJ, Wozniak DF, Koch C, Genz K, et al:. Ethanol-induced apoptotic neurodegeneration and fetal alcohol syndrome. Science 2000;**287**:1056–1060.

[28] Bittigau P, Sifringer M, Genz K, Reith E, Pospischil D, Govindarajalu S, et al: Antiepileptic drugs and apoptotic neurodegeneration in the developing brain. Proc Natl Acad Sci U S A 2002;**99**:15089–15094.

[29] Stefovska VG, Uckermann O, Czuczwar M, Smitka M, Czuczwar P, Kis J, et al: Sedative and anticonvulsant drugs suppress postnatal neurogenesis. Ann Neurol 2008;**64**:434–445.

[30] Young C, Jevtovic-Todorovic V, Qin YQ, Tenkova T, Wang H, Labruyere J, et al: Potential of ketamine and midazolam, individually or in combination, to induce apoptotic neurodegeneration in the infant mouse brain. Br J Pharmacol 2005;**146**:189–197.

[31] Jevtovic-Todorovic V, Hartman RE, Izumi Y, Benshoff ND, Dikranian K, Zorumski CF, et al: Early exposure to common anesthetic agents causes widespread neurodegeneration in the developing rat brain and persistent learning deficits. J Neurosci 2003;**23**:876–882.

[32] Mintz CD, Barrett KM, Smith SC, Benson DL, Harrison NL: Anesthetics interfere with axon guidance in developing mouse neocortical neurons in vitro via a gamma-aminobutyric acid type a receptor mechanism. Anesthesiology 2013;**118**:825–833.

[33] Fredriksson A, Ponten E, Gordh T, Eriksson P: Neonatal exposure to a combination of N-methyl-D- aspartate and gamma-aminobutyric acid type a receptor anesthetic agents potentiates apoptotic neurodegeneration and persistent behavioral deficits. Anesthesiology 2007;**107**:427–436.

[34] Thompson ME: Preventing neurotoxicity: don't forget high-dose narcotic anesthetic. Pediatr Anesth 2014;**24**:1109–1114

[35] Niu L, Cao B, Zhu H, Mei B, Wang M, Yang Y, et al: Impaired in vivo synaptic plasticity in dentate gyrus and spatial memory in juvenile rats induced by prenatal morphine exposure. Hippocampus. 2009;**19**:649–657

[36] De Graaf J, van Lingen RA, Valkenburg AJ, Weisglas-Kuperus N, Groot Jebbink L, Wijnberg-Williams B, et al: Does neonatal morphine use affect neuropsychological outcomes at 8 to 9 years of age? Pain. 2013;**154**:449–458.

[37] Li J, Xiong M, Nadavaluru PR, Zuo W, Ye JH, Eloy JD, et al: Dexmedetomidine attenuates neurotoxicity induced by prenatal propofol exposure. J Neurosurg Anesthesiol. 2016;**28**:51–64.

[38] Graham J. Forstadt LA. Bulletin#4356, Children and brain development: what we know about how children learn. Available from: https://extension.umaine.edu/publications/4356e/

[39] Stages of brain development. Available from: http://www.brainwave.org.nz/wp-content/uploads/2012/05/stages-in-brain-dev.pdf

[40] Early childhood brain development sets the stage for learning throughout life, experts say. Available from: http://www.cleveland.com/healthfit/index.ssf/2015/10/brain_development_is_an_intricate_choreographed_dance_with_many_opportunities_for_missteps_photos.html.

[41] Bourgeois JP. Neonatal synaptic big bang. In: Lagercrantz H, Hanson MA, Ment LR, Donald MP, editors. The newborn brain: neuroscience and clinical applications. 2nd ed. NewYork: Cambridge University Press; 2010. p. 71–85

[42] de Lima AD, Opitz T, Voigt T: Irreversible loss of a subpopulation of cortical interneurons in the absence of glutamatergic network activity. Eur J Neurosci 2004; **19**:2931–2943.

[43] Yu D, Liu B: Developmental anesthetic neurotoxicity: from animals to humans? J Anesth 2013;**27**:750–756

[44] Veyckemans F: Excitation phenomena during sevoflurane anesthesia in children. Curr Opin Anesthesiol 2001;**14**:339–343

[45] Harrison JL: Postoperative seizures after isoflurane anesthesia. Anesth Analg 1986;**65**:1235–1236

[46] Zeiler SR, Kaplan PW: Propofol withdrawal seizures (or not). Seizure 2008;**17**:665–667.

[47] Beal MF: Does impairment of energy metabolism result in excitotoxic neuronal death in neurodegenerative illnesses. Ann Neurol 1992;**31**:119–130

[48] Choi DW: Calcium-mediated neurotoxicity: relationship to specific channel types and role in ischemic damage Trends Neurosci. 1988;**11**:465–469

[49] Choi DW: Glutamate neurotoxicity and diseases of the nervous system. Neuron 1988;**1**:623–634

[50] Head BP, Patel HH, Niesman IR, Drummond JC, Roth DM, Patel PM: Inhibition of p75 neurotrophin receptor attenuates isoflurane-mediated neuronal apoptosis in the neonatal central nervous system. Anesthesiology 2009;**110**:813–825

[51] Elmore S: Apoptosis: a review of programmed cell death. Toxicol Pathol 2007;**35**: 495–516

[52] Hays SR, Deshpande JK: Newly postulated neurodevelopmental risks of pediatric anesthesia: theories that could rock our world. J Urol 2013;**189**:1222–1228

[53] Reddy SV: Effect of general anesthetics on the developing brain. J Anaesthesiol Clin Pharmacol. 2012;**28**:6–10.

[54] Twaroski D, Bosnjak ZJ, Bai X. MicroRNAs: new players in anesthetic-induced developmental neurotoxicity. Pharm Anal Acta. 2015;**6**:357.

[55] Twaroski DM, Yan Y, Olson JM, Bosnjak ZJ, Bai X: Down-regulation of microRNA-21 is involved in the propofol-induced neurotoxicity observed in human stem cell-derived neurons. Anesthesiology 2014;**121**:786–800.

[56] Huang C, Zhang X, Zheng J, Chen C, Chen Y, Yi J: Upregulation of miR-137 protects anesthesia-induced hippocampal neurodegeneration. Int J Clin Exp Pathol 2014;**7**:5000–5007.

[57] Mintz CD, Wagner M, Loepke AW: Preclinical research into the effects of anesthetics on the developing brain: promises and pitfalls. J Neurosurg Anesthesiol. 2012;**24**:362–367.

[58] Luo L: Actin cytoskeleton regulation in neuronal morphogenesis and structural plasticity. Annu Rev Cell Dev Biol. 2002;**18**:601–635

[59] Jevtovic-Todorovic V: Anesthesia and the developing brain: are we getting closer to understanding the truth? Curr Opin Anaesthesiol. 2011;**24**:395–399

[60] Jin H, Hu Z, Dong M, Wu Y, Zhu Z, Xu L: Ketamine induces tau hyperphosphorylation at serine 404 in the hippocampus of neonatal rats. Neural Regen Res. 2013;**8**:1590–1596.

[61] Guilarte TR, Chen MK: Translocator protein 18 kDa (TSPO): molecular sensor of brain injury and repair. Pharmacol Ther 2008;**118**:1–17.

[62] Perera F, Herbstman J: Prenatal environmental exposures, epigenetics and disease. Reprod Toxicol. 2011;**31**:363–373.

[63] Olsen EA, Brambrink AM: Anesthesia for the young child undergoing ambulatory procedures: current concerns regarding harm to the developing brain. Curr Opin Anesthesiol 2013;**26**:677–684

[64] Pellegrini L, Bennis Y, Velly L, Grandvuillemin I, Pisano P, Bruder N, et al: Erythropoietin protects newborn rat against sevoflurane-induced neurotoxicity. Paediatr Anaesth. 2014;**24**:749–759.

[65] Vutskits L, Davis PJ, Hansen TG: Anesthetics and the developing brain: time for a change in practice? A pro/con debate. Pediatr Anesth 2012;**22**:973–980

[66] Sander RD, Davidson A: Anesthetic-induced neurotoxicity of the neonate: time for clinical guidelines? Pediatr Anesth 2009;**19**:1141–1146

[67] Flick RP, Katusic SK, Colligan RC, Wilder RT, Voigt RG, Olson MD, et al: Cognitive and behavioral outcomes after early exposure to anesthesia and surgery. Pediatrics. 2011;**128**:e1053–e1061.

[68] Sprung J, Flick RP, Katusic SK, Colligan RC, Barbaresi WJ, Bojanić K, et al: Attention-deficit/hyperactivity disorder after early exposure to procedures requiring general anesthesia. Mayo Clin Proc. 2012;**87**:120–129.

[69] Flick RP, Lee K, Hofer RE, Beinborn CW, Hambel EM, Klein MK, et al: Neuraxial labor analgesia for vaginal delivery and its effects on childhood learning disabilities. Anesth Analg. 2011;**112**:1424–1431

[70] Sprung J, Flick RP, Wilder RT, Katusic SK, Pike TL, Dingli M, et al: Anesthesia for cesarean delivery and learning disabilities in a population-based birth cohort. Anesthesiology. 2009;**111**:302–310.

[71] DiMaggio C, Sun LS, Li G: Early childhood exposure to anesthesia and risk of developmental and behavioral disorders in a sibling birth cohort. Anesth Analg. 2011;**113**:1143–1151

[72] Meyer P, Langlois C, Soëte S, Leydet J, Echenne B, Rivier F, et al: Unexpected neurological sequelae following propofol anesthesia in infants: three case reports. Brain Dev 2010;**32**:872–878

[73] Fresofol product information. Available from: http://www.fresenius-kabi.com.au/files/Fresofol_PI.pdf

[74] Gleich SJ, Flick R, Hu D, Zaccariello MJ, Colligan RC, Katusic SK, et al: Neurodevelopment of children exposed to anesthesia: design of the mayo anesthesia safety in kids (MASK) study. Contemp Clin Trials 2015;**41**:45–54

[75] Sun LS, Li G, DiMaggio CJ, Byrne MW, Ing C, Miller TL, et al: Feasibility and pilot study of the pediatric anesthesia neurodevelopment assessment (PANDA) project. J Neurosurg Anesthesiol. 2012;**24**:382–388.

[76] Miller TL, Park R, Sun LS: Report of the third PANDA symposium on "Anesthesia and Neurodevelopment in Children". J Neurosurg Anesthesiol. 2012;**24**:357–361

[77] Byrne MW, Ascherman JA, Casale P, Cowles RA, Gallin PF, Maxwell LG: Elective procedures and anesthesia in children: pediatric surgeons enter the dialogue on neurotoxicity questions, surgical options, and parental concerns. J Neurosurg Anesthesiol. 2012;**24**:396–400.

[78] Miller TL, Park R, Sun LS: Report of the fourth PANDA symposium on "anesthesia and neurodevelopment in children". J Neurosurg Anesthesiol. 2014;**26**:344–348.

[79] Jevtovic-Todorovic V: Pediatric anesthesia neurotoxicity: an overview of the 2011 SmartTots panel. Anesth Analg 2011;**113**:965–968

[80] Davidson AJ, Disma N, de Graaff JC, Withington DE, Dorris L, Bell G, et al: Neurodevelopmental outcome at 2 years of age after general anaesthesia and awake-regional anaesthesia in infancy (GAS): an international multicentre, randomised controlled trial. Lancet. 2016;**387**:239–250

[81] Nemergut ME, Aganga D, Flick RP: Anesthetic neurotoxicity: what to tell the parents? Pediatr Anesth 2014;**24**:120–126

8

Medulloblastoma

Asifur Rahman

Abstract

Among the pediatric brain tumors, medulloblastoma (MB) is the most common solid variety and entirely occur in the posterior fossa with tendency to seed into CSF spaces. Despite innovations in technological developments and understanding of tumor biology, modern imaging facilities, advances in surgical practices, and newer chemotherapeutic and radiation techniques, this malignant type of tumor continues to be a formidable entity. Even though, the outcome in terms of survival rate is better than any time before, the overall result is still disappointing. With advances in management strategy, chances of survival with good quality of life have been amplified, where newer targeted therapies and rehabilitation plays an immense role. While the adverse effects of surgery and adjuvant therapies are still on play, researchers are trying ceaselessly to minimize those to give maximum wellbeing to these unfortunate children.

Keywords: medulloblastoma, surgery, radiotherapy, chemotherapy, molecular subgroup

1. Introduction

Medulloblastomas are a group of highly undifferentiated, rapidly growing, extremely malignant formidable solid tumor of childhood with worst estimated prognosis. Maximal safe resection, craniospinal irradiation (CSI) and chemotherapy remain the mainstays of first-line treatment of these aggressive embryonal tumors which are the most frequent primary malignant brain cancer in children.

The name "medulloblastoma" was first adapted by Harvey Cushing in 1930. Initially these tumors were termed as spongioblastoma indifferentiale, spongioblastoma multiforme, spongioblastoma cerebelli or simply spongioblastoma by different authors. Cushing presumed this subset of tumors to be originating from one of the five pluripotent stem cells, the medulloblast, thought to populate the primitive neural tube [1–5]. It has meanwhile been established that the concept of embryonal cell identified as medulloblast does not exist [6, 7]. Hence the term medulloblastoma that Cushing erroneously coined, which is so strongly concreted to the nomenclature, is actually a misnomer [7].

Medulloblastomas were considered as one of the most disappointing maladies in neurosurgery until the 1960s as survival was still equally poor as was in the early periods of neurosurgery when posterior fossa tumors were most daunting. Overall, improved diagnostic, surgical, and radiation technologies, newer and more effective chemotherapy regimens have led to dramatically improved patient outcomes with advanced research [8]. Multidisciplinary approach being the keystone of success for this formidable disease, significant clinical challenge still remains because of acute onset, rapid growth, rapid clinical course and early fatal termination leading to great number of morbidity and mortality despite aggressive therapeutic strategies [2, 3, 9, 10].

Survival of medulloblastoma patients have become better over the last few decades nonetheless in patients with relapse, the outcome is still miserable. Long-term survival rates have progressively improved from 22% by 1950s to 85% in 2015 with current approaches [11–14]. This significant development has resulted from combination of systemic chemotherapy and improvement in supportive care measures in addition to the regular treatment with surgery and radiotherapy [15–19]. Advances in genetic profiling with emergence of newer agents and development of newer strategies targeting the key molecular alterations have improved the outcomes further [20]. Efforts to improve survival results, dose reduction or elimination of radiation or trial with less offensive chemotherapeutic agents are going on to standardize the treatment of medulloblastoma.

2. Epidemiology

2.1. Incidence

Generally it is recognized that medulloblastoma is the most common malignant brain tumor in children. However, recent data shows that as a group, high-grade gliomas are marginally more prevalent. Approximately 350 new pediatric cases of medulloblastoma are diagnosed in the United States every year and that represents about 30% of pediatric brain tumors and 7–10% of all brain tumors [2, 6, 8, 9, 21–23].

2.2. Age

There are characteristic bimodal peaks, having a higher incidence in children between 3 and 4 years of age and between 8 and 10 years of age. About 70% of childhood medulloblastomas occur in this age range of the first decade. However, medulloblastoma has been reported in a 2-week-old infant and a 55-year-old adult [6, 9]. About 1–3% of cases are reported in adults, mostly before the age of 40 years [8, 24, 25].

2.3. Sex

Curiously enough, Cushing found medulloblastomas to be three times more common in males than females and since then most published reports indicate a continuing male predominance. On an average the male to female ratio is 2:1 [2, 8, 9].

2.4. Location

The typical medulloblastoma develops in the midline of the posterior fossa [9, 25]. Some 70–80% of medulloblastomas have been found in the midcerebellum with or without extension into the lateral cerebellar hemispheres. Medulloblastomas typically arise from the medullary velum and fill the cavity of the fourth ventricle and has the propensity to spread throughout the brain and spine via the cerebrospinal fluid (CSF) and about one third of the cases infiltrate the dorsal brainstem [8, 26].

3. Etiology

The etiologies of medulloblastoma are still obscure for most patients. Though Parental pesticide use and parental occupational contact with hydrocarbons, exposure to N-nitroso compounds and metals have been associated with higher incidence in some studies [25].

For development of medulloblastoma, the most ventured postulation in the earlier literatures was cell misplacements during early embryonic development where genetic factors play vital role [9]. This has been proven true with time with the advancement of genetic studies. Association between several familial cancer syndromes in children with medulloblastomas like TP53 germline mutation syndromes, Gorlin syndrome, and Turcot syndrome also supports predisposition of hereditary factors [8].

Studies have identified Human Cytomegalovirus (HCMV) protein pp65 immunoreactivity in medulloblastomas, but the oncogenic role of HCMV is still debated. Yet HCMV is believed to play role as a significant oncomodulator and based on that researchers are on the quest to utilize the potential of HCMV as a novel immunotherapeutic agent [25, 27–29].

4. Pathology

4.1. General

The World Health Organization (WHO) defines medulloblastoma as "a malignant, invasive embryonal tumor of the cerebellum with preferential manifestation in children, predominantly neuronal differentiation and an inherent tendency to metastasize via cerebrospinal (CSF) pathways" [30]. Although it is generally agreed that cerebellar medulloblastoma is an embryonic tumor, its origin is still a matter of speculation [9].

4.2. Macroscopic pathology

Macroscopically these midline globular, soft tumors are fairly well demarcated, and are apparently encapsulated. The marked vascularity gives them a dark, dirty brownish-red hue and occasionally they have extensive areas of necrosis. Consistency may vary from suckable to rubbery or to even firm sometimes. Calcifications are seen occasionally while hemorrhage in medulloblastoma is an extremely rare occurrence. Often marked edema of a wide zone of the neighboring tissue is also seen. They overlie the fourth ventricle as they develop in the midline in the roof of the fourth ventricle to occupy it, but most of the floors of the fourth ventricle in the great majority of cases are typically free. They usually block the aqueduct of Sylvius, with significant dilatation. These have a tendency to invade the meninges. Commonly they grow downward through the foramen magnum from the primary location between the tonsils of the cerebellum [1–3, 9]. CSF dissemination into the subarachnoid spaces often lead to local or widespread leptomeningeal metastases in the spinal axis or over the surface of the cerebral hemispheres or cerebellum and this also may cause characteristic pearly gray sheets of tumor in the meninges. Furthermore, widespread implantation of tumor can be found throughout the ventricles [9, 31].

4.3. Microscopic pathology

Generally medulloblastomas are categorized as small blue-cell tumors, based on presence of their deeply basophilic nuclei [25]. Histologically, these tumors comprise of densely packed rounded or pear-shaped or sometimes spindle-shaped cells having large ovoid nuclei containing plentiful network of chromatin with scanty cytoplasm and for the most part consisting of numerous embryonic glia fibrillae [1, 3, 8]. These are highly cellular tumors forming uniform sheets of cells, interposed with occasional thin-walled blood vessels. Low magnification reveals that the cells appear as a loose structureless mass, but the nuclei sometimes may form pseudo-rosettes or may show a palisade arrangement. Extensive areas of necrosis, numerous hemorrhagic foci and great vascularity often come across too [1, 3, 9]. Thin-walled blood vessels with delicate connective tissue confined to their walls can be demonstrated by special staining with Perdrau's stain [9].

4.4. Electron microscopic examination

The electron microscopic picture is a mosaic of cells, processes, and fibers. The tumor cells are arranged in a tightly packed mass as also seen in light microscopy. Both the glial and neuronal cells can be recognized on electron microscopic analysis [9].

4.5. Immunohistochemistry

Immunohistochemistry can help in diagnosis of medulloblastoma and can provide information augmenting the plan for further management. Mitosis is seen in up to 80% of tumors, as assessed by positive staining with the Ki-67/MIB1 antibody. Medulloblastomas are frequently positive for vimentin and synaptophysin staining [32].

4.6. Genetic aspects

With the advent of genetic profiling and molecular analysis, evolving evidences point to the fact that the different precursor cell populations that form the cerebellum are vulnerable to mutations in signal pathways that regulate their functions; these mutations modify normal development pathways and may result in the development of distinct variants of medulloblastoma [33].

5. Classification

From the very beginning of history of this special type of tumor, these has been tried to be classified in different ways. With the advent and development of molecular biology and incorporation of that with genetic profiling has taken the classification beyond the level of mere histological classification. The molecular subgroupings are helpful in prediction of course of the disease and outcome as well as choosing therapeutic options. Recently the treatment plan is devised in accordance with the classification that integrates both histological and the molecular subgroupings to have the best possible outcome on the basis of a personalized treatment for individual patients.

5.1. Histological classification

Histopathological classification of medulloblastoma has evolved with time. Rubinstein and Northfield [34] initially identified three variants of medulloblastoma: pigmented papillary medulloblastoma, medullomyoblastoma, and desmoplastic medulloblastoma. With newer technologies, newer histological types were being introduced. To alleviate the confusions, the World Health Organization (WHO) in 1976 developed a common classification of brain tumors in an effort to combine the various systems in use till then and the WHO publication "Histological Typing of Tumours of the Central Nervous System" in 1979 outlined and illustrated the new classification system [30, 35, 36]. Since then modifications, additions and characterization of classification of medulloblastoma has evolved a lot throughout the newer classifications of medulloblastoma of the WHO editions of classifications gradually in 1993 [35], 2000 [37, 38] and 2007 [30]. The present histological classification that is in practice has the following types:

1. **Classic medulloblastoma:** Most common histologic subtype (66%). Composed of sheets of densely packed, small to medium-sized, round to oval-shaped, blue cells (basophilic) with a high nuclear to cytoplasmic ratio and high mitotic and apoptotic activity. Reticulin staining shows a lack of nodular desmoplasia.

2. **Large cell/anaplastic medulloblastoma**: Large cell medulloblastomas have monomorphic cells with large, round, prominent nuclei, high mitotic activity, and frequent apoptosis, while the anaplastic medulloblastoma are characterized by hallmarks of anaplasia. Large cell and anaplastic medulloblastomas have a significant degree of cytologic overlap and are differentiated only by the degree of anaplasia.

3. **Desmoplastic/nodular medulloblastoma**: Widespread desmoplasia, characterized by presence of nodular, reticulin-poor "pale islands" of neurocytic differentiation surrounded by densely packed, mitotically active cells having pleomorphic and hyperchromatic nuclei. Reticulin staining highlights internodular desmoplasia.

4. **Medulloblastoma with extensive nodularity (MBEN)**: Similar to nodular type but has an expanded lobular architecture with more prominent reticulin-free zones that are more elongated and rich in neutrophil-like tissue. Reticulin staining highlights internodular desmoplasia. Advanced neurocytic differentiation in islands with strong nuclear NeuN expression is also seen.

Two other histologic types of medulloblastomas are also recognized but are not considered to be distinct variants. They are the Myogenic differentiation type and the Melanotic medulloblastoma. All the histopathological types have significant predictability of prognoses in accordance with the clinico-pathological characteristics of each tumor type as outlined in the WHO classification [6, 8, 30, 34].

5.2. Genetic classification and subgroups

Research in the molecular study has led to understanding of embryonal tumors of the CNS. This reflection has basically been driven by genomic studies characterizing prevalent genetic profiles and biological features. These have led to tumor reclassification, sub-typing and detection of novel entities [10, 39, 40]. Over the last two decades, individual molecular subgroups have been identified for medulloblastoma based on cytogenetic profiles. Each group is named for the cellular pathway activation or genomic alterations it exhibits and each subgroup is associated with distinct prognostic character and survival outcomes [8]. In 2010, in Boston, an international group of medulloblastoma authorities, came to a consensus to categorize medulloblastomas into four distinct subgroups: Wingless (Wnt), Sonic hedgehog (Shh), Group 3, and Group 4 based on their unique set of demographic and clinical features, genetics, gene expression, genome-wide transcriptomic and DNA methylomic profiles [41, 42]. Prediction of outcome and clinical behavior is more precise with the known molecular subgroups than the histopathology or clinical staging. [6, 43–45]. These molecular subgroups are distinct from the histologic subtypes, albeit there are certain areas of considerable overlap (**Figure 1**).

5.2.1. Wingless pathway tumors (Wnt pathway/Wnt-MB)

The Wingless pathway (also termed as the β-catenin pathway) comprises of secreted glycoproteins which are secreted to act through signal transduction to regulate various parts of embryonic development. Uncontrolled activation of Wnt pathway signaling results in accumulation of β-catenin, encoded by the CTNNB1 gene, leading to aberrant up regulation of transcription and ensues oncogenesis [46]. Wnt pathway tumors are the least common of the four molecular subgroups that represents merely about 10% of sporadic medulloblastomas [47]. Genetic features of this subgroup are characterized by the aberrations like monosomy 6, CTNNB1 mutations, and nuclear β-catenin positivity by immunohistochemistry [47]. This subgroup of medulloblastomas is more common in children and in adults than in infants. The outcomes of these medulloblastomas are outstanding and 5-year overall survival rate is 95% in children and 100% in adults [6, 10, 42]. TP53 mutations are invariably present in both the Wnt and Shh subgroup medulloblastomas [6, 42, 48]. As Wnt-MB has uniformly good prognosis, treatment regimen can be de-escalated with reduced dose of craniospinal radiation, reduced-intensity of chemotherapy, or a combination of both in patients without metastatic disease [49].

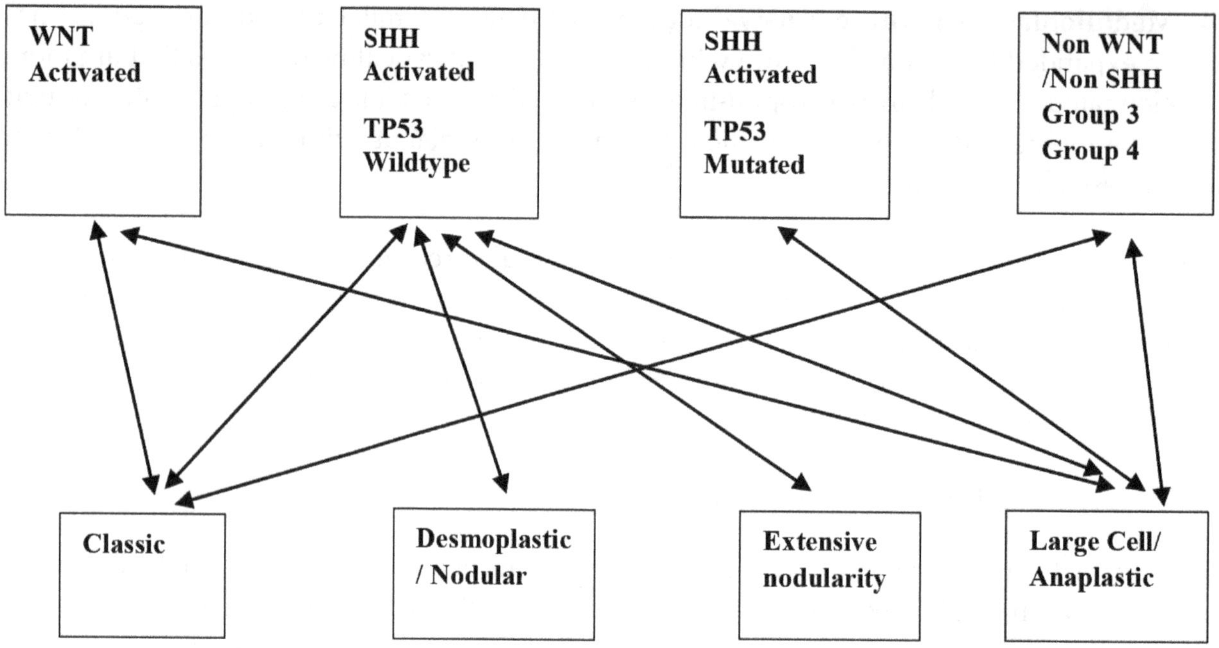

Figure 1. WHO 2016 classification of medulloblastoma subtypes, characterized by genetic and histological features.

5.2.2. Sonic hedgehog pathway tumors (Shh pathway/Shh-MB)

The Shh group of medulloblastomas is named after the Sonic Hedgehog signaling pathway, which is thought to drive this type of tumor initiation [42]. Medulloblastomas categorized by activation of Shh signaling are heterogeneous and are linked with a variety of genetic aberrations and outcomes, unlike the Wnt-MB [50]. As a whole, Shh subgroup tumors comprises nearly 30% of medulloblastomas overall [42, 48, 50].

Medulloblatomas of the Shh subgroup results from genetic predisposition of alteration of the sonic hedgehog pathway in the form of germline mutations in the patched-1 gene (PTCH1) or the suppressor of fused gene (SUFU). Loss of function PTCH1 and SUFU mutations lead to truncation of their associated protein products, leading to failure of their tumor suppressor effects and activation of Shh signaling with resultant tumorigenesis. Somatic mutations in PTCH1 and SUFU are also associated with sporadic medulloblastomas characterized by activation of the Shh pathway, along with PTCH2, MYC, SMO, GLI1 and GLI2 mutations [6, 42, 51, 52]. Deletion of chromosome 9q seems to be restricted to Shh medulloblastomas, which is fitting as the PTCH gene is located at chromosome 9q22 [42].

Clinical outcomes of individuals with Shh-MB can be divided into favorable and poor survival groups depending on TP53 mutation status which is particularly critical [48]. Patients with Shh/TP53 mutant variety medulloblastomas have extremely poor outcome than those with Shh/TP53 wild-type tumors as mutant TP53 has been associated with high rate of anaplasia and MYCN amplification, which are equally disastrous cellular events [48, 53]. Because of its clinical impact, TP53 mutation status has been incorporated into the 2016 WHO classification for CNS tumors and is part of routine assessment in all Shh-activated medulloblastomas [40].

Survival for Shh subgroup medulloblastomas is similar to Group 4 medulloblastomas and intermediate between that of Wnt and Group 3 medulloblastomas and varies significantly based on age and histologic subtype [10, 42, 48].

5.2.3. *Non-Wnt/Shh tumors*

The non-Wnt/Shh tumor subgroup encompasses Group 3 and Group 4, in which the underlying genetic predisposition of mutations have yet not been recognized [49]. These types are associated with a higher incidence of tumor dissemination and approximately 30% of patients have metastasis at the time of diagnosis [6]. Despite these similarities, features of Group 3 and Group 4 subgroup medulloblastomas vary regarding the demographic, clinical, transcriptional, and genetic differences between them and these advocate that they are actually distinct entities with molecular diversity [42, 54].

5.2.3.1. *Group 3 MB*

Nearly 30% of medulloblastomas are of the Group 3 subgroup and histologically mostly are of the "classic" variety of medulloblastomas [6, 55–57]. These tumors genetically are more likely to have high-level expression and amplification of MYC, MYCN and OTX2 with imbalance of chromosome 17 [42, 49, 51, 58]. Group 3 tumors show gain of chromosome 1q, and/or loss of chromosome 5q and chromosome 10q more than Group 4 tumors [42]. They occur more frequently in infants and children, and has the worst outcome among all molecular subgroups, with 10-year overall survival of 39% in infants and 50% in children [6, 42, 49, 51, 59].

5.2.3.2. *Group 4 MB*

About 35% of medulloblastomas overall are of Group 4 subgroup and the peak incidence for this subgroup is in late childhood and early adolescents [6, 42]. The prognosis of Group 4 tumors is similar to Shh subgroups tumors and is intermediate between those of Wnt and Group 3 subgroup tumors. Patients with metastatic disease or MYC amplifications in this Group have significantly poorer outcomes [49, 50]. Though isochromosome 17q is also seen in Group 3 tumors, it is more common in Group 4 tumors. Another prominent cytogenetic alteration among Group 4 tumors is loss of the X chromosome, which is found in 80% of females with Group 4 medulloblastoma [42].

Recently, the discovery of seven novel molecular subgroups has permitted to categorize patients further to envisage better disease subclassification and outcome predictions. These subgroup dependent grouping stratified patients into four clinical risk groups for 5-year progression-free survival: favorable risk (91% survival); standard risk (81% survival); highrisk (42% survival); and very high-risk (28% survival) [41]. Another study recommended total of 12 subgroups based on the integration of transcriptomic and methylation data. In that analysis medulloblastoma encompasses 12 subtypes; 2 Wnt, 4 Shh, 3 Group 3, and 3 Group 4 groups. These subtypes of each subgroup are clinically and biologically pertinent [54].

5.3. Integrated classification

In 2016, for the first time, the molecular characteristics was incorporated into the WHO classification for the diagnosis of CNS tumors. This integration of histological features with genetic information has considerably transformed the diagnostic work-up and reporting of tumors of the CNS. Nonetheless, this remains perplexing in embryonal tumors due to their de novo tumor heterogeneity that is being faced [10]. This integrated diagnosis is presented in a layered format; that includes the histological diagnosis, WHO grade, molecular genetic information and ultimately the integrated diagnosis. The value of this approach is clearly illustrated in embryonal tumors, in particular medulloblastoma, where the combination of molecular and histological data provides discrete diagnostic information [40]. In this new concept of a "layered diagnosis" brain tumors that are diagnosed purely morphologically are incorporated with molecular characteristics for an "integrated diagnosis" at the peak diagnostic level [60]. In the layered integrated classification, a patient would be labeled as having medulloblastoma of a definite histological subtype, the WHO grade and the molecular subgroup [61].

6. Staging

There is no well-established staging system for medulloblastoma for prediction from which treatment plan and outcome prediction can be made. In 1969, Chang et al. suggested an operative staging system for medulloblastomas adapting the TNM classification for other tumors [62]. According to the size and extent of primary tumor, T category was divided into four main groups with subdivisions of T3 (T1, T2, T3a, T3b or T4) and the M category had five groups (M0, M1, M2, M3 and M4) based on the degree of tumor spread in the CSF pathway or extra-CNS metastases [9]. Overall, M staging has remained more useful in prognostic evaluation, while the T staging is less valuable as a prognostic indicator [63]. Several studies have stratified the patients into "high-risk" and "average" or "standard-risk" groups depending on age of the patient, residual disease after surgery, pathologic variant, and M staging [8, 64]. This risk stratification is a good predictor of outcome. Standard-risk and high-risk categories have long term survival rates of approximately 85% and 70%, respectively [6].

7. Presentation

Because of its origin in the posterior fossa, the presenting symptoms of medulloblastoma are often vague complaints and understandably the diagnosis may be delayed. Presentation depends on various elements of the tumor subject to location, size, duration, compression on the surrounding structures. As these arise from the vicinity of cerebellum and brainstem, often the first feature to appear is instability of gait. Being a midline posterior fossa lesion, trunkal ataxia appears first and appendicular ataxia gradually ensues as the tumor grows bigger to compress the cerebellar hemispheres, and other common cerebellar signs follow with time. When the tumor is big enough to compress the brainstem, long tract signs begin to appear and add more difficulty in movement of the patients. As the tumor grows further, especially downwards, the lower cranial nerves start to get involved and lower cranial nerve palsies manifest. If the tumor grows bigger to occupy and block the Aqueduct of Sylvius, hydrocephalus ensues. Hydrocephalus may also result from blockage of the fourth ventricular outlets, by compression, by the growing tumor, individually or in combination. Hydrocephalus in turn may lead to features of raised Intracranial Pressure (ICP) resulting in headache, nausea, vomiting, irritability, lethargy, behavior alteration, personality change and impaired memory or attention, etc. Raised ICP occasionally gives rise to possibility of having seizure and 6th nerve palsy. Respiratory and cardiac manifestations may be evident, resulting from compromise of the respiratory and cardiac centers in the brainstem. Alteration of level of consciousness, starting from disorientation to deep coma, may result either from raised ICP or from compression on the brainstem. Papilledema or even visual impairment from raised ICP is not very uncommon, especially when presented in late stage.

Medulloblastoma is a very rapidly growing tumor and tends to follow a rapid progression in a very short period of time. The median time between onset of symptom until diagnosis (symptom interval) is 3.3 months (65 days) [65]. Rarely, patients may have symptoms for up to 6 months before diagnosis and younger patients have significantly longer interval to diagnosis while more aggressive subgroups of medulloblastoma have a shorter pre-diagnostic interval [66].

8. Diagnosis and differentials

The Accurate diagnosis of pediatric tumors is essential to ensure balance between achieving a long-term cure and avoiding treatment related disability in survivors. The tentative diagnosis of medulloblastoma is relatively straight cut one from the age of the patient, history and neurological examination findings. Nonetheless, there are other maladies that are to be kept in mind. The two commonest differential diagnosis of a posterior fossa mass in children are pilocytic astrocytoma and ependymoma. Other lesions to be considered are atypical teratoid/rhabdoid tumors, exophytic brainstem glioma and choroid plexus papilloma as well as teratoma in infants and hemangioblastoma in patients with Von Hippel-Lindau syndrome. Metastasis is the first to be thought in adults as that is the most frequently encountered posterior fossa lesion [6, 10].

9. Investigation work ups

A variety of diagnostic studies are used to confirm the clinical diagnosis of medulloblastoma and to localize the tumor exactly. The first-line diagnostic test for medulloblastoma is brain imaging.

Up until introduction of CT scan in 1971, air studies (pneumoencephalography and ventriculography) were most reliable and almost accurate in the diagnosis of medulloblastoma in all age groups. Angiography also yielded useful results regardless of age. With advent of MRI, CT scan has become an adjunct to that. Skull x-ray studies, once useful for the detection of brain tumors, is now rarely of value. Nucleotide brain scans and bone scans, myelographic examination, CSF cytology were also helpful in diagnosing a moderate number of cases [6, 8, 9, 67, 68].

9.1. Computerized tomography (CT)

CT is often used as the first-line diagnostic imaging because of its readily availability, fastness in imaging and comparatively cheaper price [8]. This is a good tool for early diagnosis with state of hydrocephalus, serial evaluation of tumor, postoperative assessment of extent of tumor removal, detection of residual and recurrent tumor, and tumor deposits in the CSF pathways as well as convenient follow-up studies [4, 15, 42]. Medulloblastomas appear typically hyperdense and sharply demarcated lesion near the fourth ventricle in the plain CT scan with a surrounding hypodense zone of edema which show better delineation with contrast enhancement showing moderate to marked increase in density (**Figure 2**). Cystic components may also be seen. Leptomeningeal tumor deposits appear as areas of increased density in the subarachnoid space. Calcification may be seen in about 10–20% of medulloblastomas [5, 62].

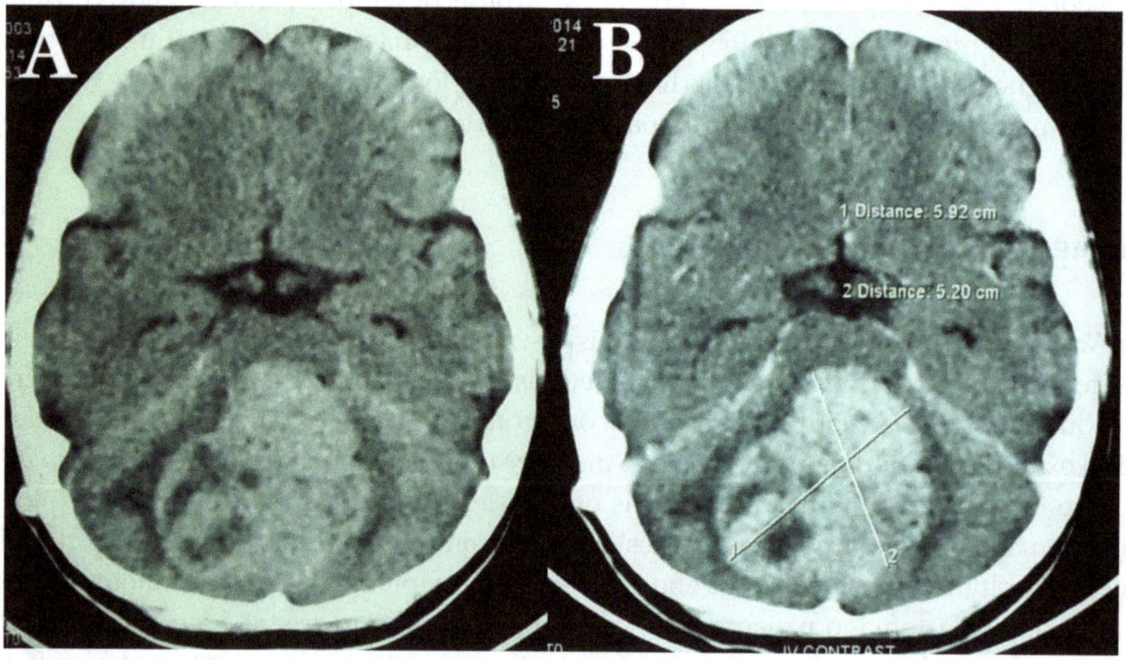

Figure 2. Plain axial CT scan (A) showing hyperdense and sharply demarcated lesion near the fourth ventricle with surrounding hypodense area of edema which with contrast enhancement (B) is well demarcated by increased density.

9.2. Magnetic resonance imaging (MRI)

The relationship between the tumor and the surrounding brain structures can be vividly demonstrated in MRI with and without gadolinium. Screening MRI of the whole spinal axis is capable of displaying and evaluating tumor dissemination, when present and pre-operative whole spine MRI is preferred [20, 21].

Different sequences of MRI can provide different information to help in diagnosis and treatment planning. Medulloblastomas are hypointense to gray matter on T1-weighted imaging (T1WI) with heterogeneous gadolinium enhancement in 90% of cases, while they are generally iso to hyperintense to gray matter on T2-weighted imaging (T2WI). The heterogeneity in T1WI and T2WI results from cyst formation, calcification or necrosis. Diffusion-weighted imaging (DWI) shows restricted diffusion and in fluid-attenuated inversion recovery (FLAIR) imaging, medulloblastomas are generally hyperintense to surrounding brain (**Figure 3**). MR spectroscopy (MRS) shows elevated choline peaks and decreased creatine and N-acetyl acetate peaks, with occasional elevation in lactic acid and lipid peaks [62].

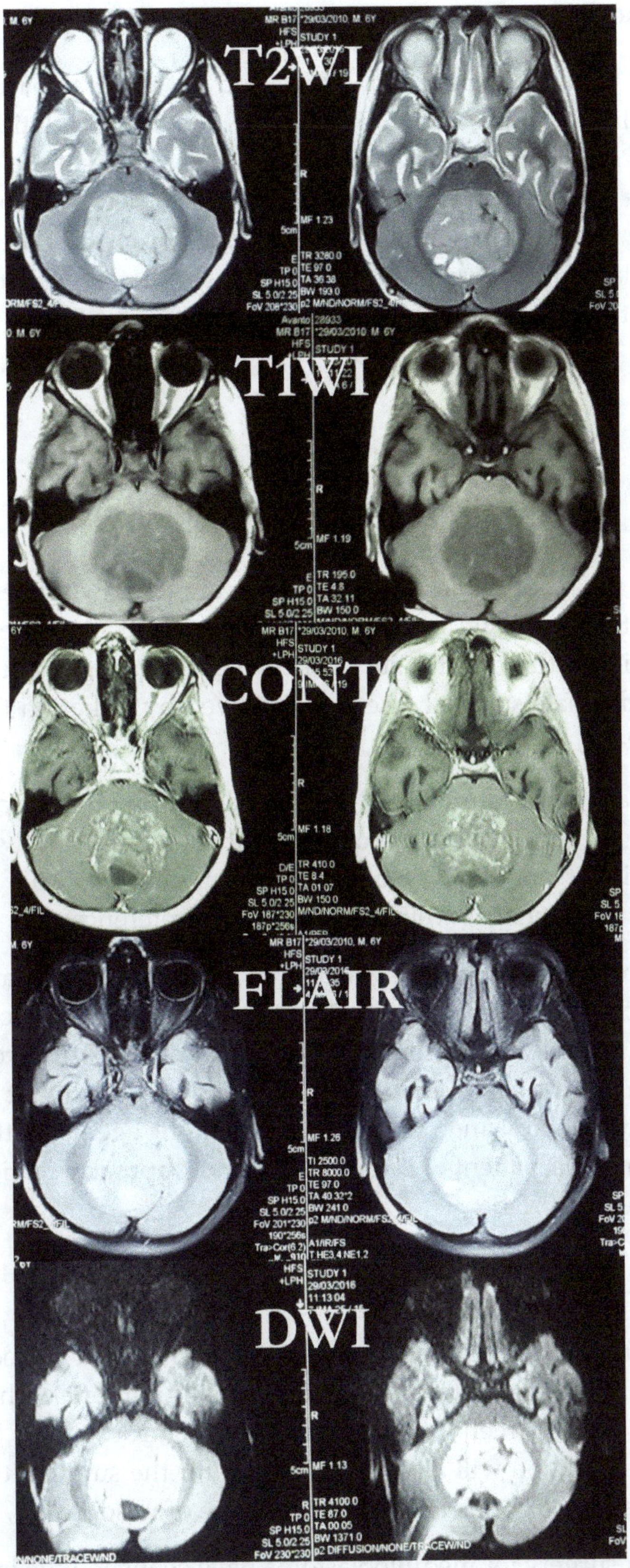

Figure 3. Medulloblastomas in T2-weighted imaging (T2WI), T1-weighted imaging (T1WI), with gadolinium enhancement (CONT), fluid-attenuated inversion recovery (FLAIR) (D) and diffusion-weighted imaging (DWI) in axial planes.

9.3. Molecular diagnosis

Molecular diagnosis is of immense importance and an integral part of the management protocol as it is invaluable in prediction of outcome and in formulation of dose of therapy, especially in cases of selection of agents for targeted therapy. As these state of the art assays are accessible merely in few laboratories of the first-world neuropathological institutions, it is often very difficult to come to an integrated diagnosis for most of the centers in the world. Nonetheless, molecular antibodies specifically targeting mutated proteins should be available in nearly all neuropathological laboratories.

10. Treatment

10.1. General

Treatment strategies for medulloblastomas have advanced slowly over the past 5 decades. Generally based on the histology and clinical factors, especially, disease dissemination at presentation and residual tumor after surgical resection, management of medulloblastoma has evolved to maximal safe surgical resection followed by radiation therapy and adjuvant chemotherapy [20, 22–24, 26, 69].

Adjuvant chemotherapy is recommended for all patients as this improves outcomes significantly. Following surgery, risks of recurrence and of neurocognitive effects of radiation therapy, doses of radiation and the type of chemotherapy protocol vary depending on extent of disease and age of the patient as well as institutional preferences [20, 29].

Though the medulloblastoma subgroups (Wnt, Shh, Groups 3 and 4) have distinct molecular and clinical profile, current adjuvant chemotherapy that are in practice are for the nontargeted ones. However, significant improvements, approximately 70% 5-year survival rate with these combined therapies are achieved at the high cost of the quality of life, resulting mostly from the effects of radiotherapy and nonspecific, antimitotic agents on the developing brains of young medulloblastoma patients [27–31]. A general approach carries significant risk of over or under-treatment. [30, 34].

10.2. Surgery and surgical techniques

In March 1925, Cushing first succeeded in gross total removal of a medulloblastoma [1, 2]. Since then, the first-line treatment for medulloblastoma is surgery with the aim of maximal safe resection, along with treatment of any concomitant hydrocephalus [8]. But Cushing also cautioned that "the temptation will always be present for the surgeon to attempt an enucleation, a conservative attitude in this respect is the course of wisdom" [1, 8].

The basic principles of surgery for medulloblastoma have changed little in the modern era, but technological revolutions in surgical technique and supportive care have made surgery safer. Development of surgical skill and other facilities has dramatically reduced the perioperative mortality from 25.2% during the period of Cushing to less than 1% in expert hands at the present time [70]. With recent technological advancements the goal of surgery is always a complete excision, but practically it can safely be accomplished only in about one fourth of cases [71].

Most surgeons prefer the prone position than to the sitting position to minimize the risk of air embolism, frontal pneumocephalus, and systemic hypotension. The straight vertical skin incision employed by almost all neurosurgeons today was described first by Naffziger in 1928 [70]. A wide craniectomy or craniotomy extending from the transverse sinuses to the foramen magnum is performed with or without removal of the posterior arch of C1. The dura is usually opened in a Y-shaped manner extending down to the level of C1 when the posterior arch is removed. The tumor may be readily evident as a red, semi circumscribed mass peeping into the vallecula when the tumor is large. The dorsal surface of the tumor is exposed and even though not truly encapsulated, medulloblastomas often have a clear interface between the tumor and surrounding brain where a dissection plane can be created. The tumor is excised in piece meal fashion either through the telovaler approach or by splitting the vermis (**Figure 4**). With the goal

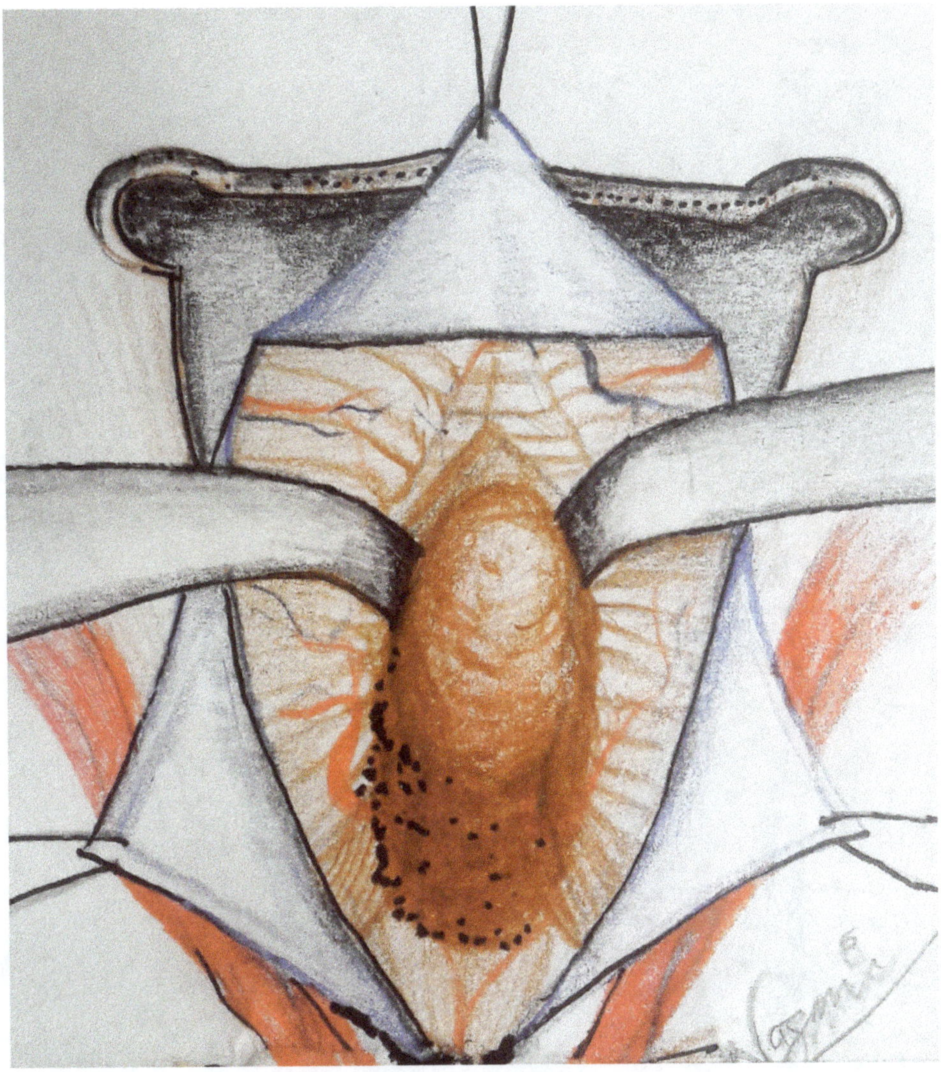

Figure 4. Schematic diagram showing the exposure of medulloblastoma after splitting the vermis in the midline.

of maximal safe resection, gross total resection can often be accomplished. Superiorly, the tumor is often projected into the aqueduct, filling it and obstructing the CSF pathway. The part projecting into the aqueduct can be meticulously removed with gentle suction, reestablishing the CSF flow (**Figure 5**). The part of the tumor that is attached to the brain stem or peduncles, is carefully removed, keeping a thin mantle leaving behind to ensure not to injure any vital structure. To alleviate the post-operative morbidity or mortality, immediate postoperative care of the patient is of immense importance. This is a factor that can make enormous difference in outcome.

Whether preoperative shunting should be done to relieve hydrocephalus prior to tumor surgery remains controversial. A ventriculoperitoneal (VP) shunt permanently or an external ventricular drain (EVD) as a temporary measure can be employed to treat hydrocephalus, if present at the time of diagnosis [8, 26, 71]. An EVD can be placed in the operating room, just prior to posterior fossa craniotomy, if the hydrocephalus is not treated preoperatively. About 20% of patients require long-term treatment of hydrocephalus with a VP shunt insertion or an endoscopic third ventriculostomy (ETV), when the hydrocephalus persists even after tumor removal [8, 71]. There is high possibility that a preoperative shunt

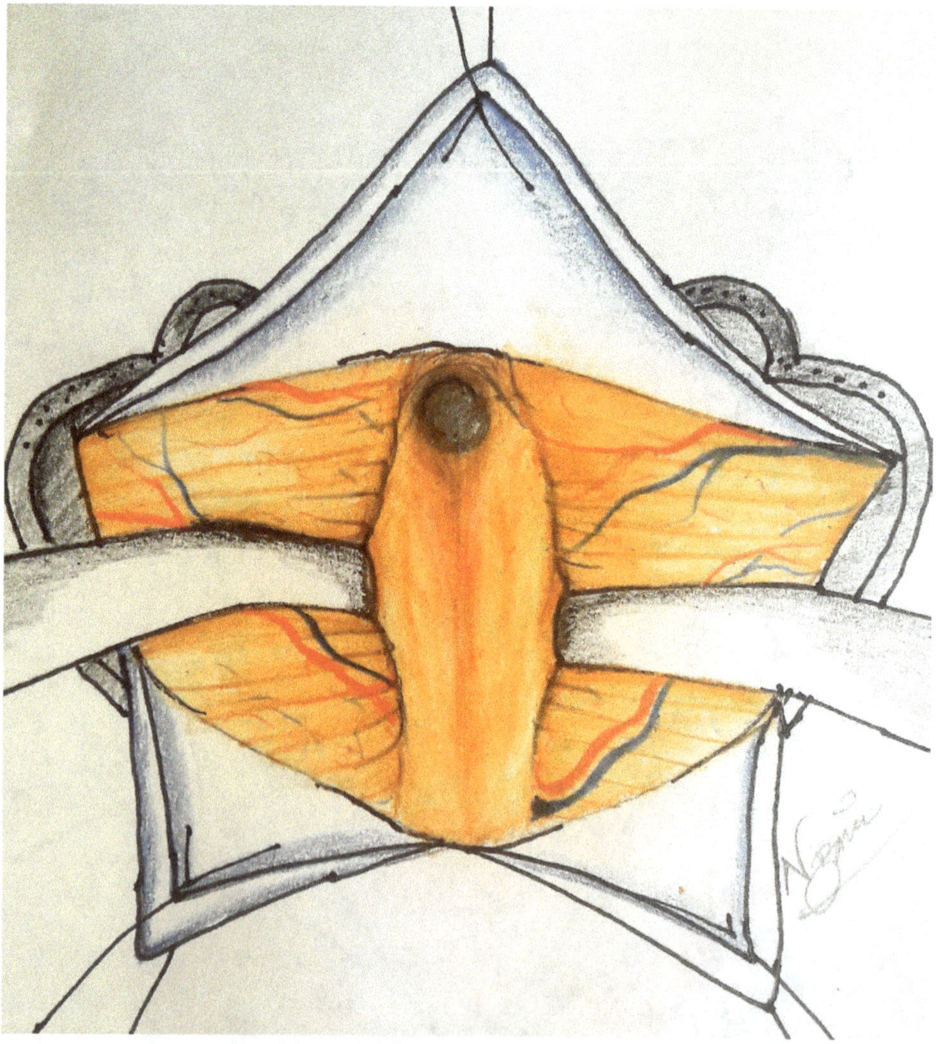

Figure 5. Schematic diagram of expanded aqueduct after removal of the medulloblastoma extending into the aqueduct.

may serve as a pathway of dissemination of the medulloblastoma, which has a tendency to spread by the CSF pathways. The use of millipore filters has been described to prevent dissemination [26, 70].

10.2.1. Complications of surgery

Clinical or subclinical venous air embolism, which is more common in sitting position, can happen in the prone position as well. With the goal of complete resection, major complications during tumor removal are usually caused by damage to the brain stem and injury to the lower cranial nerves. Aspiration pneumonia and respiratory failure often follows if the post-operative lower cranial nerve injuries are not handled meticulously. Though described frequently, cerebellar mutism, a commonly described complication of posterior fossa surgery, is less likely to occur now a days with microsurgical techniques. Meningitis, pseudomeningocele, postoperative tumor bed hematoma, epidural hematoma, subdural hematoma are among the other less often encountered complications.

10.3. Radiotherapy

Radiotherapy has been an adjunct of the treatment modality for medulloblastomas since the early twentieth century as these tumors are very responsive to radiotherapy. The survival rate has improved dramatically after the introduction of radiotherapy. Post-operative craniospinal irradiation (CSI) with or without boost to the posterior fossa are the customary protocol, as chosen by different centers [8, 72].

10.3.1. Treatment for average-risk patients ≥3 years of age

Post-operative radiotherapy dose for average risk medulloblastoma patients aged ≥3 years initially was set as 36 Gy CSI and 54 Gy boost for the posterior fossa (PF) because of high risk of local recurrence. Dose adjustment to 23.4–24 Gy CSI with the addition of adjuvant chemotherapy has been made with successful result [66, 73, 74]. Reduction in the posterior fossa radiation volume, in the form of 3-Dimensional conformal radiotherapy (3D CRT) has enabled to restrict the boost volume to the tumor bed plus a margin without compromising local control that minimizes morbidity associated with full PF irradiation by shielding normal vital structures [74–76]. Intensity-modulated radiotherapy (IMRT) or proton beam therapy similarly can reduce exposure to the heart and liver during CSI [72, 77–79].

10.3.2. Treatment for high-risk patients ≥3 years of age

The usual radiotherapy schedule for high-risk medulloblastoma patients of 3 years or more consists of standard dose regimen of 36 Gy CSI with a boost to both the posterior fossa and focal sites of metastasis of 55.8 Gy. Adjuvant chemotherapy, consisting of concurrent vincristine followed by maintenance chemotherapy with Lomustine, Vincristine, and Cisplatin has shown progression-free survival of 67% in M1, M2 and M3 stage [66, 80]. Outcomes for high-risk patients are equally poor even with inclusion of some neoadjuvant agents in addition to conventional chemotherapeutic agents [81–83].

10.3.3. Treatment of infants and children <3 years of age

As patients younger than 3 years are in risk of poor outcome of neurocognitive function following CSI, delay or omission of radiotherapy is recommended for this group of patients. M0 patients following gross total resection have commendable outcome with only chemotherapy after surgery [84].

10.3.4. Radiation hazards

The long-term sequelae of radiation therapy are well described, among which the most common ones are endocrinopathies, neurocognitive and neurosensory impairment following craniospinal irradiation depending on age of patient and radiation dose [85, 86]. Cancer survivors with a history of cranial irradiation have more tendency to have cerebrovascular disease and an increased risk of second malignancies in the radiation field [6]. Skin reactions, hair loss, growth problems, nausea and vomiting, chronic otitis media and/or otitis externa, myelosuppression are other commonly encountered side effects [71].

10.4. Chemotherapy and combined radio-chemo therapy

As medulloblastoma is a highly radiosensitive tumor, chemotherapy for this formidable tumor has been an adjunct in the treatment strategy for years. Various combinations of chemotherapeutic agents are used in conjunction with radiotherapy. The toxic effect of different chemotherapeutic agents have forced their use to be restricted in different circumstances. Now a days, the newer drugs are more soothing to the patients with better acceptability, tolerance and efficacy.

Penetrability of the blood-brain barrier of a drug is the most important feature for a chemotherapeutic agent to be a worthy regimen for brain tumors. Vincristine, Cisplatin, Cyclophosphamide, Lomustine, Etoposide, Methotrexate, Temozolomide, and Carboplatin are the commonly used effective chemotherapeutic agents for medulloblastomas [8, 87].

For average-risk medulloblastoma patients two common chemotherapy regimens are practiced. One is with a combination of Cisplatin, Lomustine, and Vincristine, while the second one comprises of a combination of Cisplatin, Cyclophosphamide, and Vincristine. These two regimens do not have significant difference in outcome regarding event-free survival (EFS) and overall survival (OS) [68]. Among conventional chemotherapeutics, Temozolomide-containing regimens have shown most promising activity. Two studies, one in monotherapy [88] and another in combination with Irinotecan [89], have shown the best results in a relatively large population, although follow up for disease-free survival is short. Its tolerable toxicity profile and synergies with other chemotherapeutics and targeted agents make it an attractive compound to serve as backbone for new strategies [20].

As children under the age of 3 years has worse long term cognitive effects, they are not commonly treated with the radiotherapy. To compensate this more intense chemotherapy is initiated instead [87]. In the last few decades, with the intension to avoid radiation and to have an equally better outcome in younger patients, protocols have been developed consisting of intense systemic chemotherapy, followed by a consolidation cycle with myeloablative chemotherapy along with autologous stem cell rescue (AuHCR) as an alternative management in these patients under the age of 3 years [90]. The 5 year EFS and OS varies between patients with localized disease, and patients with disseminated disease as well as between patients with desmoplastic, classical and anaplastic MB [91].

10.4.1. Side effects of chemotherapy

Adverse effects of adjuvant chemotherapy have been significant and needs to be modified in a good number of patients because of adverse reactions [92, 93]. The commonnest side effect of chemotherapy is hematologic toxicity in the form of leukothrombocytopenia. Other common adverse effects being anemia, somnolence, peripheral neuropathy, headaches, constipation, paresthesias, mucositis, nausea and vomiting, immune compromise and bone marrow suppression, renal toxicities with electrolyte abnormalities, hepatotoxicity, infertility [8, 71]. Some drugs carry the risk of development of treatment-related cancers which is 4.2% at 10 years [94]. Vincristine and cisplatin is known to cause various types of neurotoxicity particularly peripheral neuropathy and ototoxicity [95].

11. Recurrence

The majority of treatment failures develop within the first 2–3 years, and then the failure rate tends to decrease. Tumor recurrence occurs most frequently in the posterior fossa and that may or may not be associated with subarachnoid dissemination in the craniospinal axis [8, 9]. Inadequate post-operative dose of the radiotherapy and large volume of residual tumor are the major causes of recurrence. Commonly the outcomes in patients with relapsed disease are grave, with five-year survival rate of only about 25% and which has not improved much, even with development in treatment strategies [96–98]. Repeat surgical resection, re-irradiation, stereotactic radiosurgery, high-dose chemotherapy with AuHCR, low-dose oral Etoposide, the use of biologically targeted agents, singly or in combination, have been tried and success in control was more for localized recurrence than for disseminated recurrence [97–107]. At recurrence medulloblastomas often change towards a more anaplastic pathological variant. Interestingly Shh tumors tend to recur locally while Groups 3 and 4 recur almost entirely with metastases [10, 20, 44].

12. Metastasis

Medulloblastomas exhibit a strong propensity to metastasize through CSF pathways and tend to form tumors of variable size along ventricular surfaces, in subarachnoid space, or along nerve roots or may grow en plaque on surface of brain or spinal cord or may deposit in the ventricles [25]. Dissemination through the CSF route may be augmented by ventricular or spinal punctures or by manipulations of the lesion during operation. VP shunting has frequently been reported to cause extraneural metastases to the peritonium. Invasion of the meninges is not very uncommon [2, 9]. Extra CNS metastases have been reported to be in the bone marrow, lymph nodes, and viscera. Though very rare, metastasis to skin, liver, lung, mediastinum and retroperitoneal structures has also been reported [8, 9].

13. Surveillance

Surveillance is important as relapses encountered on surveillance imaging can be better dealt with and show improved survival as paralleled to those identified by reemergence of the clinical symptoms [108]. Though consensus about the schedule is debated, generally clinical and radiographic follow-up is recommended at three-month intervals during the first year after completion of scheduled therapy, at three to four-month intervals in the second year, every 6 months during the third year, and annually thereafter [109–112] (**Figure 6**). It is generally

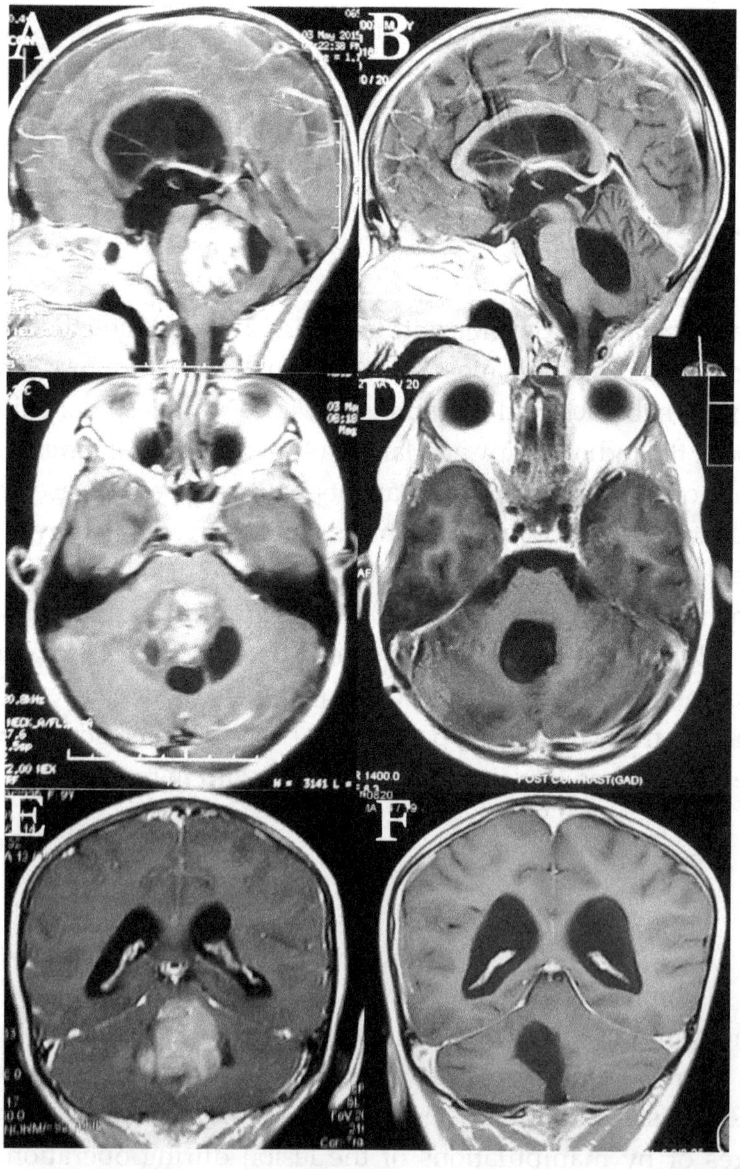

Figure 6. Preoperative contrast enhanced MRI in sagittal (A), axial (C) and coronal (E) planes and 1 year post-operative contrast enhanced MRI following radiotherapy in sagittal (B), axial (D) and coronal (F) planes of a 9 years old boy.

agreed that surveillance imaging of the brain should be complemented with full spinal MRI as it often might prove to be crucial and beneficial for the patient [110]. It is also recommended that, endocrine screening and neuropsychological testing be performed in those who were treated with craniospinal irradiation [6].

14. Medulloblastoma in adults

Medulloblastoma is much less common in adults, accounting for less than 1% - 3% of primary CNS tumors [24, 113, 114]. The annual incidence of medulloblastoma is 1–1.5 cases per million in the general adult population and 80% occur before the end of the fourth decade [24, 113–115]. Treatment protocols are limited for adults and they are treated by heterogeneous ways using various chemo-radiotherapy regimens with surgery with post-operative CSI being the mainstay of treatment [115]. As late relapse is common among adult medulloblastoma patients, long-term follow-up is warranted. Spinal seeding at presentation is a poor prognostic factor for recurrence [114, 115]. Adult medulloblastomas are clinically similar to that in the pediatric population, but lateral location and desmoplastic type is more frequent in adults as opposed to the pediatric age group. Adult medulloblastomas are thus, more amenable to complete resection and better outcome is expected because of their locations and histopathological variants respectively [24, 113–116]. Relapse following complete treatment is relatively late in adults as compared to children and they have a relatively prolonged time from relapse to death [116]. As most treatment recommendations for adults are extrapolated from the experience in pediatric patients, a protocol from the time of diagnosis includes: increasing the intensity to identify metastasis; increasing the radiotherapy dose to the primary site; adding chemotherapy following radiotherapy in medically fit patients; and following-up the patients with PET or bone scan every 6 months for at least 3 years [117, 118].

15. Outcome

Though the outcomes need to be judged cautiously because of the marked heterogeneity between studies, overall outcome of medulloblastoma patients has improved tremendously over the last decades. Still, outcome in a good number of patients with metastatic disease, adverse molecular or cytogenetic features, infants and relapsed or refractory patients remains depressing.

Many factors play role in outcome of medulloblastoma patients and outcomes have been variable in different series. The outcome has gradually improved from survival from onset to death of 8–9 months in 1930s to 54% 3-year survival in 1950s, about 75% 5-year survival in 1980s [71]. Till the last decade the five-year EFS and OS has raised to 81 ± 2.1 and 86 ± 9%, respectively [68]. Among the factors that play role in poor outcome, the noteworthy are younger age, larger residual tumor volume after surgery, inadequate dose of radiotherapy, presence of metastatic disease at diagnosis, presence of hydrocephalus, anaplastic or large cell histology, insufficient chemotherapy, MYC amplification or expression, 17p loss or 1q gain, and tumors of

Group 3 or Shh subgroup with TP53 mutations. On the contrary, patients having monosomy 6, mutation of CTNNB1, and trkC expression demonstrate a favorable outcome [6, 9, 33, 41, 49, 59]. Generally, OS for children with medulloblastoma are reported as 50–60%, whereas for average-risk and high-risk patients OS is 70–80 and 30–40% respectively [8, 119].

16. Newer therapies/future

The future of medulloblastoma treatment lies on the basis of its genetic coding and molecular subgroupings. A few drugs have been tested preliminarily and that made the researchers as well as the patients optimistic. Endeavor is going on to determine whether the intensity of treatment can be reduced safely, keeping the optimum efficacy, to mitigate the treatment-related long term developmental and cognitive morbidity without affecting survival rates, thus improving the quality of life for medulloblastoma survivors [6, 10]. The molecular biology of the subgroups have emerged to be the key elements of success in future and, with the early success and the potential utility of molecular biomarkers in prognostication and prediction, researchers are in search of more personalized and tailored therapies for the patients [8, 42, 49].

Of the different pathways of tumor origin and progression, the sonic hedgehog (Shh) pathway is a front-runner in research in this perspective. Smoothened (SMO), is an intriguing protein in developmental processes involving the hedgehog signaling pathway [120]. Assuming the role of SMO in the Shh pathway in tumorogenesis, molecules that target SMO are under intensive research and preliminary success have been achieved in some clinical trials [42, 121]. Of these, smoothened inhibitor Vismodegib showed promising result in studies with varying outcomes, having both short-term and long-lasting response, especially in standard-risk Shh medulloblastoma patients [122–125]. Trial with another SMO inhibitor Sonidegib, in cases of patients with relapsed disease also reveals promise for future [123]. Blocking GLI1 with Arsenic trioxide [126], combining SMO inhibitors with PI3K inhibitors [124], or inhibition of PIN1 by either Juglone or the flavonoids Epigallocatechin gallate and Quercetin [127], have attained certain levels of success as these aberrations are frequently encountered in this subset of patients [20]. Quercetin has been found to be a probable worthy radio-sensitizer [127]. Saridegib and Erismodegib are other potent SMO inhibitors under trial that seem to have potential in regression of tumor and inhibition of tumor progression [128].

For Non-WNT/Non-SHH medulloblastomas comprising molecular subgroups 3 and 4, Gemcitabine, a nucleoside analog, and Pemetrexed, a folate antimetabolite are currently being investigated in combination to evaluate their role in prognosis [20, 49]. Combination of these two drugs have been found to be active, particularly against Group 3 medulloblastomas [129]. These were tried separately previously in medulloblastoma patients but only combination of Gemcitabine with Oxaliplatin was found to have promising results with a disease control rate (DCR) of 50% [130]. On the other hand, the combination of Vorinostat and Retinoic acid was found to have a 5-month disease stabilization in patients with Group 4 medulloblastomas [131].

Temozolomide-containing regimens are well tolerable and have good antitumor activity against relapsed/refractory medulloblastomas [20]. Evaluation of temozolomide and

Irinotecan in a study with short follow-up has shown to have good prospect with a DCR of 73% [89]. Trials with multiagent oral antiangiogenic regimen like Bevacizumab, Cilengitide, Lenalidomide and Thalidomide either in monotherapy or in combination with Vincristine, Irinotecan, Temozolomide or Temsirolimus in patients with medulloblastoma yielded only short-lasting disease stabilizations with a tolerable toxicity profile [132–137].

Tyrosine kinase inhibitors (TKIs) like imatinib, sorafenib, lapatinib, nilotinib, dasatinib, ponatinib and bafetinib have shown to block the migration and invasion properties of MB cells which may prove to be effective alternative agents in the treatment of medulloblastomas [128].

In order to reduce treatment related side effects, newer radiotherapy techniques are being evaluated. IMRT and helical tomotherapy have been evaluated, but results were not very pleasing [24].

Immunotherapy is another novel therapeutic approach that is being evaluated for the treatment of medulloblastoma. The target antigens that have been identified are cancer testis antigens (CTAs), MAGE and GAGE proteins. MAGE-4, MAGE-A and GAGE expression have been found in 50, 62 and 84% of medulloblastomas respectively [138, 139]. MAGE antigens, are a promising targets for immunotherapy in patients with medulloblastoma as it has paved the way of immunotherapy already by targeting successfully in some other tumors [140, 141]. Vaccinations against EGFRvIII in combination with GM-CSF, is another potential immunotherapeutic approach, which have already been tested in other brain tumors [142].

In the post-surgery treatment process, delivery of anticancer drugs across the BBB remains a challenge. A number of methods have been tried to facilitate effective drug delivery across the BBB to the brain. Of those, a very promising technique is Nanoparticles (NP) encapsulating magnetic materials such as iron oxide. Upon entering the systemic circulation, through NPs a drug can be directed remotely to the disease site. The addition of receptor-specific ligands to magnetic NPs for active targeting can significantly increase their efficacy [128].

17. Rehabilitation

Quality of life and psychosocial outcomes following treatment of medulloblastoma are progressively recognized as crucial issues in decision-making regarding therapy. Long-term outcome was less emphasized than survival previously as survival was nominal in the earlier period of history of medulloblastoma, though the thought of prolongation of life and making it worth living was always there with the encouragement to persist in efforts [2]. Over the past decades, survival has improved significantly, and expectantly will continue to improve with the development of molecularly targeted agents and other modalities of treatment. With time, thoughts regarding quality of life is becoming increasingly vital both in decision-making concerning therapy and in the design of future treatment protocols where quality of life is the prime target next to survival [6]. Treatment-related endocrinologic, cognitive, and psychological sequelae, especially in Infants and very young children with medulloblastoma remain a difficult therapeutic challenge which can be tackled prudently with rehabilitation programs. For that it is an obvious need to develop active rehabilitative programs and special educational assistance for the children who survive the multi-modality therapy [71]. Optimum therapy has led to long-term survival in patients of medulloblastoma and it is expected to be increased with time with the anticipated need of more intense and dedicated rehabilitation regime for this group of patients. Thus the long-term survivors of medulloblastoma badly require multifaceted medical rehabilitation care involving team of subspecialists including oncologist, neurologist, endocrinologist, psychologist, psychiatrist and physiotherapist to overcome the challenges that they have to face in the longer run [8, 64].

18. Conclusion

Medulloblastomas have been neurosurgeons' nightmare for years. MB, a highly aggressive tumor of the cerebellum, treated with a combination of surgery, craniospinal irradiation and chemotherapy, still remains a challenge. Enriched knowledge of histological and molecular subgroups with their aberrant signaling pathways has provided novel therapeutic targets for MB to regress their growth and has enhanced both the prognostic and therapeutic implications. Efforts to modify and refine the MB treatment strategy are ongoing as toxicity and off-target effects of various newer drugs are yet not under total control. Regardless of marked advancements in overall survival for medulloblastoma patients over the past decades, substantial successes remain to be achieved, especially concerning improvement in survival, mitigating treatment-related morbidities as well as improving quality of life for survivors. These have led to modifications of therapies and research, with the emphasis on novel, less toxic and more targeted agents for the best possible survival with least long-term adverse consequences for a worthwhile post-therapy quality of life. The combination of molecular pharmacology, neurogenetics, cell biology, and biophysics will ultimately drive the utmost hope of a cure for medulloblastoma. With the advancement of modern research, medulloblastoma, once a dreaded and hopeless entity, is looming to be a potentially curable disease.

Acknowledgements

I am very grateful to my colleagues Dr. Abu Saleh Mohammad Abu Obaida and Dr. Muhtamim Chowdhury for their critical advices in preparing this chapter. I am immensely indebted to my colleague Dr. Nazmin Ahmed for her beautiful schematic diagrams that have made this chapter colorful.

Author details

Asifur Rahman

Address all correspondence to: bijoun14@yahoo.com

Department of Neurosurgery, Bangabandhu Sheikh Mujib Medical University, Shahbag, Dhaka, Bangladesh

References

[1] Bailey P, Cushing H. Medulloblastoma cerebelli: A common type of midcerebellar glioma of childhood. Archives of Neurology and Psychiatry. 1925;**14**(2):192-224

[2] Cushing H. Experiences with the cerebellar medulloblastomas. Acta Pathologica, Microbiologica, et Immunologica Scandinavica. 1930;**7**(1-2):1-86

[3] Globus JH, Strauss I. Spongioblastoma multiforme: A primary malignant form of brain neoplasm: Its clinical and anatomic features. Archives of Neurology and Psychiatry. 1925;**14**(2):139-191

[4] Ribbert H. Über das Spongioblastom und das Gliom. Virchows Archiv. 1918;**225**(2):195-213

[5] Strauss I, Globus J. Spongioblastoma with unusually rapid growth following decompression. Neurological Bulletin. 1918;**1**:273

[6] Millard NE, De Braganca KC. Medulloblastoma. Journal of Child Neurology. 2016;**31**(12):1341-1353

[7] Rorke LB. Presidential address: The cerebellar medulloblastoma and its relationship to primitive neuroectodermal tumors. Journal of Neuropathology & Experimental Neurology. 1983;**42**(1):1-15

[8] Quinlan A, Rizzolo D. Understanding medulloblastoma. Journal of the American Academy of PAs. 2017;**30**(10):30-36

[9] Chin HW, Maruyama Y, Young AB. Medulloblastoma: Recent advances and directions in diagnosis and management—Part I. Current Problems in Cancer. 1984;**8**(11):1-54

[10] Pickles JC, Hawkins C, Pietsch T, Jacques TS. CNS embryonal tumours: WHO 2016 and beyond. Neuropathology and Applied Neurobiology. 2018;**44**(2):151-162

[11] Farwell JR, Dohrmann GJ, Flannery JT. Medulloblastoma in childhood: An epidemiological study. Journal of Neurosurgery. 1984;**61**(4):657-664

[12] Packer RJ, Sutton LN, Goldwein JW, Perilongo G, Bunin G, Ryan J, et al. Improved survival with the use of adjuvant chemotherapy in the treatment of medulloblastoma. Journal of Neurosurgery. 1991;**74**(3):433-440

[13] Paterson E, Farr R. Cerebellar medulloblastoma: Treatment by irradiation of the whole central nervous system. Acta Radiologica. 1953;**39**(4):323-336

[14] Ramaswamy V, Remke M, Adamski J, Bartels U, Tabori U, Wang X, et al. Medulloblastoma subgroup-specific outcomes in irradiated children: Who are the true high-risk patients? Neuro-Oncology. 2015;**18**(2):291-297

[15] Allen J, Donahue B, Mehta M, Miller DC, Rorke LB, Jakacki R, et al. A phase II study of preradiotherapy chemotherapy followed by hyperfractionated radiotherapy for newly diagnosed high-risk medulloblastoma/primitive neuroectodermal tumor: A report from

the Children's oncology group (CCG 9931). International Journal of Radiation Oncology, Biology, Physics. 2009;**74**(4):1006-1011

[16] Jakacki RI, Burger PC, Zhou T, Holmes EJ, Kocak M, Onar A, et al. Outcome of children with metastatic medulloblastoma treated with carboplatin during craniospinal radiotherapy: A Children's oncology group phase I/II study. Journal of Clinical Oncology. 2012;**30**(21):2648-2653

[17] Lannering B, Rutkowski S, Doz F, Pizer B, Gustafsson G, Navajas A, et al. Hyperfractionated versus conventional radiotherapy followed by chemotherapy in standard-risk medulloblastoma: Results from the randomized multicenter HIT-SIOP PNET 4 trial. Journal of Clinical Oncology. 2012;**30**(26):3187-3193

[18] Taylor RE, Bailey CC, Robinson K, Weston CL, Ellison D, Ironside J, et al. Results of a randomized study of preradiation chemotherapy versus radiotherapy alone for non-metastatic medulloblastoma: The International Society of Paediatric Oncology/United Kingdom Children's Cancer study group PNET-3 study. Journal of Clinical Oncology. 2003;**21**(8):1581-1591

[19] von Hoff K, Hinkes B, Gerber NU, Deinlein F, Mittler U, Urban C, et al. Long-term outcome and clinical prognostic factors in children with medulloblastoma treated in the prospective randomised multicentre trial HIT '91. European Journal of Cancer. 2009;**45**(7):1209-1217

[20] Bautista F, Fioravantti V, Carceller F, Madero L, Lassaletta A, Moreno L. Medulloblastoma in children and adolescents: a systematic review of contemporary phase I and II clinical trials and biology update. Cancer medicine. 2017;**6**(11):2606-2624

[21] McNeil DE, Coté TR, Clegg L, Rorke LB. Incidence and trends in pediatric malignancies medulloblastoma/primitive neuroectodermal tumor: A SEER update. Pediatric Blood & Cancer. 2002;**39**(3):190-194

[22] Ostrom QT, De Blank PM, Kruchko C, Petersen CM, Liao P, Finlay JL, et al. Alex's lemonade stand foundation infant and childhood primary brain and central nervous system tumors diagnosed in the United States in 2007-2011. Neuro-Oncology. 2014;**16**(suppl_10):x1-x36

[23] Ostrom QT, Gittleman H, Fulop J, Liu M, Blanda R, Kromer C, et al. CBTRUS statistical report: Primary brain and central nervous system tumors diagnosed in the United States in 2008-2012. Neuro-Oncology. 2015;**17**(Suppl 4):iv1

[24] Brandes AA, Bartolotti M, Marucci G, Ghimenton C, Agati R, Fioravanti A, et al. New perspectives in the treatment of adult medulloblastoma in the era of molecular oncology. Critical Reviews in Oncology/Hematology. 2015;**94**(3):348-359

[25] Packer RJ, Cogen P, Vezina G, Rorke LB. Medulloblastoma: Clinical and biologic aspects. Neuro-Oncology. 1999;**1**(3):232-250

[26] Park TS, Hoffman HJ, Hendrick EB, Humphreys RP, Becker LE. Medulloblastoma: Clinical presentation and management: Experience at the hospital for sick children, Toronto, 1950-1980. Journal of Neurosurgery. 1983;**58**(4):543-552

[27] Baryawno N, Rahbar A, Wolmer-Solberg N, Taher C, Odeberg J, Darabi A, et al. Detection of human cytomegalovirus in medulloblastomas reveals a potential therapeutic target. The Journal of Clinical Investigation. 2011;**121**(10):4043

[28] Hortal AM, Vermeulen JF, Van Hecke W, Bovenschen N. Oncogenic role of cytomegalovirus in medulloblastoma? Cancer Letters. 2017;**408**:55-59

[29] Libard S, Popova SN, Amini R-M, Kärjä V, Pietiläinen T, Hämäläinen KM, et al. Human cytomegalovirus tegument protein pp65 is detected in all intra-and extra-axial brain tumours independent of the tumour type or grade. PLoS One. 2014;**9**(9):e108861

[30] Louis DN, Ohgaki H, Wiestler OD, Cavenee WK, Burger PC, Jouvet A, et al. The 2007 WHO classification of tumours of the central nervous system. Acta Neuropathologica. 2007;**114**(2):97-109

[31] Bailey P. Further notes on the cerebellar medulloblastomas: The effect of roentgen radiation. The American Journal of Pathology. 1930;**6**(2):125

[32] Crawford JR, MacDonald TJ, Packer RJ. Medulloblastoma in childhood: New biological advances. The Lancet Neurology. 2007;**6**(12):1073-1085

[33] Gulino A, Arcella A, Giangaspero F. Pathological and molecular heterogeneity of medulloblastoma. Current Opinion in Oncology. 2008;**20**(6):668-675

[34] Rubinstein L, Northfield D. The medulloblastoma and the so-called "arachnoidal cerebellar sarcoma" a critical re-examination of a nosological problem. Brain. 1964;**87**(2):379-412

[35] Kleihues P, Burger PC, Scheithauer BW. The new WHO classification of brain tumours. Brain Pathology. 1993;**3**(3):255-268

[36] Rorke LB, Gilles FH, Davis RL, Becker LE. Revision of the World Health Organization classification of brain tumors for childhood brain tumors. Cancer. 1985;**56**(S7):1869-1886

[37] Eberhart CG, Kepner JL, Goldthwaite PT, Kun LE, Duffner PK, Friedman HS, et al. Histopathologic grading of medulloblastomas. Cancer. 2002;**94**(2):552-560

[38] Kleihues P, Louis DN, Scheithauer BW, Rorke LB, Reifenberger G, Burger PC, et al. The WHO classification of tumors of the nervous system. Journal of Neuropathology & Experimental Neurology. 2002;**61**(3):215-225

[39] Gajjar A, Pfister SM, Taylor MD, Gilbertson RJ. Molecular insights into pediatric brain tumors have the potential to transform therapy. Clinical Cancer Research. 2014;**20**(22):5630-5640

[40] Louis DN, Perry A, Reifenberger G, Von Deimling A, Figarella-Branger D, Cavenee WK, et al. The 2016 World Health Organization classification of tumors of the central nervous system: A summary. Acta Neuropathologica. 2016;**131**(6):803-820

[41] Schwalbe EC, Lindsey JC, Nakjang S, Crosier S, Smith AJ, Hicks D, et al. Novel molecular subgroups for clinical classification and outcome prediction in childhood medulloblastoma: A cohort study. The Lancet Oncology. 2017;**18**(7):958-971

[42] Taylor MD, Northcott PA, Korshunov A, Remke M, Cho Y-J, Clifford SC, et al. Molecular subgroups of medulloblastoma: The current consensus. Acta Neuropathologica. 2012; **123**(4):465-472

[43] Gibson P, Tong Y, Robinson G, Thompson MC, Currle DS, Eden C, et al. Subtypes of medulloblastoma have distinct developmental origins. Nature. 2010;**468**(7327):1095-1099

[44] Ramaswamy V, Remke M, Bouffet E, Faria CC, Perreault S, Cho Y-J, et al. Recurrence patterns across medulloblastoma subgroups: An integrated clinical and molecular analysis. The Lancet Oncology. 2013;**14**(12):1200-1207

[45] Wang X, Dubuc AM, Ramaswamy V, Mack S, Gendoo DM, Remke M, et al. Medulloblastoma subgroups remain stable across primary and metastatic compartments. Acta Neuropathologica. 2015;**129**(3):449-457

[46] Northcott PA, Korshunov A, Pfister SM, Taylor MD. The clinical implications of medulloblastoma subgroups. Nature Reviews Neurology. 2012;**8**(6):340-351

[47] Ellison DW, Kocak M, Dalton J, Megahed H, Lusher ME, Ryan SL, et al. Definition of disease-risk stratification groups in childhood medulloblastoma using combined clinical, pathologic, and molecular variables. Journal of Clinical Oncology. 2010;**29**(11):1400-1407

[48] Zhukova N, Ramaswamy V, Remke M, Pfaff E, Shih DJ, Martin DC, et al. Subgroup-specific prognostic implications of TP53 mutation in medulloblastoma. Journal of Clinical Oncology. 2013;**31**(23):2927-2935

[49] Staedtke V, Dzaye OD, Holdhoff M. Actionable molecular biomarkers in primary brain tumors. Trends in Cancer. 2016;**2**(7):338-349

[50] Kool M, Korshunov A, Remke M, Jones DT, Schlanstein M, Northcott PA, et al. Molecular subgroups of medulloblastoma: An international meta-analysis of transcriptome, genetic aberrations, and clinical data of WNT, SHH, Group 3, and Group 4 medulloblastomas. Acta Neuropathologica. 2012;**123**(4):473-484

[51] Shih DJ, Northcott PA, Remke M, Korshunov A, Ramaswamy V, Kool M, et al. Cytogenetic prognostication within medulloblastoma subgroups. Journal of Clinical Oncology. 2014;**32**(9):886-896

[52] Smith MJ, Beetz C, Williams SG, Bhaskar SS, O'Sullivan J, Anderson B, et al. Germline mutations in SUFU cause Gorlin syndrome-associated childhood medulloblastoma and redefine the risk associated with PTCH1 mutations. Journal of Clinical Oncology. 2014;**32**(36):4155-4161

[53] Rausch T, Jones DT, Zapatka M, Stütz AM, Zichner T, Weischenfeldt J, et al. Genome sequencing of pediatric medulloblastoma links catastrophic DNA rearrangements with TP53 mutations. Cell. 2012;**148**(1):59-71

[54] Cavalli FM, Remke M, Rampasek L, Peacock J, Shih DJ, Luu B, et al. Intertumoral heterogeneity within medulloblastoma subgroups. Cancer Cell. 2017;**31**(6):737-754 (e6)

[55] Cho Y-J, Tsherniak A, Tamayo P, Santagata S, Ligon A, Greulich H, et al. Integrative genomic analysis of medulloblastoma identifies a molecular subgroup that drives poor clinical outcome. Journal of Clinical Oncology. 2010;**29**(11):1424-1430

[56] Kool M, Koster J, Bunt J, Hasselt NE, Lakeman A, Van Sluis P, et al. Integrated genomics identifies five medulloblastoma subtypes with distinct genetic profiles, pathway signatures and clinicopathological features. PLoS One. 2008;**3**(8):e3088

[57] Northcott PA, Korshunov A, Witt H, Hielscher T, Eberhart CG, Mack S, et al. Medulloblastoma comprises four distinct molecular variants. Journal of Clinical Oncology. 2010;**29**(11):1408-1414

[58] Hatten ME, Roussel MF. Development and cancer of the cerebellum. Trends in Neurosciences. 2011;**34**(3):134-142

[59] Pfister S, Remke M, Benner A, Mendrzyk F, Toedt G, Felsberg J, et al. Outcome prediction in pediatric medulloblastoma based on DNA copy-number aberrations of chromosomes 6q and 17q and the MYC and MYCN loci. Journal of Clinical Oncology. 2009;**27**(10):1627-1636

[60] Banan R, Hartmann C. The new WHO 2016 classification of brain tumors—What neurosurgeons need to know. Acta Neurochirurgica. 2017;**159**(3):403-418

[61] Louis DN, Perry A, Burger P, Ellison DW, Reifenberger G, Deimling A, et al. International Society of Neuropathology-Haarlem consensus guidelines for nervous system tumor classification and grading. Brain Pathology. 2014;**24**(5):429-435

[62] Chang CH, Housepian EM, Herbert C. An operative staging system and a megavoltage radiotherapeutic technic for cerebellar medulloblastomas. Radiology. 1969;**93**(6): 1351-1359

[63] Dufour C, Beaugrand A, Pizer B, Micheli J, Aubelle M-S, Fourcade A, et al. Metastatic medulloblastoma in childhood: Chang's classification revisited. International Journal of Surgical Oncology. 2012;**2012**:1-6

[64] Packer RJ, Vezina G. Management of and prognosis with medulloblastoma: Therapy at a crossroads. Archives of Neurology. 2008;**65**(11):1419-1424

[65] Wilne S, Collier J, Kennedy C, Jenkins A, Grout J, Mackie S, et al. Progression from first symptom to diagnosis in childhood brain tumours. European Journal of Pediatrics. 2012;**171**(1):87-93

[66] Ramaswamy V, Remke M, Shih D, Wang X, Northcott PA, Faria CC, et al. Duration of the pre-diagnostic interval in medulloblastoma is subgroup dependent. Pediatric Blood & Cancer. 2014;**61**(7):1190-1194

[67] Fouladi M, Gajjar A, Boyett JM, Walter AW, Thompson SJ, Merchant TE, et al. Comparison of CSF cytology and spinal magnetic resonance imaging in the detection of leptomeningeal disease in pediatric medulloblastoma or primitive neuroectodermal tumor. Journal of Clinical Oncology. 1999;**17**(10):3234-3237

[68] Packer RJ, Gajjar A, Vezina G, Rorke-Adams L, Burger PC, Robertson PL, et al. Phase III study of craniospinal radiation therapy followed by adjuvant chemotherapy for newly diagnosed average-risk medulloblastoma. Journal of Clinical Oncology. 2006;**24**(25):4202-4208

[69] Müller W, Afra D, Schröder R, Slowik F, Wilcke O, Klug N. Medulloblastoma: Survey of factors possibly influencing the prognosis. Acta Neurochirurgica. 1982;**64**(3):215-224

[70] Sutton LN, Phillips PC, Molloy PT. Surgical management of medulloblastoma. Journal of Neuro-Oncology. 1996;**29**(1):9-21

[71] Chin HW, Maruyama Y, Young AB. Medulloblastoma: Recent advances and directions in diagnosis and management—Part II. Current Problems in Cancer. 1984;**8**(12):1-51

[72] Yuh GE, Loredo LN, Yonemoto LT, Bush DA, Shahnazi K, Preston W, et al. Reducing toxicity from craniospinal irradiation: Using proton beams to treat medulloblastoma in young children. The Cancer Journal. 2004;**10**(6):386-390

[73] Gajjar A, Chintagumpala M, Ashley D, Kellie S, Kun LE, Merchant TE, et al. Risk-adapted craniospinal radiotherapy followed by high-dose chemotherapy and stem-cell rescue in children with newly diagnosed medulloblastoma (St Jude Medulloblastoma-96): Long-term results from a prospective, multicentre trial. The Lancet Oncology. 2006; **7**(10):813-820

[74] Merchant TE, Kun LE, Krasin MJ, Wallace D, Chintagumpala MM, Woo SY, et al. Multi-institution prospective trial of reduced-dose craniospinal irradiation (23.4 Gy) followed by conformal posterior fossa (36 Gy) and primary site irradiation (55.8 Gy) and dose-intensive chemotherapy for average-risk medulloblastoma. International Journal of Radiation Oncology Biology Physics. 2008;**70**(3):782-787

[75] Fukunaga-Johnson N, Lee JH, Sandler HM, Robertson P, McNeil E, Goldwein JW. Patterns of failure following treatment for medulloblastoma: Is it necessary to treat the entire posterior fossa? International Journal of Radiation Oncology Biology Physics. 1998;**42**(1):143-146

[76] Wolden SL, Dunkel IJ, Souweidane MM, Happersett L, Khakoo Y, Schupak K, et al. Patterns of failure using a conformal radiation therapy tumor bed boost for medulloblastoma. Journal of Clinical Oncology. 2003;**21**(16):3079-3083

[77] Clair WS, Adams J, Bues M, Fullerton B, La Shell S, Kooy H, et al. Advantage of protons compared to conventional X-ray or IMRT in the treatment of a pediatric patient with medulloblastoma. International Journal of Radiation Oncology Biology Physics. 2004;**58**(3):727-734

[78] Panandiker AP, Ning H, Likhacheva A, Ullman K, Arora B, Ondos J, et al. Craniospinal irradiation with spinal IMRT to improve target homogeneity. International Journal of Radiation Oncology Biology Physics. 2007;**68**(5):1402-1409

[79] Parker W, Filion E, Roberge D, Freeman CR. Intensity-modulated radiotherapy for craniospinal irradiation: Target volume considerations, dose constraints, and competing risks. International Journal of Radiation Oncology Biology Physics. 2007;**69**(1):251-257

[80] Packer RJ, Sutton LN, Elterman R, Lange B, Goldwein J, Nicholson HS, et al. Outcome for children with medulloblastoma treated with radiation and cisplatin, CCNU, and vincristine chemotherapy. Journal of Neurosurgery. 1994;**81**(5):690-698

[81] Kortmann R-D, Kühl J, Timmermann B, Mittler U, Urban C, Budach V, et al. Postoperative neoadjuvant chemotherapy before radiotherapy as compared to immediate radiotherapy followed by maintenance chemotherapy in the treatment of medulloblastoma in childhood: Results of the German prospective randomized trial HIT'91. International Journal of Radiation Oncology Biology Physics. 2000;**46**(2):269-279

[82] Taylor RE, Bailey CC, Robinson KJ, Weston CL, Walker DA, Ellison D, et al. Outcome for patients with metastatic (M2-3) medulloblastoma treated with SIOP/UKCCSG PNET-3 chemotherapy. European Journal of Cancer. 2005;**41**(5):727-734

[83] Zeltzer PM, Boyett JM, Finlay JL, Albright AL, Rorke LB, Milstein JM, et al. Metastasis stage, adjuvant treatment, and residual tumor are prognostic factors for medulloblastoma in children: Conclusions from the Children's Cancer group 921 randomized phase III study. Journal of Clinical Oncology. 1999;**17**(3):832

[84] Grill J, Sainte-Rose C, Jouvet A, Gentet J-C, Lejars O, Frappaz D, et al. Treatment of medulloblastoma with postoperative chemotherapy alone: An SFOP prospective trial in young children. The Lancet Oncology. 2005;**6**(8):573-580

[85] Gurney JG, Kadan-Lottick NS, Packer RJ, Neglia JP, Sklar CA, Punyko JA, et al. Endocrine and cardiovascular late effects among adult survivors of childhood brain tumors. Cancer. 2003;**97**(3):663-673

[86] Packer RJ, Gurney JG, Punyko JA, Donaldson SS, Inskip PD, Stovall M, et al. Long-term neurologic and neurosensory sequelae in adult survivors of a childhood brain tumor: Childhood cancer survivor study. Journal of Clinical Oncology. 2003;**21**(17):3255-3261

[87] De Braganca KC, Packer RJ. Treatment options for medulloblastoma and CNS primitive neuroectodermal tumor (PNET). Current Treatment Options in Neurology. 2013;**15**(5): 593-606

[88] Cefalo G, Massimino M, Ruggiero A, Barone G, Ridola V, Spreafico F, et al. Temozolomide is an active agent in children with recurrent medulloblastoma/primitive neuroectodermal tumor: An Italian multi-institutional phase II trial. Neuro-Oncology. 2014;**16**(5):748-753

[89] Grill J, Geoerger B, Gesner L, Perek D, Leblond P, Cañete A, et al. Phase II study of irinotecan in combination with temozolomide (TEMIRI) in children with recurrent or refractory medulloblastoma: A joint ITCC and SIOPE brain tumor study. Neuro-Oncology. 2013; **15**(9):1236-1243

[90] Dhall G, Grodman H, Ji L, Sands S, Gardner S, Dunkel IJ, et al. Outcome of children less than three years old at diagnosis with non-metastatic medulloblastoma treated with chemotherapy on the "head start" I and II protocols. Pediatric Blood & Cancer. 2008;**50**(6):1169-1175

[91] Dhall G, Ji L, Haley K, Grimm JP, Gilles FH, Gardner SL, et al. Outcome of infants and young children with newly diagnosed medulloblastoma treated on head start III protocol. Journal of Clinical Oncology.. 2011;**29**(15_suppl):2011

[92] Van Eys J, Chen T, Moore T, Cheek W, Sexauer C, Starling K. Adjuvant chemotherapy for medulloblastoma and ependymoma using iv vincristine, intrathecal methotrexate, and intrathecal hydrocortisone: A southwest oncology group study. Cancer Treatment Reports. 1981;**65**(7-8):681

[93] Pezzotta S, Knerich R, Butti G. Chemotherapy for medulloblastoma in children current status and future prospects. Pediatric Neurosurgery. 1982;**9**(3-4):294-298

[94] Packer RJ, Zhou T, Holmes E, Vezina G, Gajjar A. Survival and secondary tumors in children with medulloblastoma receiving radiotherapy and adjuvant chemotherapy: Results of Children's oncology group trial A9961. Neuro-Oncology. 2012;**15**(1):97-103

[95] Trobaugh-Lotrario AD, Smith AA, Odom LF. Vincristine neurotoxicity in the presence of hereditary neuropathy. Pediatric Blood & Cancer. 2003;**40**(1):39-43

[96] Bowers DC, Gargan L, Weprin BE, Mulne AF, Elterman RD, Munoz L, Giller CA, Winick NJ. Impact of site of tumor recurrence upon survival for children with recurrent or progressive medulloblastoma. Journal of neurosurgery. 2007;**107**(1 Suppl):5-10

[97] Dunkel IJ, Boyett JM, Yates A, Rosenblum M, Garvin JH Jr, Bostrom BC, et al. High-dose carboplatin, thiotepa, and etoposide with autologous stem-cell rescue for patients with recurrent medulloblastoma. Children's Cancer group. Journal of Clinical Oncology. 1998;**16**(1):222-228

[98] Dunkel IJ, Gardner SL, Garvin JH, Goldman S, Shi W, Finlay JL. High-dose carboplatin, thiotepa, and etoposide with autologous stem cell rescue for patients with previously irradiated recurrent medulloblastoma. Neuro-Oncology. 2010;**12**(3):297-303

[99] Kadota RP, Mahoney DH, Doyle J, Duerst R, Friedman H, Holmes E, et al. Dose intensive melphalan and cyclophosphamide with autologous hematopoietic stem cells for recurrent medulloblastoma or germinoma. Pediatric Blood & Cancer. 2008;**51**(5):675-678

[100] Wetmore C, Herington D, Lin T, Onar-Thomas A, Gajjar A, Merchant TE. Reirradiation of recurrent medulloblastoma: Does clinical benefit outweigh risk for toxicity? Cancer. 2014;**120**(23):3731-3737

[101] Bakst RL, Dunkel IJ, Gilheeney S, Khakoo Y, Becher O, Souweidane MM, et al. Reirradiation for recurrent medulloblastoma. Cancer. 2011;**117**(21):4977-4982

[102] Yamada A, Moritake H, Kamimura S, Yamashita S, Takeshima H, Nunoi H. Proposed strategy for the use of high-dose chemotherapy with stem cell rescue and intrathecal topotecan without whole-brain irradiation for infantile classic medulloblastoma. Pediatric Blood & Cancer. 2014;**61**(12):2316-2318

[103] Aguilera D, Mazewski C, Fangusaro J, MacDonald TJ, McNall-Knapp RY, Hayes LL, et al. Response to bevacizumab, irinotecan, and temozolomide in children with relapsed medulloblastoma: A multi-institutional experience. Child's Nervous System. 2013;**29**(4):589-596

[104] Ashley DM, Meier L, Kerby T, Zalduondo FM, Friedman HS, Gajjar A, et al. Response of recurrent medulloblastoma to low-dose oral etoposide. Journal of Clinical Oncology. 1996;**14**(6):1922-1927

[105] Gururangan S, Krauser J, Watral MA, Driscoll T, Larrier N, Reardon DA, et al. Efficacy of high-dose chemotherapy or standard salvage therapy in patients with recurrent medulloblastoma. Neuro-Oncology. 2008;**10**(5):745-751

[106] Guruangan S, Dunkel IJ, Goldman S, Garvin JH, Rosenblum M, Boyett JM, et al. Myeloablative chemotherapy with autologous bone marrow rescue in young children with recurrent malignant brain tumors. Journal of Clinical Oncology. 1998;**16**(7): 2486-2493

[107] Milker-Zabel S, Zabel A, Thilmann C, Zuna I, Hoess A, Wannenmacher M, et al. Results of three-dimensional stereotactically-guided radiotherapy in recurrent medulloblastoma. Journal of Neuro-Oncology. 2002;**60**(3):227-233

[108] Saunders DE, Hayward RD, Phipps KP, Chong WK, Wade AM. Surveillance neuroimaging of intracranial medulloblastoma in children: How effective, how often, and for how long? Journal of Neurosurgery. 2003;**99**(2):280-286

[109] Bartels U, Shroff M, Sung L, Dag-Ellams U, Laperriere N, Rutka J, et al. Role of spinal MRI in the follow-up of children treated for medulloblastoma. Cancer. 2006;**107**(6):1340-1347

[110] Perreault S, Lober RM, Carret A-S, Zhang G, Hershon L, Décarie J-C, et al. Surveillance imaging in children with malignant CNS tumors: Low yield of spine MRI. Journal of Neuro-Oncology. 2014;**116**(3):617-623

[111] Perreault S, Lober RM, Carret A-S, Zhang G, Hershon L, Décarie J-C, et al. Relapse patterns in pediatric embryonal central nervous system tumors. Journal of Neuro-Oncology. 2013;**115**(2):209-215

[112] Sethi RV, Giantsoudi D, Raiford M, Malhi I, Niemierko A, Rapalino O, et al. Patterns of failure after proton therapy in medulloblastoma; linear energy transfer distributions and relative biological effectiveness associations for relapses. International Journal of Radiation Oncology Biology Physics. 2014;**88**(3):655-663

[113] Greenberg HS, Chamberlain MC, Glantz MJ, Wang S. Adult medulloblastoma: Multiagent chemotherapy. Neuro-Oncology. 2001;**3**(1):29-34

[114] Chan AW, Tarbell NJ, Black PM, Louis DN, Frosch MP, Ancukiewicz M, et al. Adult medulloblastoma: Prognostic factors and patterns of relapse. Neurosurgery. 2000;**47**(3): 623-632

[115] Abacioglu U, Uzel O, Sengoz M, Turkan S, Ober A. Medulloblastoma in adults: Treatment results and prognostic factors. International Journal of Radiation Oncology Biology Physics. 2002;**54**(3):855-860

[116] Menon G, Krishnakumar K, Nair S. Adult medulloblastoma: Clinical profile and treatment results of 18 patients. Journal of Clinical Neuroscience. 2008;**15**(2):122-126

[117] Mokhtech M, Morris CG, Indelicato DJ, Rutenberg MS, Amdur RJ. Patterns of failure in patients with adult medulloblastoma presenting without extraneural metastasis. American Journal of Clinical Oncology. 2017;**14**:50

[118] Riffaud L, Saikali S, Leray E, Hamlat A, Haegelen C, Vauleon E, et al. Survival and prognostic factors in a series of adults with medulloblastomas. Journal of Neurosurgery. 2009;**111**(3):478-487

[119] Rutkowski S, von Hoff K, Emser A, Zwiener I, Pietsch T, Figarella-Branger D, et al. Survival and prognostic factors of early childhood medulloblastoma: An international meta-analysis. Journal of Clinical Oncology. 2010;**28**(33):4961-4968

[120] Chidambaram A, Gerrard B, Hanson M, Dean M. Chromosomal localization of the human and murine orthologues of the Drosophila smoothened gene. Genomics. 1998;**53**(3):416-417

[121] Wang C, Wu H, Evron T, Vardy E, Han GW, Huang X-P, et al. Structural basis for smoothened receptor modulation and chemoresistance to anticancer drugs. Nature Communications. 2014;**5**:4355

[122] Gajjar A, Stewart CF, Ellison DW, Kaste S, Kun LE, Packer RJ, et al. Phase I study of vismodegib in children with recurrent or refractory medulloblastoma: A pediatric brain tumor consortium study. Clinical Cancer Research. 2013;**19**(22):6305-6312

[123] Geoerger B, Aerts I, Casanova M, Chisholm JC, Hargrave DR, Leary S, et al. A phase I/II study of LDE225, a smoothened (Smo) antagonist, in pediatric patients with recurrent medulloblastoma (MB) or other solid tumors. American Society of Clinical Oncology. 2012;**2012**:9519

[124] Robinson GW, Orr BA, Wu G, Gururangan S, Lin T, Qaddoumi I, et al. Vismodegib exerts targeted efficacy against recurrent sonic hedgehog-subgroup medulloblastoma: Results from phase II Pediatric brain tumor consortium studies PBTC-025B and PBTC-032. Journal of Clinical Oncology. 2015;**33**(24):2646-2654

[125] Rudin CM, Hann CL, Laterra J, Yauch RL, Callahan CA, Fu L, et al. Treatment of medulloblastoma with hedgehog pathway inhibitor GDC-0449. New England Journal of Medicine. 2009;**361**(12):1173-1178

[126] DeSouza R-M, Jones BR, Lowis SP, Kurian KM. Pediatric medulloblastoma – Update on molecular classification driving targeted therapies. Frontiers in Oncology. 2014;**4**:176

[127] Bomgaars L, Geyer J, Franklin J, Dahl G, Park J, Winick N, et al. Phase I trial of intrathecal liposomal cytarabine in children with neoplastic meningitis. Journal of Clinical Oncology. 2004;**22**(19):3916-3921

[128] Kumar V, McGuire T, Coulter DW, Sharp JG, Mahato RI. Challenges and recent advances in medulloblastoma therapy. Trends in Pharmacological Sciences. 2017;**38**(12):1061-1084

[129] Morfouace M, Shelat A, Jacus M, Freeman BB, Turner D, Robinson S, et al. Pemetrexed and gemcitabine as combination therapy for the treatment of Group 3 medulloblastoma. Cancer Cell. 2014;**25**(4):516-529

[130] Geoerger B, Chisholm J, Le Deley M-C, Gentet J-C, Zwaan CM, Dias N, et al. Phase II study of gemcitabine combined with oxaliplatin in relapsed or refractory paediatric solid malignancies: An innovative therapy for children with Cancer European consortium study. European Journal of Cancer. 2011;**47**(2):230-238

[131] Fouladi M, Park JR, Stewart CF, Gilbertson RJ, Schaiquevich P, Sun J, et al. Pediatric phase I trial and pharmacokinetic study of vorinostat: A Children's oncology group phase I consortium report. Journal of Clinical Oncology. 2010;**28**(22):3623-3629

[132] Chintagumpala M, Blaney SM, Bomgaars LR, Aleksic A, Kuttesch JF, Klenke RA, et al. Phase I and pharmacokinetic study of thalidomide with carboplatin in children with cancer. Journal of Clinical Oncology. 2004;**22**(21):4394-4400

[133] MacDonald TJ, Stewart CF, Kocak M, Goldman S, Ellenbogen RG, Phillips P, et al. Phase I clinical trial of cilengitide in children with refractory brain tumors: Pediatric brain tumor consortium study PBTC-012. Journal of Clinical Oncology. 2008;**26**(6):919-924

[134] Piha-Paul SA, Shin SJ, Vats T, Guha-Thakurta N, Aaron J, Rytting M, et al. Pediatric patients with refractory central nervous system tumors: Experiences of a clinical trial combining bevacizumab and temsirolimus. Anticancer Research. 2014;**34**(4):1939-1945

[135] Robison NJ, Campigotto F, Chi SN, Manley PE, Turner CD, Zimmerman MA, et al. A phase II trial of a multi-agent oral antiangiogenic (metronomic) regimen in children with recurrent or progressive cancer. Pediatric Blood & Cancer. 2014;**61**(4):636-642

[136] Venkatramani R, Malogolowkin M, Davidson TB, May W, Sposto R, Mascarenhas L. A phase I study of vincristine, irinotecan, temozolomide and bevacizumab (vitb) in pediatric patients with relapsed solid tumors. PLoS One. 2013;**8**(7):e68416

[137] Warren KE, Goldman S, Pollack IF, Fangusaro J, Schaiquevich P, Stewart CF, et al. Phase I trial of lenalidomide in pediatric patients with recurrent, refractory, or progressive primary CNS tumors: Pediatric brain tumor consortium study PBTC-018. Journal of Clinical Oncology. 2010;**29**(3):324-329

[138] Kasuga C, Nakahara Y, Ueda S, Hawkins C, Taylor MD, Smith CA, et al. Expression of MAGE and GAGE genes in medulloblastoma and modulation of resistance to chemotherapy. Pediatrics. 2008;**1**(4):305-313

[139] Oba-Shinjo SM, Caballero OL, Jungbluth AA, Rosemberg S, Old LJ, Simpson AJ, et al. Cancer-testis (CT) antigen expression in medulloblastoma. Cancer Immunity Archive. 2008;**8**(1):7

[140] Atanackovic D, Altorki NK, Stockert E, Williamson B, Jungbluth AA, Ritter E, et al. Vaccine-induced CD4+ T cell responses to MAGE-3 protein in lung cancer patients. The Journal of Immunology. 2004;**172**(5):3289-3296

[141] Kim S, Castro F, Gonzalez D, Maciag P, Paterson Y, Gravekamp C. Mage-b vaccine delivered by recombinant listeria monocytogenes is highly effective against breast cancer metastases. British Journal of Cancer. 2008;**99**(5):741

[142] Kim W, Liau LM. Dendritic cell vaccines for brain tumors. Neurosurgery Clinics. 2010;**21**(1):139-157

9

Pre and Postoperative Management of Pediatric Patients with Congenital Heart Diseases

Eva Miranda Marwali, Beatrice Heineking and Nikolaus A. Haas

Abstract

Stabilization during preoperative cardiac surgery especially in neonates has an important role to predict outcome for pediatric congenital heart surgery. We tried to elaborate general guidelines on how to diagnose and some anticipations for emergency treatments tailored by the type of congenital heart disease in neonates. Stabilization consists of medical treatment including emergent prostaglandin institution in some types of duct dependent lesion. The role of interventional catheterization such as patent ductus arteriosus (PDA) stent, balloon pulmonary valvotomy, etc. as modalities for stabilization before surgery was also elaborated. Some general and specific guidelines based on the type of surgeries for postoperative management were also discussed.

Keywords: pediatric, congenital heart disease, preoperative stabilization, postoperative management

1. Initial treatment of critically ill neonates with cardiac defects

In the following paragraphs of this chapter, the general features of various congenital heart defects, their clinical symptoms and treatment principles for the management of congenital heart defects that become symptomatic in neonates will be discussed. In this context, the special measures for the initial treatment of the most common defects are presented [1–8, 11].

1.1. Epidemiology

Based on many epidemiological studies, the actual incidence of congenital heart defects is 8–11 per 1000 live births independent of ethical background, social welfare or medical standards.

As a rule thumb nearly half of these children require any form of surgical or interventional intervention within the first year of life. With adequate management, more than 90% of these children can reach adulthood and lead a relatively normal life.

1.2. Symptoms

It is typical for the different congenital heart defects to present and become manifest at different times in early life. Of most importance are the very early phase when the patent ductus arteriosus closes for all ductal-dependent cardiac defects; the next important timeframe of clinical manifestation is the reduction in pulmonary vascular resistance (PVR) for defects with left-to-right shunt.

Note

Typical leading symptoms for the presentation of congenital heart defects in neonates are as follows:

- Heart failure or cardiogenic shock (usually in the first or second week of life if there is left heart obstruction; for shunt defects typically not until after the drop in pulmonary resistance at the age of 2–8 weeks)
- Cyanosis

Additional important clinical symptoms that may lead to the diagnosis of a congenital heart defect in neonates are the presence of a murmur on auscultation or any form of arrhythmia (rarely as the primary symptom of a congenital heart defect).

1.2.1. Heart failure

The characteristic clinical signs of heart failure in neonates are as follows:

- Tachypnea, dyspnea, thoracic retractions
- Rarely but possible pulmonary edema mainly due to overflow
- Tachycardia
- Hepatomegaly
- Failure to thrive, difficulty in feeding, increased sweating, abnormal sleepiness
- Pallor, prolonged capillary refill time

It is evident that the clinical symptoms of neonatal heart failure are unspecific and may be similar to the clinical symptoms of sepsis. Therefore, many neonates with heart failure are treated for suspected sepsis.

In particular, cardiac defects with left-sided obstruction (coarctation of the aorta, critical aortic stenosis, hypoplastic left heart syndrome), or typically become manifest as early as the first 1–2 weeks of life with the clinical symptoms of cardiogenic shock caused by early duct closure.

1.2.2. Cyanosis

- Cyanosis is a clinical sign that becomes evident when about 5% of the hemoglobin is deoxygenated. In neonates with polycythemia (Hb >20 g/dl), this may be present even without hypoxemia, in patients with anemia this may be overseen. To avoid this, pulse oximetry at all four limbs is the standard of care.
- *Neonatal screening*: Cyanosis in a newborn should be picked up by a neonatal screening program that measures saturation by pulse oximetry at all four extremities at the first day of life. It should be standard of care that all newborns should have this screening test. If the saturation is >95% and the control 12 h later is again >95%, a cyanotic heart defect can be ruled out. If the saturation is ≤95%, additional examinations (today—ECHO as the preferred method of choice) are needed.
- *Hyperoxia test*: The hyperoxia test is a more historical test and no longer useful in the times of ECHO. It was used to try and distinguish between cardiac and pulmonary cyanosis. In patients with pulmonary cyanosis, the oxygen saturation increases markedly after oxygen is given, while oxygen saturation is usually not significantly improved in those with cyanotic heart defects. This test lacks specificity and sensitivity to rule out or confirm cardiac defects. Both pre- and postductal oxygen saturation should be measured.
- Cardiac cyanosis can be the result of either reduced lung perfusion due to a right-to-left shunt, complete venous mixing in patients with total anomalous pulmonary venous return or intracardiac mixing of systemic and pulmonary venous blood. Methemoglobinemia is another rare cause for cyanosis. In addition, cyanosis can be caused by abnormality in the central nervous system (e.g., after cerebral hemorrhage or in cases with central apnea in premature neonates, etc.)

Note

All newborns should have a neonatal screening for congenital heart defects immediately after birth and 12 h later. Today ECHO is the main diagnostic tool for secondary investigation and to rule out or confirm congenital heart defects.

If the diagnosis can not be immediately confirmed by echocardiography, an attempt of treating the neonate with intravenous prostaglandin E1 is justified.

The hyperoxia test is no longer standard of care. If there is no adequate increase in oxygen saturation in a cyanosed neonate, a congenital heart defect with ductal dependent lung perfusion must be assumed.

1.2.3. Heart murmur

As innocent murmurs are unlikely in this age group, a heart murmur in a neonate is always suggestive of a congenital heart defect. Usually, stenosis of the semilunar valves or AV valve insufficiency present immediately after birth due to a loud systolic murmur, the typical VSD murmur in a large VSD, for example, can often be not auscultated until after the pulmonary resistance has dropped and the pressure gradient between the left and right ventricles increases. In addition, in many critical heart defects, there might be no indicative heart murmur at all (e.g., d-TGA simplex, coarctation of the aorta).

1.2.4. Arrhythmias

Arrhythmias often present in neonates without structural heart defects (i.e., atrial flutter, congenital AV block) and therefore are rarely the first symptom of a congenital heart defect. An AV block may occur in association with an l-TGA or heterotaxy syndromes. Supraventricular tachycardia due to accessory conduction pathways occurs more frequently with an Ebstein anomaly. The most common arrhythmia in a newborn is atrial flutter that requires immediate electrical cardioversion after diagnosis with adenosine but usually presents without additional defects.

1.3. Hemodynamic situation

The congenital heart defects that become symptomatic in neonates can be divided into five groups (**Table 1**).

Group	Examples
Cardiac defects with ductal-dependent systemic circulation (left heart obstructions)	Critical aortic stenosis, hypoplastic left heart syndrome, interrupted aortic arch, critical coarctation of the aorta
Cardiac defect with ductal-dependent pulmonary circulation (right heart obstructions)	Critical pulmonary stenosis, pulmonary atresia with intact ventricular septum, pulmonary atresia with VSD, pronounced form of Tetralogy of Fallot, severe Ebstein's anomaly, tricuspid atresia with pulmonary atresia or high-grade pulmonary stenosis
Cardiac defects with parallel circulation	d-TGA—transposition of the great arteries
Cardiac defects with complete intracardiac mixing of blood	Total anomalous pulmonary venous connection, univentricular heart
Cardiac defects with a large left-to-right shunt symptomatic usually after 4–6 weeks	Large VSD, complete AVSD, large PDA, aortopulmonary window, Truncus arteriosus communis, univentricular hearts with unobstructed pulmonary blood flow

Table 1. Classification of congenital heart defects which become symptomatic in the neonatal period.

In a ductal-dependent defect survival depends on the persistence of a patent ductus arteriosus. In general, ductal-dependent systemic circulation must be distinguished from ductal-dependent pulmonary circulation. In patients with ductal-dependent systemic circulation, there is a high-grade obstruction of the structures of the left heart (mitral valve, aortic valve, arch and coarctation). To ensure sufficient systemic perfusion, the systemic circulation must be supplied with blood from the pulmonary circulation across the patent ductus arteriosus like in utero. In ductal-dependent pulmonary circulation, there is a high-grade right heart obstruction leading to cyanosis. Perfusion of the pulmonary circulation depends mainly on the blood supply from the aorta across the patent ductus arteriosus.

In parallel circulations (d-TGA), survival depends on additional shunts (especially a sufficiently large atrial shunt) between the two circulations to enable mixing of the cyanosed and the arterialized blood.

In cardiac defects with complete intracardiac mixing of blood, the resulting cyanosis is often only relatively mild; when excessive pulmonary blood flow due to the lack of pulmonary stenosis is often present simultaneously, this leads to pulmonary recirculation of the saturated blood. Heart failure usually develops as a result of the excessive pulmonary blood flow after 4–6 weeks.

Based on this principle, congenital heart defects with a large left-to-right shunt do not become clinically symptomatic until the age of about 4–6 weeks; at that time, the PVR has dropped and the shunt between the systemic and pulmonary circulation increases dramatically. If left-sided heart obstruction is, however, also present (e.g., VSD with CoA), the symptoms may develop as early as the first week of life.

1.4. Diagnostic measures

1.4.1. Oxygen saturation

As a standard of care, oxygen saturation should always be measured in children both preductally (right hand) and postductally (lower limb). If there is a defect with ductal-dependent systemic circulation, the (postductal) oxygen saturation measured in the feet may be lower than the (preductal) saturation in the right hand.

The brachiocephalic trunk branches off from the aortic arch well before the ductus arteriosus; therefore, it is safe to assume that the saturation measured in the right hand is equivalent to preductal saturation (except in the rare cases of a lusoric artery).

1.4.2. Blood gas analysis (BGA)

As metabolic acidosis is the typical finding in severe heart failure and cardiogenic shock, routine (arterial) BGA is recommended on multiple occasions. In addition, all BGA should measure lactate as surrogate of cardiac output and thereby tissue perfusion.

1.4.3. Echocardiography (ECHO)

As mentioned before, today echocardiography is the diagnostic method of choice in all patients with a presumed cardiac defect or impaired circulatory situation. ECHO allows an accurate diagnosis of all significant cardiac defects that become symptomatic in the neonatal period. As modern standard of care, every neonatal unit must have ECHO and support of a pediatric cardiologist available on a 24/7 basis.

1.4.4. Hyperoxia test

In the time of ECHO, this test has only anecdotic relevance and lacks sensitivity and specificity. This test has been used to distinguish between cardiac or pulmonary central cyanosis. After breathing 100% oxygen for a few minutes, the cyanosis disappears or should be clearly reduced in pulmonary cyanosis and there is a relevant increase in arterial partial oxygen pressure. In cardiac cyanosis, the partial oxygen pressure should remain largely unchanged as the cardiac right-to-left shunt or inadequate pulmonary perfusion cannot be compensated by the administration of oxygen.

Note

Today in any case, echocardiography examination is preferable to a hyperoxia test and must be available in every neonatal unit on a 24/7 basis.

1.4.5. Pulse and blood pressure in all limbs

All neonates with suspected cardiac defect should have a pulse and blood pressure measurement at all 4 limbs. If a difference in blood pressure between the right arm (preductal) and the lower limbs (postductal) is then manifest or the peripheral pulses in the lower limbs cannot be palpated, this is a hint and leading findings of coarctation of the aorta or an interrupted aortic arch. This examination is helpful to assess systemic circulation.

Note

In a large patent ductus arteriosus, there may be no difference in blood pressure between the upper and lower halves of the body even with relevant coarctation of the aorta or interrupted aortic arch. The saturations, however, vary substantially.

1.5. Treatment

According to the different anatomic variations and physiologic situation, there is a substantial difference in the management of these children. The treatment principles for the various groups of congenital heart defects are presented below and based on the pathophysiology, the specific treatments of the individual heart defects in the neonatal period are described in this context.

1.5.1. Cardiac defects with ductal-dependent systemic circulation

In ductal-dependent systemic circulation, we should reestablish the prenatal circulation. Therefore, attempts must be made to provide as much blood as possible from the pulmonary circulation to supply the systemic circulation via the patent ductus arteriosus. As a result of this strategy, a saturation of 75–85% is adequate and saturations >85% that indicate excessive pulmonary blood flow should be avoided. The treatment principles of ductal-dependent systemic circulation are as follows:

- Provide patency of the ductus arteriosus with a continuous prostaglandin E1 infusion (initial dosage 20–50 ng/kg/min, to be reduced after ECHO assessment; caveat: Apnoea).
- Lower systemic vascular resistance:
    - By reducing afterload: i.e., with sodium nitroprusside infusion
    - If catecholamines are needed: Use preferably milrinone and/or dobutamine (vasodilatation effects); avoid vasoconstrictive effects of other catecholamines (dopamine, noradrenaline)

- Increase pulmonary resistance, increase pulmonary artery pressure:
  - Avoid intubation, extubate early
  - Avoid additional oxygen
  - Aim for mild metabolic acidosis (pH 7.35)
  - Aim for mild hypoventilation (pCO_2 around 60 mmHg)
- In case of pulmonary edema caused by congestion and pulmonary overflow, give intravenous diuretics (1–2 mg/kg furosemide), ensure high PEEP (i.e., 10–15 cm H_2O) and reduce prostaglandin E1 to a minimum (e.g., 10 ng/kg/min)

Note

The administration of oxygen ($SatO_2$ >85%) as a general measure and hyperventilation in children with ductal-dependent systemic circulation can lead to an acute decompensation of the hemodynamic situation.

1.5.2. Cardiac defects with ductal-dependent pulmonary circulation

The situation is reversed in ductal-dependent pulmonary circulation, but the prenatal situation should be achieved too. Again a saturation of 75–85% is adequate and saturations >85% should be avoided as they indicate inadequate pulmonary perfusion. The following measures can be useful to allow more blood to flow from the systemic circulation to the pulmonary circulation via the patent ductus arteriosus if needed:

- Secure patency of the ductus arteriosus via a prostaglandin E1 infusion (initial dosage 20–50 ng/kg/min).
- Lower pulmonary vascular resistance:
  - Aim for mild metabolic alkalosis (use buffering) (pH 7.45–7.5)
  - Adjust ventilation for mild hyperventilation (pCO_2 around 35 mmHg)
  - Increase FiO_2
- Increase systemic vascular resistance and support systemic pressure by:
  - Noradrenaline infusion
  - Possibly also adrenaline infusion
  - Use volume more generously
  - Do not use dopamine
- Maintain rather high dosage of prostaglandin E1.

Excursus: Prostaglandin

Prostaglandin E1 is given to maintain patency or reopen the ductus arteriosus in neonates with ductal-dependent defect. Due to its short half-life, it must be administered continuously intravenous. The initial dosage in a patient with a nearly closed duct is between 50 and 100 ng/kg/min. Based on the actual effect, this dosage can be reduced gradually to a minimum of 5–10 ng/kg/min,

The most common side effects are as follows:

- Apnea (administer in readiness for intubation)
- Bradycadia
- Vasodilatation (pulmonary and systemic), hypotension
- Fever
- Edema
- (Cortical hyperostosis, periostitis only after long-term administration)

Practical tip: When a prostaglandin infusion is required, always a second venous access should be inserted to ensure safe prostaglandin administration immediately via other access if the first one is dislocated. The second access can also be used for volume substitution in case of acute hypotension.

1.5.3. Cardiac defects with parallel circulations

The only example of this cardiac defect is a transposition of the great arteries (d-TGA) together with its variations. The management of this situation is described in the specific treatment section.

1.5.4. Cardiac defects with complete intracardiac mixing of blood

The different cardiac defects (i.e., univentricular hearts) in this group are also described in the following treatment section.

1.5.5. Cardiac defects with a large left-to-right shunt

When the pulmonary resistance drops after the first 4–6 weeks of life, the left-to-right shunt and thereby pulmonary blood flow will increase dramatically. Consequently, heart failure may develop caused by increased volume load, which must be treated medically (diuretics, ACE inhibitors, beta blockers, possibly digoxin or cathecholamines) until corrective surgery is performed. As additional oxygen will lower the pulmonary resistance and increase excessive pulmonary blood flow, no additional oxygen should be administered.

1.6. Specific treatment of the most common symptomatic heart defects in the neonatal period

1.6.1. Left ventricle outflow tract obstruction lesion (i.e., critical aortic stenosis, coarctation of the aorta and interrupted aortic arch)

The initial management of these children has some common features:

- Shock therapy, including intubation and ventilation (high PEEP (>10 cm H_2O) if there is pulmonary edema)
- Prostaglandin E1: initial dosage 50–100 ng/kg/min
- Oxygen: avoid excessive administration, use PEEP to improve oxygenation. (note: oxygen lowers pulmonary resistance and thus increases pulmonary blood flow)
- Use diuretics (furosemide), to manage pulmonary edema and lower preload
- Use catecholamines (dobutamine, adrenaline, NOT dopamine), preferably milrinone depending on blood pressure and myocardial function. (If there is a subvalvular stenosis, catecholamines should be administered with particular caution due to a possible increase in the obstruction.)
- Assess by ECHO and reduce afterload (e.g., sodium nitroprusside)
- Aim for moderate metabolic acidosis (target pH 7.35)
- Administer as little volume as possible; preferably only after cardiac function has recovered or is assessed to be stable in echocardiography

1.6.1.1. Critical aortic stenosis (AoS)

1.6.1.1.1. Hemodynamic situation

Due to the severe obstruction of the aortic valve, the left ventricular function usually is markedly impaired and cannot provide sufficient cardiac output for the systemic circulation which is supplied with blood from the pulmonary artery via the patent ductus arteriosus (i.e., prenatal situation). Left ventricular hypertrophy and possibly fibroelastosis have already developed in utero. This defect is often associated with other left heart obstructions (mitral stenosis, coarctation of the aorta, hypoplastic aortic arch—i.e., Shones complex). If a heart murmur is not already detected in the neonate, many patients with critical aortic stenosis present in severe cardiac shock. In addition, there is differential cyanosis.

In critical AoS with PDA-dependent systemic circulation (prostaglandin infusion), a left-to-right shunt at the atrial level is necessary to allow mixing of the oxygenated pulmonary venous blood via the right atrium, the right ventricle, the pulmonary artery and then the patent ductus arteriosus. A balloon atrial septostomy (Rashkind maneuver) may be necessary, if the shunt at the atrial level is not large enough,

1.6.1.1.2. Further procedure

If suspected ensure prompt transfer to a pediatric cardiac center for interventional catheterization and performance of balloon valvuloplasty (method of choice) or surgical commissurotomy (rarely required); possibly carry out an emergency Rashkind maneuver if there is a restrictive foramen ovale and inadequate left ventricular function after balloon valvuloplasty.

1.6.1.2. Coarctation of the aorta (CoA)

1.6.1.2.1. Hemodynamic situation

In patients with critical CoA, the lower half of the body is supplied with deoxygenated blood from the pulmonary artery via the PDA (differential cyanosis). When the ductus arteriosus closes, dramatic hypoperfusion of the body distal to the aortic isthmus occurs. The left ventricle has now suddenly contract against the pronounced obstruction and rapid decompensation occurs. Associations with other left heart obstructions (bicuspid aortic valve) or a VSD are common.

1.6.1.2.2. Further procedure

Again organize prompt transfer to a pediatric cardiac center for surgical correction, which is generally attempted after the hemodynamic situation has been stabilized. In some special conditions (e.g., for patients in poor general condition or with necrotizing enterocolitis—NEC), primary interventional catheterization with balloon dilatation or implantation of a coronary stent may be indicated for stabilization until surgery.

1.6.1.3. Interrupted aortic arch

1.6.1.3.1. Hemodynamic situation

There are different forms of an interrupted aortic arch and the perfusion of the lower half of the body depends however entirely on a patent ductus arteriosus (i.e., prostaglandin). A VSD is nearly always associated with this defect and other left heart obstructions occur occasionally. Again oxygen saturation should be measured preductally (right hand), as the preductal saturation reflects the situation of the perfusion and blood supply in the CNS and coronary arteries. The levels measured in the lower limbs correspond with pulmonary arterial saturation.

1.6.1.3.2. Further procedure

Prompt transfer to a pediatric cardiac center for surgical correction.

1.6.1.4. Hypoplastic left heart syndrome

1.6.1.4.1. Hemodynamic situation

In patients with a hypoplastic left heart syndrome (HLHS), both the pulmonary and systemic systems are supplied by the right ventricle. Although there are four forms of HLHS (i.e., MA and AoA, MS and AoA, MS and AoS, MA and AoS with VSD), retrograde coronary perfusion takes place in all across the ductus arteriosus with mixed blood from the pulmonary artery and retrogradely across the coarctation and ascending aorta. Within the first few hours of life, the drop in pulmonary resistance together with the manifestation of a coarctation causes the blood from the pulmonary artery to flow primarily into the pulmonary circulation. Therefore, the systemic circulation—together with the coronary arteries—is increasingly less perfused. Severe heart failure develops, which if untreated usually results in shock. As a result, there is severe metabolic acidosis but due to pulmonary recirculation, the oxygen saturation is only moderately reduced. The higher the oxygen saturation is, the more the ratio of pulmonary to systemic perfusion changes are in favor of pulmonary over perfusion and systemic underperfusion. In addition, postnatal closure of the PDA enhances this fatal circulation with underperfusion of the systemic circulation and excessive pulmonary perfusion [9].

It is important to note that oxygenated pulmonary venous blood from the left atrium can only reach the systemic circulation across a sufficiently large shunt to the right atrium (see above).

1.6.1.4.2. Initial treatment

- Shock treatment, including intubation and ventilation (but avoid ventilation if possible, as long as the pH is balanced); hyperventilation must be avoided
- Prostaglandin E1: initial dosage 50–100 ng/kg/min
- Avoid administering oxygen (additionally reduces pulmonary resistance and thus systemic perfusion), target saturation 70–85%
- Administer some furosemide (1–2 mg/kg) to lower preload or for pulmonary edema
- Catecholamine treatment is often required, but should be administered with restraint (can increase the myocardial oxygen consumption), give milrinoneor dobutamine if needed, do not use dopamine
- Possibly reduce afterload (e.g., sodium nitroprusside)
- For severe acidosis, large amounts of NaBic are often required to manage acidosis (doses up to 10 ml/kgbw of NaBic are common!)
- Aim for moderate metabolic acidosis (target pH 7.35, avoid over-buffering)
- As little volume as possible should be administered; preferably only after cardiac function has recovered or is assessed to be stable in echocardiography

1.6.1.4.3. Further procedure

If the atrial defect is restrictive (leading symptom: severe cyanosis, oxygen saturation <65%, seriously ill child), pulmonary congestion has developed and an emergency balloon atrial septostomy (Rashkind maneuver) may be needed.

The patient should be transferred quickly to a pediatric cardiac center for surgery after stabilization (usually a Norwood procedure as the first step of three-stage Fontan palliation).

1.6.2. Right ventricle outflow tract obstruction lesion (critical pulmonary stenosis and pulmonary atresia with intact ventricular septum or ventricular septal defect, tetralogy of fallot, tricuspid atresia with pulmonary stenosis and Ebstein anomaly)

The initial treatment of this group of patients has some common features:

- Prostaglandin E1 infusion: initial dosage 50–100 ng/kg/min
- Initially more generous oxygen therapy (lowers pulmonary resistance)
- Initially more generous volume therapy (i.e., 20 ml/kg bw)
- Try to achieve mild metabolic alkalosis (use over-buffering) (pH 7.45–7.5)
- Possibly ventilation and mild hyperventilation (pCO_2 around 35 mmHg)
- Possibly use an increase in systemic resistance (noradrenaline)

1.6.2.1. Critical pulmonary stenosis

1.6.2.1.1. Hemodynamic situation

A critical pulmonary stenosis is a high-grade obstruction of the pulmonary valve with subsequent hypoxemia. As the right ventricle cannot drain into the pulmonary circulation, secondary hypoxia occurs due to a right-to-left shunt across the foramen ovale/ASD. The musculature of the RV is severely hypertrophic and the RV and tricuspid valve may sometimes be hypoplastic. To ensure oxygenation, the pulmonary circulation is supplied with blood from the aorta via the PDA.

1.6.2.1.2. Further procedure

After diagnosis and prostaglandin infusion organize transfer to a pediatric cardiac center for interventional catheter balloon valvuloplasty.

1.6.2.2. Pulmonary atresia with intact ventricular septum

1.6.2.2.1. Hemodynamic situation

In pulmonary atresia with intact ventricular septum, which can be judged as extreme form of pulmonary stenosis, the right ventricle cannot drain its blood normally to the PA. The majority of blood from the right ventricle either flows back into the right atrium due to tricuspid regurgitation. In addition in some cases, the right ventricle may be connected with the coronary arteries via myocardial sinusoids. In the latter case, the coronary arteries may have other problems and are stenotic so that coronary perfusion may depend on blood flow from the right ventricle (right ventricular dependent coronary circulation (RVDCC). Usually there is suprasystemic pressure in the right ventricle and the right ventricle is hypoplastictic various degrees. Again, the pulmonary circulation is supplied with blood from the aorta via the PDA to ensure oxygenation.

1.6.2.2.2. Further procedure

After stabilization, organize transfer to a pediatric cardiac center. In most cases, cardiac catheterization is needed to rule out myocardial sinusoids and coronary anomalies. In some cases, it is possible to open the right ventricular outflow tract by interventional catheterization or implant a stent into the PDA. Otherwise interim palliative surgery (opening the right ventricular outflow tract or aortopulmonary shunt) must be performed accordingly.

1.6.2.3. Tricuspid atresia

1.6.2.3.1. Hemodynamic situation

In tricuspid atresia, that may give an example for all univentricular heart defects, there is no continuity between the right atrium and ventricle, so the right atrium can drain into the left atrium only across a right-to-left shunt at atrial level. There are various forms of tricuspid atresia depending on the variations of obstructions of the right ventricular outflow tract or pulmonic valve. The RV is usually perfused from the LV across a VSD that is almost always present. The RV is hypoplastic to various extents. Oxygen saturation is identical in the aorta and pulmonary artery because of the complete mixing of blood.

Frequently stenosis and even atresia of the pulmonary artery occur and may have a negative effect on the blood flow to the pulmonary circulation. If there is atresia or a high grade stenosis of the pulmonary artery, perfusion of the lungs depends on a patent ductus arteriosus (see above). In addition, the great vessels can be in normal position or in transposition.

If there is no pulmonary stenosis and blood flow to the pulmonary circulation is unobstructed, the main symptom that may develop later on is heart failure (tachypnea, hepatomegaly, pallor, possible pulmonary edema), but this constellation is much less common.

Initial treatment if there is no pulmonary stenosis (leading symptom: heart failure):

- Anticongestive treatment (diuretics, milrinone, rarely catecholamines)
- Restrictive volume therapy
- Restrictive oxygen therapy

1.6.2.3.2. Further procedure

Transfer to a pediatric cardiac center should be organized. If there is a restrictive atrial shunt (rare), an interventional catheter balloon atrial septostomy (Rashkind maneuver) may be needed. If there is inadequate pulmonary perfusion, a palliative aortopulmonary shunt is placed. The separation of circulations is performed later as multistep procedure (Fontan procedure).

1.6.2.4. Tetralogy of Fallot

1.6.2.4.1. Hemodynamic situation

In tetralogy of Fallot, there is a typical combination of a large VSD with overriding of the aorta, a subpulmonary and pulmonary stenosis, often combined with supravalvular stenosis of various degrees and a marked hypertrophy of the right ventricle. Cyanosis is determined by the extent of the obstruction of the right ventricular outflow tract and thereby pulmonary blood flow. In most cases, this obstruction is only mild at birth, but becomes more significant during the first few weeks of life due to the increase in the infundibular stenosis. If there is pronounced stenosis of the right ventricular outflow tract (functional pulmonary atresia), the children may already develop symptoms with cyanosis or hypoxic spells even in the neonatal period. Hypercyanotic spells occur if there is a sudden increase in subpulmonary muscular obstruction of the RVOT (i.e., agitation) or an acute drop in peripheral vascular resistance (i.e., after feeding).

Treatment of a hypoxic-hypercyanotic spell:

- Immediate sedation (e.g., ketamine IV 2–5 mg/kg, alternatively opiates, benzodiazepines)
- Oxygen therapy
- Increase in systemic resistance by
  - pressing the child's flexed knee against the chest ("jack-knife position")
  - if necessary infusion of vasoconstrictors (noradrenaline)
  - generous volume bolus (e.g., 20–50 ml/kg)
- Compensation of metabolic acidosis by buffering
- Possibly beta blockers (e.g., propranolol IV 0.01–0.1 mg/kg very slowly under monitor guidance)

1.6.2.4.2. Further procedure

Rapid transfer to a pediatric cardiac center is urgently needed. In most circumstances, interventional management can improve the hemodynamic situation (i.e., balloon dilatation of the pulmonary valve, stenting of the right ventricular outflow tract, stenting of a PDA). Only in few cases, early surgical correction is required today. In special situations (e.g., very small children), an aortopulmonary shunt is first placed as a palliative measure to ensure lung perfusion.

1.6.2.5. Pulmonary atresia with ventricular septal defect

1.6.2.5.1. Hemodynamic situation

From the hemodynamic aspect, this disease is an extreme form of Tetralogy of Fallot. Pulmonary perfusion is, however, dependent on a patent ductus arteriosus (prostaglandin infusion) or aortopulmonary collaterals.

1.6.2.5.2. Further procedure

After stabilization with prostaglandin infusion, a rapid transfer to a pediatric cardiac center should be organized. In cases with only membranous valvular atresia, an attempt can be made to open the valve by interventional catheterization (or with stent placement). In addition placing a stent in the PDA may help to achieve catch-up growth of the pulmonary vessels, which are almost always hypoplastic. If this intervention is not possible, an aortopulmonary shunt is placed as surgical palliation. After catch-up growth of the pulmonary vascular system, a continuity between the pulmonary vessels and the right ventricle is created surgically later (e.g., with a valved conduit).

1.6.2.6. Ebstein's anomaly

1.6.2.6.1. Hemodynamic situation

In Ebstein's anomaly, there is apical displacement of the tricuspid valve into the right ventricle combined with moderate to severe tricuspid regurgitation and reduced flow from the small right ventricle to the pulmonary artery. The right atrium is markedly too massively dilated. A pronounced Ebstein's anomaly can already be symptomatic in the neonatal period. Cyanosis occurs due to a right-to-left shunt at the atrial level caused by minimal antegrade flow to the pulmonary artery. In addition, the gross dilatation of the heart may compress the lungs and impair pulmonary function.

The disease may often complicated by accessory pathways (Wolf-Parkinson-White syndrome).

Besides initial treatment stated above, in Ebstein's anomaly:

- If there is heart failure, possibly catecholamines and diuretics
- If there is supraventricular tachycardia, it should be terminated with a vagal maneuver, adenosine, amiodarone, possibly cardioversion

1.6.2.6.2. Further procedure

The goal of surgical treatment is to reconstruct the tricuspid valve and close the ASD. If there is insufficient lung perfusion, it may be necessary to place an aortopulmonary shunt. If there is pronounced hypoplasia of the right ventricle, the univentricular Fontan pathway may be the only option. The overall prognosis is unfavorable for children who become symptomatic already in the neonatal period. These children require urgent transfer to a pediatric cardiac center.

1.6.3. d-transposition of the great arteries (d-TGA)

1.6.3.1. Hemodynamic situation

In d-TGA, there is parallel connection of the pulmonary and systemic circulations; the systemic venous blood is directed back into the aorta and the pulmonary venous blood is pumped back to the pulmonary artery. Survival is only possible if shunts between the two circulatory systems do exist. The most important is a patent foramen ovale or ASD as shunt at atrial level, so oxygenated blood can reach the systemic circulation via the right ventricle across this left-to-right shunt. A PDA has a favorable effect on oxygenation because PDA blood flow increases lung perfusion and as a result the volume load and pressure in the left atrium is increased, so the left-to-right shunt at atrial level increases and more oxygenated blood can reach the systemic circulation [10].

Oxygen application may act indirectly by reducing pulmonary resistance and thus increasing pulmonary perfusion and thereby left atrial volume load and pressure (caution: uncontrolled administration of oxygen can also lead to closure of the ductus arteriosus when used without prostaglandin).

In addition to improve mixing between the two circulations, especially in "poor mixers," an attempt should be made to improve mixed venous saturation.

If there is an associated large VSD, cyanosis is usually less pronounced.

Initial treatment:

- Prostaglandin E1 infusion: initial dosage 50 ng/kg/min
- Generous volume therapy
- Aim for mild metabolic alkalosis (over-buffering) (pH 7.45–7.5, lowers pulmonary resistance)
- Oxygen therapy for severe cyanosis in neonates (caution: induces closure of the ductus arteriosus)
- If possible avoid intubation, ventilation and relaxation (lowers oxygen consumption and therefore increases mixed venous saturation. On the other hand, ventilation increases the intrathoracic pressure, which can impair mixing of the blood)
- Consider the improve cardiac output and thus mixed venous saturation by milrinone
- Generous treatment of anemia (improves oxygen supply)

1.6.3.2. *Further procedure*

If there is a restrictive shunt at the atrial level, a bedside interventional catheter balloon atrial septostomy (Rashkind maneuver) should be performed as soon as possible before transfer to a pediatric cardiac center. The surgical standard treatment is an arterial switch operation (Jatene procedure) within the first 2 weeks of life.

1.6.4. *Truncus arteriosus communis*

1.6.4.1. *Hemodynamic situation*

In a truncus arteriosus communis (TAC), only one vessel (common trunk) arises from the heart. The systemic and pulmonary circulation and the coronaries are here supplied from this trunk only. A VSD is almost always present. Since the blood follows the path of least resistance and tends to flow into the pulmonary circulation, there is usually excessive pulmonary blood flow after the drop in pulmonary resistance between the second and eighth weeks of life. In this situation, clinical signs of heart failure are already present in the first weeks of life. Due to the significant pulmonary recirculation, there is often only astonishingly mild cyanosis, although the trunk vessel contains only mixed blood.

Initial treatment:

- Oxygen lowers pulmonary resistance and thus increases blood flow to the pulmonary circulation, leading to excessive pulmonary blood flow and increasing heart failure—therefore, use oxygen restrictively
- Treatment of heart failure: diuretics, possibly catecholamines (dobutamine) or phosphodiesterase inhibitor (milrinone), afterload reducer (ACE inhibitor, possibly sodium nitroprusside)
- If associated with an interrupted aortic arch: prostaglandin E1 infusion: initial dosage 50–100 ng/kg/min

1.6.4.2. Further procedure

Organize transfer to a pediatric cardiac center. The definitive correction with a Rastelli procedure is generally performed within the first weeks of life depending on the clinical signs of heart failure.

1.6.5. Total anomalous pulmonary venous connection (TAPVC)

1.6.5.1. Hemodynamic situation

Depending on the location of the anomalous connection of the pulmonary veins, we distinguish between supracardiac, cardiac, infracardiac and mixed forms. Please note that an infracardiac total anomalous pulmonary venous connection is regularly associated with an obstruction at the connection site.

In a total anomalous pulmonary venous connection, all pulmonary veins drain into the systemic venous system and oxygenated blood is guided from there into the right atrium. The perfusion of the systemic circulation thus depends on a right-to-left shunt at the atrial level that is necessary for survival.

In a TAPVC without obstruction of the pulmonary vein, the hemodynamic situation is similar to that of a large ASD (volume overload of the right atrium, ventricle and pulmonary circulation).

Initial treatment:

Total anomalous pulmonary venous connection with obstruction of the pulmonary vein:

- Oxygen therapy
- Intubation and ventilation with a high PEEP (>10 cm H_2O) for pulmonary edema

- Lower PVR: hyperventilation, generous buffering (target pH 7.45–7.5), increase oxygen supply, possibly inhaled NO or prostacyclin IV
- Diuretics, possibly catecholamines for low cardiac output (caution: catecholamines can exacerbate pulmonary edema)

1.6.5.2. Further procedure

A TAPVC with obstruction of the pulmonary vein is an absolute cardiac surgery emergency that must be surgically corrected immediately. Dilatation with or without stent implantation can treat the stenosis of the pulmonary vein in individual cases, so that the surgical repair can be performed after the child is stabilized.

If there is a restrictive atrial shunt or if surgical correction is not possible immediately, an interventional catheter balloon atrial septostomy (Rashkind maneuver) may be considered.

1.6.6. Complete atrioventricular septal defect

1.6.6.1. Hemodynamic situation

In a complete atrioventricular septal defect (AVSD, AV canal), both segments of the ventricular and atrial septum in the region of the AV valves are absent and the development of the AV valves is also impaired. This malformation results in a large left-to-right shunt that increases when the pulmonary resistance drops within the first weeks of life. Children with a complete AVSD usually develop heart failure when the pulmonary resistance drops after 2–8 weeks of life. The situation can be complicated by (mainly systemic) AV valve insufficiency.

Note

trisomy 21 is frequently associated with AVSD. All neonates with trisomy 21 must therefore have an ECHO examination at an early age.

Initial treatment:

- Avoid oxygen (excessive pulmonary blood flow is increased)
- Pharmacological treatment of heart failure: diuretics, ACE inhibitors, beta blockers, rarely catecholamines (possibly digoxin?)

1.6.6.2. Further procedure

The corrective surgery is generally performed at the age of 4–6 months and it may be necessary earlier if conservative heart failure treatment is unsuccessful.

2. Postoperative cardiac intensive care therapy

The following remarks apply primarily to those patients that are transferred immediately after surgery from the surgical operating room and their early postoperative period in the pediatric cardiac intensive care unit (PCICU).

2.1. Basics

One of the main requirements for providing good quality of care in a PCICU is to understand that the job of the intensive care physician starts far before the operated child is admitted to the PCICU. Detailed information on the case of the child is required in advance before the day of admission. The PCICU intensivist must be aware of and understand the hemodynamics of the cardiac defect (i.e., check the ECHO, cath data, etc.), possible complicating or concomitant diseases, the actual planned surgical repair or procedure and the usually possible perioperative and postoperative complications.

Every intensive care physician should be familiar with the major steps of cardiac surgery in general and the specific steps and details of the case to be admitted. These steps include the whole process of surgery from opening the thorax and the mediastinum, thereafter arterial and venous cannulation for the cardiopulmonary bypass, initiation of cardiopulmonary bypass, cardioplegic arrest and finally, the restoration of cardiac function at the end of the operation including decannulation and closure of the thorax.

To obtain this crucial understanding, every intensivist should visit the cardiac theatre on a regular basis and observe about 50 surgeries per year. In complex cases, the intensivist should work together in the time after decannulation or weaning of the bypass with the anesthetist before admission of the patient to the PCICU.

2.2. Preparation of the bed place

The majority of patients will be admitted on a planned and forseable basis. Before the patient is transferred to the PCICU, a careful and standardized preparation of the bed/place must be completed to avoid unnecessary misunderstanding and streamline the admission process. This preparation may vary from unit to unit but generally includes the following:

- Preparation of the ventilation equipment, adjustment of the settings to the estimated patient-specific parameters, checking of the ventilation bag and mask, oxygen delivery, suction equipment and catheters. In addition, it must be determined by contacting the operating theatre or by assessment of the preoperative information whether iNO (nitric oxide) ventilation is required and possible with the ventilation equipment
- Medication plan: The prepared medication plan should be tailored to the patients' age and weight and include the medication and calculated dosages for the presumed standardized postoperative treatment (i.e., sedation, pain therapy, antibiotics, catecholamines, vasodilators, diuretics, fluid therapy and infusions). The perfusors and flushing solutions should be purged and primed before the patient is transferred to the PCICU

- Monitoring: The bedside monitor is checked beforehand and the patient-specific alarms according to reference values for age and disease are set
- Administrative tasks: Unit specific paperwork is prepared and an X-ray order for the first postoperative X-ray and laboratory order for the first laboratory tests should be prepared

2.3. Postoperative transfer of the patient to the ICU

In order to understand the physiology of the patient, a detailed handover from the different disciplines treating the patient during surgery is necessary. The checklist in **Table 2** contains some common and useful questions that the intensive care physician should discuss with the surgeons, anesthesiologists and cardiac technicians/perfusionists at transfer. The information is crucial and may have direct impact on the subsequent PCICU management.

Surgical aspects
- What were the intraoperative findings? Compared to before?
- What surgical technique was performed? Any problems?
- What drainages were placed intraoperatively (e.g., pleural drainage, mediastinal drainage)?
- What is the assessment of postoperative result?
- Was an intraoperative transesophageal echocardiography performed and what were the findings (residual gradient, valve insufficiency, residual shunt, myocardial function)?
- Did any intraoperative arrhythmias occur? How were they treated?
- Did any intraoperative bleeding problems occur? How were they treated?
Anesthesiology aspects
- Tube size and brand, cuffed and uncuffed?
- Ventilation settings (FiO_2, tidal volume, rate, peak pressure and PEEP)
- Central venous catheter: location of insertion, size
- Arterial access: location, size
- Was an LA or pulmonary artery catheter placed?
- Anesthetics and cardiac medication used (cathecolamines, vasodilators, anti arrhythmics) and their dosages
- Heparinization and current coagulation levels
- Use of blood products (pack red cells, platelet concentrates, fresh frozen plasma)
Cardiopulmonary bypass
- Bypass time
- Aortic cross clamp time
- Cardiac arrest time
- Minimum temperature during bypass
- Was hemofiltration performed at the end of the bypass?

Table 2. Checklist for postoperative transfer.

2.4. Initial examination after transfer to the ICU

Immediately after the patient is admitted to the ICU, the most important clinical parameters must be assessed by the admitting physician and the nurses involved to confirm that the patient is in a stable and safe situation:

- Respiration: Is the chest moving? How are thorax/chest movements? Symmetrical lung expansion? Adequate expansion? How is the Oxygen saturation? FiO2?
- Circulation: Palpation of peripheral pulses (femoral, brachial), visual check of pressure parameters on the monitor (arterial blood pressure, CVP, if inserted pulmonary artery pressure or LA pressure) and check of capillary filling time (normal<2–3 s)
- Diuresis: Is the urine bag filled? How much? Is the bladder filled despite urine catheter? Does the urine look clear or hemolytic? Does the patient appear edematous (puffy) or rather dehydrated?
- Bleeding: Are the drains connected to suction? How much is in the bag and how quick is it filling? Are the secretions dark red (venous blood), bright red (arterial blood), yellowish or clear (serous), warm (fresh) or cold (older)?
- Neurology: is the patient sedated/anesthetized, what is the status of the pupils, are there spontaneous movements and is the patient breathing against the ventilator?
- Body temperature
- Assessment of catheters, lines and cables inserted

During this gross examination to assess the patient's stability, the patient is connected to the bedside monitor system and other equipment. The arterial and central venous accesses are connected with the pressure transducers, set to zero and activated again. The patient is also connected to the ventilator and the drainages set to suction (in general, the suction pressure is set at around 15 cm H_2O). In addition, the external pacemaker is checked for proper function.

In parallel, the first blood samples are taken and include an arterial and central venous blood gas analysis, an ACT and a survey of different pathology markers to asses organ function. The first blood gas analysis including electrolyte status provides information on the ventilation situation, the hemodynamic status (lactate, central venous saturation) and electrolyte metabolism (especially potassium). A standard limb ECG is then recorded, a chest X-ray arranged and finally, an initial exploratory echocardiography (ECHO) performed as a standard in every patient.

2.5. Further postoperative management

2.5.1. Fluid intake

As capillary leak is a normal reaction to bypass and the subsequent inflammatory process induces edema of all organs, the amount of free water intake should be limited postoperatively. Therefore, fluid intake is ideally reduced to 30–50% of the normal maintenance on the first postoperative day and then increased day by day to 75 and finally 100% on the following days.

Patients, however, who underwent cardiac surgery without cardiopulmonary bypass (e.g., resection of an aortic coarctation, PDA ligature) do not require any restriction of postoperative fluid intake.

As soon as the children are able to drink, oral fluid intake should not be restricted any more.

2.5.2. *Ventilation*

The majority of patients are ventilated after cardiac surgery when they arrive in the PCICU. Pulmonary function is affected by a large variety of preoperative, intraoperative and postoperative factors. Important examples to be considered are listed below:

- Preoperative factors:
    - Preexisting excessive pulmonary blood flow (wet lung, congestion)
    - Preexisting pulmonary hypertension (left-to-right shunt)
    - External compression of the airways, for example, due to vascular rings or prominent pulmonary arteries
- Intraoperative factors:
    - Atelectasis due to surgical manipulation in the thorax or lack of ventilation during the bypass
    - Edema development due to the effect of cardiopulmonary bypass and SIRS
        - Trauma of the lung
- Postoperative factors:
    - Swollen mucosa (SIRS)
    - Atelectasis
    - Lung edema as a result of a postoperative increased lung perfusion. Typical examples are after a shunt procedure or operative opening of circulation in the lungs in pulmonary atresia or severe stenosis ("reperfusion edema")
    - Impaired respiratory mechanics due to postoperative diaphragmatic paresis
    - Pain-related reduction in respiratory capacity (surgery drains)
    - Respiratory depression caused by drugs
    - Pneumothorax, pleural effusions
        - Bleeding through MAPCAS

2.5.3. *Settings of the ventilator*

Volume-controlled ventilation is the ventilation of choice in every cardiac patient after cardiac surgery. In many ventilators, a setting with a pressure control combination (i.e., PRVC-mode) can be chosen. Hereby markedly, lower rates are usually used (e.g., 20/min for neonates) in the sedated patient. The tidal volume is usually set to 10–15 ml/kg. A relatively long inspiration time is usually selected initially. The PEEP is around 5–10 mmHg and an FiO_2 value is selected at which oxygen saturation of over 95% can be achieved. When the patients waking up, the volume controlled mode is combine with a SIMV mode.

In spontaneous breathing patients, the following values can be used as references for the age-specific respiratory rate:

- Neonates: 40/min
- Infants: 25–30/min
- Toddlers: 25/min
- School-age children: 20/min
- Adolescents: 15/min

Again, in the controlled situation, the rate settings used are much slower.

The following situations are important variants from these initial settings of the ventilator:

- *Univentricular heart*: In univentricular hearts, the balance between systemic and pulmonary circulation is very important to avoid pulmonary overcirculation at the cost of inadequate systemic perfusion. At an oxygen saturation of around 75–85%, a nice balance between systemic and pulmonary perfusion is achieved (Qp/Qs = 1:1). Therefore, the target oxygen saturation in these patients is approximately 80%. Uncritical oxygen administration must be avoided.

- *Fontan circulation*: In these patients, the transpulmonary blood flow is depending completely on the intrathoracic pressure and pulmonary vascular resistance. Theoretically, a high PEEP increases the intrathoracic pressure and thus reduces passive blood across the pulmonary vascular system. A lower PEEP level (<5 mmHg) is therefore often recommended for Fontan patients. On the other hand, a higher PEEP also increases the residual functional capacity and reduces atelectases, so better lung perfusion can be achieved via the Euler–Liljestrand reflex. It has been advocated earlier to ventilate Fontan patients without PEEP—this management strategy is inappropriate and no longer recommended.

- *Pulmonary hypertension*: Pulmonary vascular resistance is reduced by a low pCO_2, a high pH and a high FiO_2. To use this principle, patients with known or presumed pulmonary hypertension (i.e., large VSD, older age, truncus, etc.) should be ventilated using mild hyperventilation (Target pCO_2: 30–35 mmHg) and with higher than normal FiO_2 to achieve an oxygen saturation of around 100% and a paO_2 of more than 150 mmHg

2.5.4. Infection prophylaxis

Cardiopulmonary bypass reduces the capacity of the immune system to act against bacterial infections and so postoperative antibiotic prophylaxis is always given for children after cardiac surgery. The antibiotics used and the duration of antibiotic treatment are, however, subject of some controversy. First or second generation cephalosporins are frequently used, for example, cefazolin 30 mg/kg/dose every 8 hourly. For an uncomplicated postoperative course, many centers carry out antibiotic prophylaxis for 2–3 days (6–9 doses, until the drains are out) although hardly any evidence-based data for this procedure are available. For patients with an open sternum or peritoneal dialysis or ECMO, no additional management is required but prolonged treatment is often used in many centers. Antibiotic prophylaxis is then continued for 24 h post-chest closure or ECMO/PD removal.

2.5.5. *Sedation*

In most centers, a combination of an opiate (morphine, fentanyl) and a benzodiazepine (midazolam) is administered intravenously continuously in the initial postoperative period. Propofol is often used in older children who are sedated for only a short period. No time (2–3 days) or dose (3–8 mg/kg/h) limitation applies in these cases. Lactate levels should be checked on a routine basis.

2.5.6. *Analgesia*

Surgery itself and the drains in the body after surgery is painful procedure. To reduce postoperative pain, a fixed and standardized combination of non-steroidal analgesics (i.e., paracetamol, ibuprofen) and opiates (morphine, fentanyl) is usually used for analgesia for the first 2–3 days. Patient-controlled analgesia with a PCA pump is also applicable for older children (who can already play a video game).

2.5.7. *Kidney function*

Kidney function nearly always deteriorates in patients who have undergone cardiac surgery. The use of cardiopulmonary bypass leads to renal impairment and intraoperative fluid loading and inflammatory reactions that result in fluid retention. A negative fluid balance is therefore targeted postoperatively.

Urine excretion reflects a combination of cardiac function and cardiac output in combination with kidney function. In general, a urine excretion of at least 2 ml/kg/h after cardiac surgery is a minimum to ensure adequate fluid balance. Patients most often have a combination of pre-renal kidney failure (low cardiac output, capillary leak, volume deficit) in combination with the direct effects of SIRS on the kidney itself. In addition, a low systemic blood pressure and, in case of ascites, a high intra-abdominal pressure leads to a low perfusion pressure in the kidneys (aggressive drainage of ascites). Other less common examples of renal kidney failure are renal vein thrombosis or iatrogenic kidney damage (aminoglycosides, cyclosporin A). Post-renal kidney failure can be caused by obstructions in the region of the efferent urinary tract (e.g., obstruction of the urinary catheter or the urethra) or simply by increased intra abdominal pressure caused by capillary leak and ascites.

Suitable diuretics in the postoperative phase are primarily loop diuretics (Furosemide, ethacrynic acid). They are administered as a bolus or as a continuous infusion if the response is inadequate. The combination with theophylline sometimes enhances the effect. If excretion is insufficient or the fluid balance is clearly positive, peritoneal fluid drainage, or peritoneal dialysis should be initiated early.

2.6. Common postoperative problems and complications

Typical postoperative problems and their most common causes are summarized in **Table 3**.

Problem	Common causes
Blood pressure too high	Pain, fear, catecholamines, excessive fluid volume, result of the abrupt drug discontinuation (beta blockers, ACE inhibitors); typical postoperative problem after correction of an aortic coarctation. Rare causes: cerebral seizures, hypoglycemia (counter regulation)
Blood pressure too low	Hypovolemia, low cardiac output: limited myocardial function, pericardial effusion, arrhythmia (junctional ectopic tachycardia, AV block), excessive drainage loss, hemorrhage, excessive diuresis; vasodilators, anaphylaxis, sepsis, shock, pneumothorax
Central venous pressure (CVP) too low	Fluid deficit (excessive drainage losses, hemorrhage, excessive diuresis, volume intake too low)
Central venous pressure (CVP) too high	Tense/stiff patient (reaction to wake up, insufficient sedation in ventilation patients); impaired right ventricle function. In patients with univentricular heart, a high CVP suggests poor systemic ventricular or a relevant AV valve regurgitation. Other causes are a pericardial tamponade or pneumothorax
Arterial saturation too low	Atelectasis, hypoventilation, technical problems with the ventilation device, disconnected/obstructed tube, pneumothorax, pleural effusion, pneumonia, pulmonary edema, pulmonary hemorrhage, secretion, right to left shunt
Arterial saturation too high	In patients with univentricular hearts, saturation over 85% suggest an imbalance between pulmonary and systemic perfusion: excessive blood flow to the lungs and diminished supply to the systemic circulation
Bradycardia	Sinus bradycardia, AV block
Tachycardia	Narrow QRS complexes: sinus tachycardia, supraventricular tachycardia, JET Wide QRS complexes: ventricular tachycardia
Increase in lactate	Poor systemic perfusion, seizures, gut ischemia

Table 3. Typical postoperative problems and the most common causes.

2.6.1. Low cardiac output syndrome (LCOS)

There is a variety of factors that can result in myocardial dysfunction and subsequent low cardiac output postoperatively. Typically, they include an inflammatory reaction to cardiopulmonary bypass, myocardial ischemia and inadequate myocardial function as a result of the intraoperative clamping of the aorta, intraoperative hypothermia, a reperfusion edema, or if a surgical procedure was performed using a ventriculotomy—direct myocardial damage, coronary ischemia, inadequate cardioplegia, mechanical alteration, or an infection.

2.6.1.1. Symptoms

Typical clinical signs of low cardiac output are as follows:

- Tachycardia
- Oliguria

- Delayed capillary filling time (>3–4 s)
- Hypotension
- Decreased pulse pressure
- Reduced mixed venous saturation (Note: a difference between arterial and mixed venous saturation not <20–25% suggests sufficient cardiac output and adequate oxygen supply)
- Metabolic acidosis (BE less than −5)
- High lactate level (>3 mmol/l)

2.6.1.2. *Treatment*

The treatment of low cardiac output has to focus on the underlying causes which should be eliminated if possible. The following measures depending on the hemodynamic situation are commonly used as follows:

- Volume substitution (in case of hypovolemia)
- Inotropic support (catecholamines (i.e., adrenaline, dobutamine), phosphodiesterase inhibitors, intravenous calcium)
- Afterload reduction (sodium nitroprusside, phosphodiesterase inhibitors)
- Consider hormonal therapy for hypotensive resistance to epinephrine and vasopressors: cortisol for suspected adrenal insufficiency, IV or oral triidothyronine (T3) for euthyroid sick syndrome (low T3 levels with LCOS symptoms)
- Chronotropic support (pacemaker therapy, positive chronotropic drugs)
- Treatment of arrhythmias (amiodarone)
- Ventilation strategy
- Reduction in oxygen consumption (sedation, cooling)
- Mechanical circulatory support (ECMO, LVAD)

2.6.2. *Pulmonary hypertensive crisis*

Based on the underlying anatomy and pathophysiology, many patients may have a significant elevation of pulmonary pressures or pulmonary vascular resistance before surgery. Typical heart defects for this are those with high flow and pressure driven left-to-right shunt defects (large VSD, AVSD, Truncus, etc.) and those with unrestricted flow over a long period (i.e., >6 or 12 months of age). Postoperatively, there may be a rapid and critical increase in pulmonary arterial pressure or pulmonary vascular resistance in certain situations (i.e., agitation, external stimulation such as suctioning, pain, etc.). The result of a rapid increase in PVR is a standstill of the trans-pulmonary blood flow with secondary congestion in the right atrium (high CVP) and ventricle and drop in pressure in the left atrium and ventricle (low CO and BP). Ultimately, cardiac output collapses and the coronaries are not perfused. The following patients are at a particularly high risk for this type of crisis:

- Patients with already increased pulmonary vascular resistance preoperatively (primary pulmonary hypertension)
- Neonates within the first week of life
- Patients with pulmonary venous hypertension (e.g., within the context of a total anomalous pulmonary venous connection or mitral stenosis)
- Older children with a still uncorrected high flow and pressure shunt defects that led to an increase in pulmonary vascular resistance (e.g., complete AV canal, large VSD, truncus)

The following factors may increase pulmonary vascular resistance:

- Hypoxia
- Acidosis (pH <7.3, BE less than −5)
- High partial pressure of carbon dioxide ($paCO_2$ >50)
- Polycythemia
- Atelectasis
- Agitation

The following factors may reduce pulmonary vascular resistance:

- Oxygen administration
- Alkalosis
- Hyperventilation
- NO inhalation (nitric oxide)
- Recruitment of atelectatic lung segments

Prophylaxis of a pulmonary hypertensive crisis is crucial, the acute management as well as the prophylaxis of a pulmonary hypertensive crisis includes the following measures:

- Sufficient analgesia and sedation or relaxation for 1–2 days
- Oxygenation (paO_2 >150)
- Optimizing the ventilation (adequate PEEP)
- Slightly alkalotic pH level (target pH 7.4–7.5) and mild hyperventilation ($paCo_2$ 30–35)
- Pharmacological vasodilators (NO, iloprost, prostacyclin)
- Avoidance of unnecessary manipulations such as too frequent suctioning

2.7. Specific early postoperative problems

Cardiac defects or surgery-specific postoperative problems and complications are summarized in **Table 4**.

Cardiac defect/operation	Specific early postoperative problems and complications
ASD closure	Sinus node dysfunction, left heart failure/pulmonary edema in older children and adults
VSD closure	Pulmonary hypertensive crisis, complete AV block, JET, residual shunt
AV canal correction	Pulmonary hypertensive crisis, complete AV block, JET, AV valve stenosis or incompetence
PDA ligation	Injury to the recurrent laryngeal nerve (vocal cord paralysis) or the thoracic duct (chylothorax), accidental ligation or injury to surrounding vessels (especially left pulmonary artery, aorta
Truncus arterious correction	Pulmonary hypertensive crisis, truncus valve stenosis or incompetence, right ventricular dysfunction
Aortopulmonary window (correction)	Pulmonary hypertensive crisis, coronary ischemia
Anomalous pulmonary venous connection (correction)	Pulmonary hypertensive crisis, atrial arrhythmia, residual stenosis of the pulmonary veins or pulmonary vein anastomosis with the left ventricle, high left ventricular filling pressure due to the relatively small left atrium and ventricle
Fallot correction	Right ventricular diastolic dysfunction (poor compliance of the hypertrophic ventricle), JET, complete AV block, residual pulmonary stenosis, residual VSD, pulmonary insufficiency after a transannular patch
Pulmonary atresia with intact ventricular septum	Right ventricular dysfunction, myocardial ischemia due to right ventricle dependent coronary circulation, circular shunting due to creation of an aortopulmonary shunt and opening of right ventricular outflow tract
Aortic stenosis correction	Residual stenosis, disruption of left ventricular diastolic function, aortic insufficiency, AV block
Ross procedure	Coronary ischemia
Konno procedure	Coronary ischemia, obstruction of the right ventricular outflow tract, arrhythmias (e.g., AV block), mitral regurgitation
Subaortic stenosis (resection)	Residual stenosis, mitral valve injury, (ventricular) arrhythmia, AV block
Coarctation of the aorta (resection)	Residual obstruction, paraplegia, post-coarctectomy syndrome, unmasking an aortic valve stenosis, injury to the recurrent laryngeal nerve, chylothorax
Interrupted aortic arch (correction)	Residual obstruction, compression of the left main bronchus by the aorta, injury to the recurrent laryngeal nerve, chylothorax
Mitral stenosis correction	Pulmonary hypertensive crisis, residual stenosis, mitral regurgitation, left ventricular dysfunction
Creation of an aortopulmonary shunt	Imbalance between systemic and pulmonary perfusion, shunt leak, shunt thrombosis, pulmonary edema, coronary ischemia
Pulmonary artery banding	Cyanosis, insufficient banding (excessive pulmonary blood flow), Qp-Qs mismatch
Norwood procedure	Low cardiac output, imbalance between systemic and pulmonary perfusion, residual obstruction of the aortic arch, AV valve insufficiency, SIRS
Superior cavopulmonary anastomosis (Glenn, Hemifontan)	Cyanosis, hypertension, edema/congestion of the upper half of the body, Chylothorax
Fontan completion	Ascites, pleural effusions, edema, cyanosis, low cardiac output, arrhythmias

Cardiac defect/operation	Specific early postoperative problems and complications
TGA (switch operation)	Coronary ischemia, left ventricular dysfunction, neo aortic insufficiency, peripheral pulmonary stenosis
TGA (Mustard/Senning atrial baffle procedure)	Pulmonary or systemic venous obstruction, atrial arrhythmias
Bland-White-Garland syndrome (correction)	Myocardial dysfunction, mitral regurgitation

Table 4. Specific early postoperative problem and complications (modified from Schwartz and Millar 2009 in Roger's Handbook of Pediatric Intensive care).

2.8. Postoperative features of heart defects with a univentricular heart

The large group of heart defects with a univentricular physiology may pose great challenges to postoperative intensive care in the PCICU. These patients include those with a hypoplastic left heart syndrome, tricuspid atresia, or a double inlet left ventricle. The most important principles in the postoperative treatment of these patients are presented below. As an example, the three-stage surgical procedure for patient with a hypoplastic left heart syndrome is explained. In general, palliation in a Fontan procedure is made with the goal of achieving complete separation of the pulmonary and systemic circulation to eliminate cyanosis. The lungs are perfused passively from the vena cavae without any pumping chamber in between. The single ventricle supplies only the systemic circulation and thereby has a reduced volume load.

The three stages are as follows:

- Norwood procedure or Damus-Kaye-Stansel procedure with a shunt
- Upper cavopulmonary anastomosis (Glenn procedure, "hemi Fontan")
- Total cavopulmonary anastomosis (Fontan procedure)

2.8.1. Norwood procedure

The Norwood procedure is the first step for patients with a hypoplastic left heart syndrome toward separation of the circulatory systems by a Fontan procedure. There are several modifications of this surgical procedure (classical Norwood, Norwood-Sano-procedure). The principal goal is to form a neo-aorta from the pulmonary artery and the hypoplastic aorta that can supply the systemic circulation with blood without a pressure gradient (i.e., unobstructed systemic blood flow). To achieve this, the pulmonary artery and the hypoplastic aorta are anastomosed distal to the valves. Additional patch material is usually required for the reconstruction of the aortic arch and excision of the coarctation. In this manner, a strong vessel for systemic perfusion is created. The pulmonary artery is transected shortly before the pulmonary artery bifurcation and in most cases, pulmonary perfusion is ensured via an aortopulmonary shunt or Sano shunt (placement of a conduit through right ventricular to pulmonary artery).

To achieve the unobstructed inflow to the heart and outflow from the pulmonary veins, an atrial septectomy is also performed. There is a balance between the pulmonary and systemic circulatory systems when arterial saturation is between 75 and 85% (Qp/Qs = 1).

Typical problems after a Norwood procedure are low cardiac output, capillary leak caused by SIRS and hypoxemia.

2.8.1.1. *Low cardiac output*

As a typical result of the long bypass time required or even prolonged circulatory arrest, a systemic inflammatory response syndrome (SIRS) of various degrees occurs in these neonates. As a consequence, myocardial function is usually markedly impaired so that a certain and often higher amount of catecholamine support is always needed postoperatively. Other possible causes of inadequate systemic perfusion are increased pulmonary perfusion at the expense of systemic perfusion (Qp/Qs >1; leading symptoms: arterial saturation>85%, tachycardia, hypotension, oliguria, metabolic acidosis). To manage this situation, an attempt is made by reducing the afterload of the systemic circulation and increasing pulmonary resistance. AV valve insufficiency or arrhythmias can also cause or deteriorate low cardiac output.

2.8.1.2. *Hypoxemia*

Hypoxemia (i.e., saturation <70%) can be the result of an imbalance between pulmonary and systemic circulations to the detriment of the pulmonary circulation—for example, in an obstruction of the aortopulmonary shunt or increased pulmonary resistance.

Other causes are typical pulmonary problems such as atelectasis, a pleural effusion, edema, or pneumonia. Peripheral cyanosis occurs with low cardiac output or increased oxygen consumption (leading symptom: reduced systemic venous saturation).

2.8.2. *Superior cavopulmonary anastomosis*

The aim of a superior cavopulmonary anastomosis is to allow passive blood flow from the upper half of the body into the pulmonary circulation. The superior vena cava is anastomosed in an end-to side manor with the pulmonary artery and thereby the systemic venous blood from the upper half of the body then flows passively to the lungs without an intermediate pumping chamber and is oxygenated there. The systemic venous blood from the lower half of the body does not reach the lungs, but is mixed with the pulmonary venous blood in the heart and pumped into the systemic circulation. The systemic circulation thus contains mixed blood. The saturation of these children is usually about 80–85%.

This step leads to a complete hemodynamic unloading of the univentricular heart as the pulmonary circulation and systemic circulation are now connected in series. The Qp/Qs ratio is then 0.6–0.7; oxygen saturation is 80–85%. In comparison with older children, the head and upper limbs in young children are relatively large and therefore, the overall ratio of pulmonary perfusion is still higher in younger children. The percentage of systemic venous blood from the upper half of the body, that reaches the lungs via the cavopulmonary anastomosis and is oxygenated there, is correspondingly higher.

Typical postoperative problems are increased pressure in the superior vena cava, hypertension and hypoxemia.

2.8.2.1. *Elevated pressure in the superior vena cava*

In a superior cavopulmonary anastomosis, elevated pressure in the superior vena cava suggests an obstruction in the area of the cavopulmonary anastomosis or pulmonary circulation or elevated pulmonary vascular resistance.

The difference in pressure between the superior vena cava and atrium (transpulmonary gradient) should be <10 mmHg. A high pressure in the superior vena cava can restrict cerebral outflow and lead to marked edema in the upper half of the body (superior vena cava syndrome).

After this operation, patients should be positioned with the upper body elevated (about 45°, half sitting position). Elevated intrathoracic pressure from mechanical ventilation additionally hinders passive blood flow from the superior vena cava into the pulmonary circulation and patients should therefore be quickly extubated.

2.8.2.2. *Hypertension*

Temporary hypertension during the first few postoperative days is not unusual in these patients. The elevation of intracranial pressure that is necessary to maintain adequate cerebral perfusion pressure may be one reason. Aggressive lowering of the blood pressure should therefore be avoided but normal arterial pressures should be obtained.

2.8.2.3. *Hypoxemia*

Saturation levels below 75% following a superior cavopulmonary anastomosis can be caused by many reasons all resulting in a reduction in pulmonary perfusion. This may be due to an obstruction in the area of the anastomosis or pulmonary vessels. Another possible explanation is that blood from the upper half of the body is conducted past the alveoli, for example, if there are venovenous collaterals (connections between the systemic and pulmonary veins), the azygos vein was not ligated by the surgeon, a left sided superior vena cava has reopened or arteriovenous collaterals (connections between the pulmonary arteries and veins) have gained importance.

In the early postoperative phase, arterial saturation can often be improved by attempting mild hypoventilation. Slightly elevated pCO_2 (>50 mmHg) causes vasodilatation of the cerebral vessels, so more blood flows to the brain. Since this allows relatively more blood to reach the upper half of the body, more blood is conducted through the SVC and into the lungs and becomes oxygenated. In addition, the blood can also be slightly alkalized by administering sodium bicarbonate (target pH >7.4).

2.8.3. *Total cavopulmonary anastomosis (Fontan procedure)*

In a Fontan procedure (total cavopulmonary anastomosis), the pulmonary and systemic circulation are finally completely separated by anastomosing the inferior vena cava also with the pulmonary circulation. A tunnel is created that connects the inferior vena cava with the pulmonary artery. This tunnel may pass either through the atrium (intracardiac Fontan) or alternatively outside the heart (extracardiac tunnel). It should be standard to leave a small shunt between the Fontan tunnel and the atrium (i.e., Fontan fenestration) that functions as an overflow (right-to-left shunt) if the resistance in the pulmonary circulation is too high and not all of the systemic venous blood can enter the pulmonary circulation. This may have the disadvantage of mild hypoxemia but the positive effects (improved systemic circulation, decompression of the venous side, less ascites, edema, etc.) clearly overweigh the disadvantage of lower saturations.

When the Fontan circulation is completed, all of the systemic venous blood (exception: coronary sinus) flows passively into the pulmonary circulation without passing through a pumping ventricle. The oxygenated blood is then pumped into the systemic circulation by the univentricular heart.

Typical postoperative problems are low cardiac output, hypoxemia, effusions, arrhythmias and thrombosis.

2.8.3.1. *Low cardiac output*

In Fontan patients, low cardiac output can often occur due to low preload (hypovolemia), increased pulmonary resistance, or an obstruction in the area of the systemic venous outflow (tunnel stenosis, anastomosis stenosis). Therefore, higher volume requirements are often necessary in these patients. In addition, poor ventricular function or AV valve insufficiency and arrhythmias can also cause low cardiac output.

2.8.3.2. *Arrhythmias*

As the completion of the Fontan procedure require surgical manipulation at the atrium and the area of the sinus node, atrial arrhythmias may occur and sinus node dysfunction is typical. A pacemaker (atrial stimulation) sometimes becomes necessary.

2.8.3.3. *Hypoxemia*

Cyanosis can be the result of a relevant right-to-left shunt across a tunnel fenestration. In addition, the usual pulmonary problems (i.e., pleural effusion, atelectasis, pneumonia) can also lead to hypoxemia. Reduced pulmonary perfusion, caused by arteriovenous or venovenous collaterals can also cause hypoxemia in Fontan patients.

2.8.3.4. *Effusions*

Pleural effusions and ascites are common immediately after surgery. They can be the result of elevated venous pressure and volume load required and may lead to considerable postoperative complications.

2.8.3.5. Thrombosis

Based on the low flow in the Fontan circuit, these patients are at an increased risk of developing venous thrombosis. This risk is increased especially if there is low cardiac output. Most centers therefore recommend lifelong anticoagulation for Fontan patients. There is, however, no uniform opinion with respect to the duration or the form of anticoagulation (vitamin K antagonists or platelet aggregation inhibitors). While many different anticoagulation regimens are used in small children (no anticoagulation, aspirin, warfarin), there is a general consensus that anti-coagulation is obligatory in patients after puberty.

Acknowledgements

Parts of this book chapter are similar to a recent publication of the third author [11]. Based on the content of the scientific information, this is, however, current state-of-the-art knowledge and medical management; therefore, similarities in the text are logical necessity.

Author details

Eva Miranda Marwali[1*], Beatrice Heineking[2] and Nikolaus A. Haas[2]

*Address all correspondence to: evamarwali@yahoo.com

1 Pediatric Cardiac Intensive Care Unit, National Cardiovascular Center Harapan Kita, Jakarta, Indonesia

2 Department of Pediatric Cardiology and Pediatric Intensive Care Medicine, University Hospital of Munich, Ludwig Maxmilians University, Munich, Germany

References

[1] Allen HD, et al. Moss and Adams' heart disease in infants, children and adolescents including the fetus and young adult. Philadelphia: Lippincott Williams & Wilkins; 2008.

[2] Chang AC, et al. Pediatric cardiac intensive care. Philadelphia: Lippincott Williams & Wilkins; 1998.

[3] Cloherty JP, Eichenwald EC, Stark AR. Manual of neonatal care. Philadelphia: Lippincott Williams & Wilkins; 2008.

[4] Driscoll DJ. Fundamentals of pediatric cardiology. Philadelphia: Lippincott Williams & Wilkins; 2006.

[5] Helfaer MA, Nichols DG. Roger's handbook of pediatric intensive care. Philadelphia: Lippincott Williams & Wilkins; 2009.

[6] Keane JF, Lock JE, Fyler DC. Nadas' pediatric cardiology. Philadelphia: Saunders Elsevier; 2006.

[7] Kretz FJ, Becke K. Anesthesia and Pediatric Intensive Care Medicine. Stuttgart: Thieme; 2007.

[8] Park MK. Pediatric cardiology for practitioners. Philadelphia: Mosby Elsevier; 2008.

[9] Alsoufi B, Bennetts J, Verma S, Caldarone CA. New developments in the treatment of hypoplastic left heart syndrome. Pediatrics 2007;119:109–117.

[10] Derrick G, Cullen S. Transposition of the great arteries. Curr Treat Options Cardiovasc Med 2000;2:499–506.

[11] Haas NA, Kleideiter U. Pediatric cardiology—symptoms, diagnosis—treatment. Stuttgart, New York, Delhi, Rio de Janeiro: Thieme Verlag; 2015.

10

Neonatal Care for Anesthesiologists

Esra Caliskan

Abstract

In recent years, developments in obstetrics and neonatology have significantly improved the survival and quality life time of neonates. Therefore, anesthesiologists are more confronted with these patients due to surgical and non-surgical procedures. For a safe anesthetic approach and safe care, anesthesiologist must have necessary knowledge and equipment on the physiology of the newborn and should be better understand how immature organs respond to surgery and anesthetic. The purpose of this section is to present spot information that will allow clinicians and anesthesiologists to better understand the problems of neonatal patients and to perform safe care for these patients in the light of the physiologic characteristics of neonates. General principles of anesthetic management of neonatal patients are also reviewed and discussed.

Keywords: neonatal physiology, anesthetic management, perioperative evaluation, postoperative care, neonatal surgery

1. Introduction

Differently from the adult patients, pediatric, especially neonatal age group is a patient population that is difficult to assess. It should not be forgotten that children are not miniaturized adults. Therefore, the preoperative evaluation of the neonate is admittedly the most important part of anesthetic evaluation. The developments in the field of neonatal medicine over the past two decades have increased our probability of encountering a healthy and unhealthy neonatal population [1]. Surgical procedures especially emergency surgical conditions can be represent a significant anesthetic challenge and life threatening in neonatal period [2, 3].

Therefore, the anesthetist needs to take into account the immature function of many vital organ systems, the normal course of development, the effects of the underlying pathologic disease processes, which can frequently lead to serious physiological instability [4, 5].

In this chapter will be discussed issues that related to the anesthetic approach and postoperative care to neonatal patients.

2. Physiological feature in neonatal period

2.1. Organ and system differences in neonate

The neonatal period shows anatomical and physiological differences when compared to adult period. In this section, will be mentioned to physiological characteristics of neonates, also anatomical differences of neonates will be discussed in the part of anesthetic management.

It is important to know the anatomical airway differences between adults and children and newborns for a complete anesthesia assessment [6]. These differences can be listed as follows:

- Proportionately larger head and tongue,
- Narrower nasal passages,
- An anterior and cephalad larynx,
- A longer epiglottis,
- Shorter trachea and neck.

Because of these anatomical features, nasal breathing is dominant in neonates and infants until about 5 months of age [6].

In the newborn period, many vital organ and system functions are immature [7]. In respiratory system, high pulmonary vascular resistance (PVR) which is characteristics in fetal circulation decreases by approximately 10% after labor, but the apparent decrease occurs with the first breath [8, 9]. When the transition period to the adult circulation is examined, pulmonary blood flow, increased alveolar and arterial PO_2 appear to be important factors.

The characteristics of the neonatal respiratory system can be listed as follows: [1, 6].

- Immature hypoxic response, lower functional residual capacity (limits oxygen reserves during period of apnea, rapid desaturation in prolonged intubation attempt),
- Central control of ventilation is not fully develop,
- Peripheral feedback mechanisms are not sufficiently mature,
- Neonatal oxygen consumption 6 cc kg^{-1} per minute is twice that of resting adult (this value increases 10 cc kg^{-1} in the first week of life).

Cardiovascular system changes are also observed during neonatal period. The circulation of a newborn infant is a dynamic state which may revert to a transitional characteristic at any time. This means that the adult series circulation accompanies fetal parallel circulation [10].

The onset of spontaneous breathing is the main factor that reduces high PVR which is characteristic of fetal circulation. This decrease in pulmonary pressure is followed by an increase in systemic vascular resistance and left atrial pressure. Some clinical situations such as hypoxia and acidosis may lead to reduction of pulmonary blood flow which causes a return the fetal circulation features that is called persistent fetal circulation (PFC) [11].

Cardiac function is heart rate dependent in healthy neonates because the immature myocardium has limited compliance [2, 12].

The parasympathetic system is predominant in neonates [10], so that vagal stimulus by laryngoscopy and hypoxia may cause bradycardia. Therefore, it should be avoided bradycardia and treated aggressively when it is observed.

Liver and kidney function are also closely related to the anesthetic management of neonates. In the neonatal period, both organs have not yet completed maturation. The liver serves a critical role in carbohydrate, protein, lipid metabolism, coagulation. And is the primary site for biotransformation of drugs [13]. Hepatic oxidation, reduction and hydrolysis maturation process is rapid and these functions reaches adult rates around 6 month of ages [14]. Because of this, newborns may metabolize drugs (include anesthetic drugs) and toxins less efficiently than adults in the early months of their lives, as the pathway of degradation is immature [1]. Also, one of the changes in early infancy is the lower concentration of total serum protein, albumin and α1-acid glycoprotein. These proteins reach the adult level at about 1 year old [14].

One of the main routes of clearance of drugs and metabolites are the kidneys too. Glomerular filtration rate (GFR), active secretion and passive reabsorption are functions that determine renal excretion of drugs [15].

The kidneys also play an important role in the maintaining of acid base homeostasis and fluid electrolyte balance. GFR and reabsorption are increase age dependent manner. A neonate's kidney takes approximately 6–12 months to achieve adult performance.

In the perioperative period, fluid electrolyte balance is affected and the metabolism of commonly used anesthetic drug altered [10]. Drug metabolism and protein binding are also reduced due to immature organ (hepatic and renal) function [16].

Maturational physiologic changes are most prominent in neonatal period and infancy. The distribution of total body fluid component in neonates is different from adults. Body fluid constitute a greater proportion of body weight in the neonate (approximately 70–75%) and higher than adults. In neonate, the intracellular and extracellular fluid compartments are approximately 45 and 33% of body weight, respectively [17]. These body component changes affect volumes of distribution of drugs.

2.2. Thermoregulation

The newborn baby has a greater surface area relative to weight and a thin layer subcutaneous fat tissue [3]. These properties cause more heat loss to the environment in neonates than older children and adult. Nonshivering thermogenesis is regulated by brown fat is the primary mechanism in heat generation in the neonates [1]. Brown fat tissue is located in the posterior neck along the interscapular and vertebral regions and it is responsible for heat generation in newborns.

There are four different mechanisms of heat loss [18]:

- Evaporation,
- Convection,
- Conduction,
- Radiation,

Cold intravenous fluids, exposure to cold sterilization solutions, drying of anesthetic gases and the direct effect of anesthetic agents on temperature regulation are the factors that increase this loss.

For this reason mentioned above, caution should be exercised in serious temperature changes in the perioperative period. Hypothermia may cause undesirable effects such as acidosis, myocardial depression, and delay recovery from anesthesia [19, 20].

Maximum precautions should be taken to prevent hypothermia in the perioperative period. These precautions are mentioned in the intraoperative management section.

Characteristics of neonates and infants that differentiate them adult patients are summarized in **Table 1**.

Anatomical differences	**Physiological differences**	**Pharmacological differences**
Head and neck • Relatively larger head and tongue • Narrower nasal passage • Anterior and cephalad larynx • Relatively longer epiglottis and shorter trachea Circulation • Left ventricle –noncompliant • Transitional circulation Respiratory • Weak intercostal and diaphragmatic muscles • Increased resistance to airflow	Increasing parameters • Heart rate (dependent cardiac output) • Respiratory rate • Metabolic rate • Total body water content • Chest wall compliance • Ratio of body surface area to body weight Decreasing parameters • Blood pressure • Functional residual capacity • Lung compliance	Hepatic function • Immature biotransformation • Decreased protein, decreased binding for drug Respiratory changes • More rapid rise in *FA/FI • more rapid induction and recovery from inhaled anesthetics • Increased minimum alveolar concentration Body fluid changes • Relatively larger volume distribution for water- soluble drugs • Immature neuromuscular junction

*FA/FI: Fractional alveolar concentration/fractional inspired concentration.
Table has modified by Lange Clinical Anesthesia 2015.

Table 1. Characteristics of neonates and infants that differentiate them adult patient.

3. General principles of anesthesia in neonate

Neonatal period, which is the most vulnerable time period in terms of anesthetic risk and perioperative mortality, is a challenging period for pediatric anesthetists.

Drug interactions, physiological and anatomical differences, and knowledge of risk factors are also important to reduce these risks.

What are the risks associated with neonatal anesthesia? In addition to the neonatal differences, prematurity, congenital anomalies, asphyxia at birth, and emergency situations that required surgery are risk factors. At the same time, there is a very narrow margin of error, including airway management, vascular access and drug administration. Some of these risk factors are summarized in **Table 2**.

Therefore, a safe aesthetic approach depends on a good understanding of the variables and physiological and anatomical changes taking place in the transition from fatal to neonatal life.

Anatomical differences
Airway anomalies
Difficult airway: Micrognathia, macroglossia, cleft palate-lift
Prematurity, Immature organ and system function
Respiratory
Apnea (especially premature neonates)
Respiratory failure, mechanical ventilatory support, supplemental oxygen
Oxygenation: avoid high FiO_2 (high FiO_2, risk of retinopathy, NEC)
Cardiac
Transitional circulation
Persistent pulmonary hypertension
Immature myocardium
Parasympathetic dominance
Neurological problems
Intraventricular/periventricular hemorrhage (IVH, PVH)
Congenital syndromes and disorders (especially associated with risk of difficult airway, comorbidities of cardiac defect)
• Pierre-Robin syndrome
• Treacher-Collins syndrome (mandibulofacial dysostosis)
• Goldenhar syndrome
• Klippel-Feil syndrome
• Down syndrome
Pharmacological differences
Anesthetic drugs – dilutional changes, prolonged effect
Fluid management
Glucose: avoid hypoglycemia
Intolerance for rapid fluid infusion
Problems of vascular access
Temperature management
Prevent hypothermia
Emergency surgery

Table 2. Risk factors in neonatal anesthesia.

3.1. Effects of anesthetic drugs and inhalation anesthetics on neonates

Effective and safe drug administration in neonates should be based on detailed knowledge on the physiological characteristics of the neonates and pharmacokinetics and pharmacodynamics of given drug. Clinical pharmacology in neonates is recognized with extensive variability. The effect of anesthetic agents varies with organ maturation, body water content and metabolic differences and, coexisting disease in neonatal patient population.

Inhalation anesthesia is a commonly used anesthetic technique in neonatal population. However, intravenous and regional anesthesia methods also can be applied as anesthetic technique in this patient population. The minimum alveolar concentration (MAC) of an inhaled anesthetic is the alveolar concentration that prevents movement in 50% of patients in response to a standardized stimulus (e.g., surgical incision) and changes with age [1, 6, 21]. MAC for inhalational agents is less in neonates than in infants (up to 6 months of age [12, 21]. In newborns, cardiac and respiratory functions and blood pressure are very sensitive to volatile anesthesia. Immature myocardium and less developed compensatory mechanisms are responsible for this result. Therefore, these anesthetics can cause dose dependent cardiac and respiratory depressant effect and can be seen bradycardia, hypotension and postoperative apnea. These effects are more pronounced during the induction period [12, 22].

Intravenous anesthetic agents may be used for induction of anesthesia when inhalational anesthetics are not preferred and/or not practices.

Factors affecting the administration of intravenous anesthesia can be listed as follows:

- Larger intravascular and extracellular fluid compartments,
- Immaturity of hepatic biotransformation pathways,
- Decreased protein binding,
- Increased organ blood flow,
- Higher metabolic rate.

These factors mentioned above affect the properties of the intravenous anesthetics such as duration of effect (onset and termination), doses and toxicity limits of drugs.

An opioid agent causes fewer hemodynamic changes but it should be noted that increase the risk of postoperative apnea and late-onset re-sedation in recovery in preterm and term neonates [2, 4].

Thus, it is crucial that intravenous lines are flushed and cleared of any medication (e.g. opioid, neuromuscular blocker).

Muscle relaxant may be required for some surgical procedures (especially abdominal surgical procedures such as necrotizing enterocolitis, abdominal wall defect). The response of neonates to nondepolarizing muscle relaxant is quite variable. Neuromuscular junction is immature in preterms and this increases the susceptibility to muscle relaxants. However, the large extracellular distribution volume will dilute the drug concentration, while those metabolized in the liver will prolong the duration.

4. Anesthesia preparation in neonates before surgical procedure

4.1. Preoperative evaluation

Anesthetic management in neonatal patients can be challenging but careful preoperative assessment means that a safe and smooth preparation process for the neonates and anesthetic team. This evaluation is also an approach that encourages confidence for their parents.

A careful preoperative examination allows the anesthetist to determine the risk of anesthesia based on the general state of health of newborn. It is aimed to establish an appropriate plan for anesthesia, postoperative care and analgesia in the light of acquired information.

Preoperative assessment in neonates should include a comprehensive examination of the neonate's perinatal history (such as prematurity, apnea-hypoxic episode history, duration of oxygen dependency, neurological damage etc.), congenital anomalies, previous anesthesia applications, and general state of health (acute, chronic lung disease, cardiac pathologies, etc.) [23].

Premature, ex-premature and term neonates are highly heterogeneous group within newborn period and needs various surgical interventions. Most of them come directly from the neonatal intensive care unit (NICU) and require urgent intervention. Many unusual congenital syndromes occur in childhood. These congenital anomalies in newborn period may accompany emergency surgical procedures [24]. Congenital anomalies that may cause difficult intubation should be noted and the anesthesia plan should be made accordingly.

In addition, a more detailed examination should be performed to reveal early postnatal problems that may be seen (such as hypoglycemia, infection and sepsis, etc.).

Risk factors which are important in neonatal anesthesia are summarized in **Table 2**.

A systematic approach to preoperative evaluation will prevent important problems from being overlooked. Many healthy neonates undergoing elective simple surgery and procedures are fit and do not require compressive physical examination. However, evaluation of the head and neck (such micrognathia, limited neck mobility, macroglossia, etc.) and cardiorespiratory examination (cardiac congenital anomalies, breathing sounds, respiratory pathologies associated with increased secretion and inflammation etc.) should be performed before surgical procedures. Also in cardiac examination, previously undiagnosed murmur with pathological qualities (e.g. loud, continuous, diastolic and or/associated with a trill) may be noticeable.

Evaluation of the airway is critical to the delivery of safe anesthesia. In neonates with a syndrome associated with airway anomalies, the potential presence of a difficult airway (**Table 2**) (*e.g. Pierre-Robin, Goldenhar, Treacher-Collins Syndrome, cleft palate and lip, maxilla mandibular synechia, etc.*) can be identified preoperatively.

It is also important to identify any concomitant (such as necrotizing enterocolitis, hyaline membrane syndrome, cardiac pathologies, sepsis, etc.) disease which might increase the risk of anesthesia and surgery. Familial, genetic, and neuromuscular diseases are important for anesthetic management. The presence of these diseases should be questioned.

Body weight, height, head circumference size must be recorded in order to evaluate newborn's physical status. For example, microcephaly is associated with some genetic disorders and may cause neurological sequel, which may pose a risk for anesthesia.

In laboratory evaluation, a baseline hemoglobin measurement should be obtained for minor surgical procedures [24]. If there is no indication for emergency surgery, anemia should be treated before surgical procedure. Because, even if it is a minor surgery, anemia may precipitate postoperative apnea and bradycardia in neonate. In addition to hemoglobin, in infants with fluid and electrolyte deficit, initial electrolyte values are also important. In major surgeries (e.g. oesophageal atresia, necrotizing enterocolitis, congenital cardiac surgery, neurosurgery) full blood count, blood electrolyte values, renal function and clotting test are recommended [25].

Fasting time before elective surgery should be pointed out. Clear liquid, breast milk and formula milk intake should be prohibited at according to the recommended fasting times (2 hours for clear liquids, 4 hours for breast milk, 6 hours for formula/non-human milk) before elective surgery [12, 14, 25]. Since prolonged period of fasting time pose a risk for hypoglycemia and dehydration, dextrose containing intravenous maintenance fluids should be instituted early period.

A systematic approach the preoperative assessment is summarized in **Table 3**.

Gathering of patient information
History of neonate
Perinatal
Medical conditions (co-morbidities, congenital syndromes, genetic disease)
Medications
Previous anesthesia and surgical experience
Examination
Body weight, height
Physical observation
Airway (especially pathologies that can cause difficult intubation, micrognathia)
Respiratory System
Prematurity
Bronchopulmonary dysplasia
Laryngeal pathologies, stridor
Breathing sounds
Cardiovascular system
Auscultation of heart
Neurological (intracranial hemorrhage history-treatment, seizure activation)
Previous resuscitation history
Previous anesthesia experience
Optimize medical condition
Determination of anesthesia risk
Determination of anesthetic plan

Table 3. Systematic approach to preoperative assessment.

4.2. Preparation of the operating theater

Anesthesia preparation should be based on the information obtained from the preoperative visit. But, anesthesia preparation does not include preparation of anesthetic equipment, drugs and anesthesia station only. It also includes preparations for the operating theater, such as proper heating of the surgery room, preparations for aspiration materials and arrangements for the patient's position.

The newborn baby has a high ratio surface area to body weight and a thin layer subcutaneous fat tissue. Therefore, neonates lose heat rapidly more than older children and adult [1]. The operating room temperature must be set to maintained neonate's thermoneutral temperature in order to minimize heat loss. In addition, the following applications can be used to reduce heat loss:

- Humidify and warm inspired anesthetic gases
- Many devices such as warmed blanket, overhead radiant heater, a forced air warmer mattress, clear plastic drapes
- Using heating solution for cleansing the skin
- Warm blood and intravenous solutions
- Transport the neonate in a heated incubator

Gas resources and suction materials must be checked.

The patient position is one of the issues to be considered. Different materials such as soft foam padding, rolls and tapes can be used safely for the position.

4.3. Assessment of patient and anesthetic equipment

Proper anesthesia preparation is very important for safe anesthetic management. This is one of the goals of the preoperative visit.

4.3.1. Airway

No matter what anesthetic method is used (sedation or general anesthesia), the airway must be guaranteed in every situation. Difficult, immature airway and respiratory system can lead to airway obstruction during sedation or mask ventilation. Therefore, appropriately size face mask, oropharyngeal airway, laryngoscope blades, endotracheal tube and suction catheters must be available. The use of transparent face masks are recommended for early recognition of cyanosis, vomiting and secretions.

Endotracheal Intubation Study Group [26] demonstrated that the use of Microcuffed tracheal tubes is effective and safe in neonates and young children. But, most anesthetist prefer to use according to the clinical condition of the patient rather than routine.

The laryngeal mask airway (LMA) can be used as an alternative to endotracheal intubation in the presence of difficult airway and for some short surgical procedures. Against possibility of difficult pediatric airway, advanced airway devices (such as Glidescope, Airtraq) which allow indirect visualization of the larynx should be available [27].

4.3.2. Anesthesia devices

The anesthesia device must be pre-checked before surgical procedure and anesthesia practice. It is essential that the anesthesia ventilator has the ability to provide neonatal compliance, small tidal volume (usually in pressure controlled ventilator mode) and positive end-expiratory pressure [24]. In recent years, new generation anesthesia machines have been developed which is able to small tidal volumes [28] and to provide the ability to ventilate using pressure support ventilation (PSV) [29].

4.3.3. Monitoring

Heart rate-electrocardiography, non-invasive blood pressure, pulse oximetry, and temperature monitorizations are sufficient for basic monitorizations in a healthy newborn.

In neonates whom more risky for surgical procedures, in major surgical procedures and a special circumstances (such as congenital cardiac surgery, oesophageal atresia, congenital diaphragmatic hernia, expected ventilation-perfusion anomalies, hemodynamic changes, and acid-base imbalance), invasive arterial blood pressure and central venous pressure should be monitored.

Two oxygen saturation probes (the right arm probe – pre ductal, the leg probe - post ductal) must be plugged. This approach may provide the diagnosis as, with reverting to transitional circulation and is important to evaluate possible PDA mediated shunt development.

In last three decades, continuous monitoring of respiratory gases (inspiratory oxygen and expiratory end-tidal carbon dioxide and monitoring of gas flows) and continuous use of ventilator disconnection devices are observed routinely in most anesthesia clinic [27].

The precordial oesophageal stethoscope is a traditional and still valid method of monitoring the newborn. With this method, changes in heart rate and respiratory parameters can be identified in early phase.

5. Intraoperative management of anesthesia

5.1. Induction of anesthesia

The anesthesia station is the working area of the anesthetist. Before the surgical procedure, all drugs and equipments required for anesthetic administration should be checked. The neonate should be properly monitored and placed on a forced-air warming mattress before the induction of anesthesia. A safe intravenous access should be established for drug use and fluid therapy. The use of a topical anesthetic such as EMLA cream facilitates awake placement of intravenous cannula [30].

In addition to routine monitoring, direct observation of the neonate is also an important monitoring method. This observation allows the anesthetist to recognize early signs of certain clinic situations (such as cyanosis and pallor).

Inhalation agents or intravenous anesthetics may be used for induction of anesthesia. Although depending on the choice of anesthetist, induction with inhalation anesthetics is a more preferred method. One of the characteristics of the newborns that are different from older children and adults is that they have relatively high alveolar ventilation but low functional residual capacity [6, 14, 24]. This higher minute ventilation to FRC ratio with relatively higher blood flow to vessel rich organs contributes to a rapid increase in alveolar anesthetic concentration. These features enable rapid induction and rapid recovery in general anesthesia [6].

Inhalational induction has the advantage of protection of spontaneous ventilation (especially, important in neonates with potentially difficult airway).

With the advantages we have mentioned above, volatile anesthetics cause dose dependent cardiac and respiratory depressant effect in neonates. These effects can result bradycardia, hypotension and postoperative apnea. This hypotensive effect is also more pronounced in neonates and preterms with cardiovascular instability than older children.

Also, immature airway and respiratory system may cause airway obstruction in mask ventilation during induction phase. Laryngospasm is a frequent occurrence in neonatal anesthesia in this period [31] and if it is intervened early is usually easy to manage. However, laryngospasm, hypoventilation, hypoxia are among the causes of apnea during induction (especially in cases of late notice) [32].

In short surgical procedures, mask ventilation or laryngeal mask airway may be suitable to support respiration. However, endotracheal intubation is frequently performed in patients with emergency surgical procedures, long and major surgical interventions, conditions that requiring muscle relaxation and aspiration risk.

In situation that where inhalation anesthetics are contraindicated or not preferred, intravenous anesthetics may be used to induce and maintain anesthesia.

As we have already mentioned, total body water and extracellular fluid are increased in neonates [16]. These different fluid component affect volumes of distribution of intravenous anesthetic drugs (this means increasing the volume of distribution, especially for water-soluble drugs).

In addition, due to the immaturity of hepatic functions, duration of action will be prolonged in neonates if the drug depends on hepatic metabolism [6].

Muscle relaxant may be required for some neonatal surgical procedures. However, due to immaturity of the neuromuscular junction, neonates have an increased sensitivity to the effects of nondepolarizing neuromuscular blocking drugs [33]. For this reason, prolonged effects may occur at additional doses.

5.2. Intraoperative period

Balanced general anesthesia management is usually achieved by inhalation anesthesia supplemented with different class and wide range of drugs and/or muscle relaxants and regional techniques or achieved by total intravenous anesthesia.

Barbiturates, opioids, propofol, ketamine listed among these intravenous drugs [14]. Long-acting agents such as morphine should be avoided especially in day-case surgery or procedures and postoperative apnea risk should be kept in mind.

In neonatal patients, reduced hepatic glycogen stores, inadequate muscle glycogen reserve and gluconeogenesis enzyme activity require close monitoring of blood glucose concentration [34].

Intravenous glucose infusion may be required to maintain normoglycemia (serum glucose concentration of 40–90 mg dL [1, 24].

All maintenance fluids and blood products used intraoperatively must be warmed before use. Intravenous fluids should be titrated with an infusion pump or a fluid-adjusted burette to avoid excessive fluid loading and to give a controlled fluid.

Following the first few days of baby's life, in all newborns of gestational age, adequate intake of sodium is essential for continued normal developmental activity [1]. In full term neonates, it is not usually necessary to add sodium in maintenance fluids in the first 24 hours of life. However, sodium is added to the maintenance fluids after the second day to replace the sodium losses from the renal and gastrointestinal tract [35]. Also, non-hypotonic, dextrose-containing fluids for sodium replacement may also be used. But, hypotonic fluids should be avoided. These fluids are most common cause of potentially lethal postoperative hyponatremia [35, 36].

Intraoperative fluid requirement should also be met, depending on pre-existing fluid deficits, quality and duration of operation, and the extent of blood loss.

It should not be allowed hypothermia during the intraoperative period. Hypothermia may cause stress in the newborn, leading to postoperative respiratory insufficiency and ventilatory support [10]. On the other hand, the only stressor factor that to avoid in newborns is not hypothermia. Many stress factors (such as hypotension episodes, hypoxia, hypercapnia, acidosis, anemia) can occur during intraoperative period. These factors leads increase PVR and can cause return of the transitional circulation [Ivanova-24]. Different therapeutic maneuvers such as hyperventilation, deepening anesthesia, increased inspired oxygen, and volume expansion may also help in treatment [10].

5.3. Postoperative period and pain practices in neonate

Many neonates undergoing day-case surgery can be anesthetized using mask ventilation and/or LMA by continuing spontaneous breathing without the use of muscle relaxants and intubation.

However, in some situations (such as in major surgical procedures, urgent surgery, full stomach, etc.) endotracheal intubation must be done to secure the airway.

In these patients, in these patients there are many factors that determine postoperative extubation (including surgical conditions).

In major surgeries, (such as NEC, oesophageal atresia, diaphragmatic hernia) endotracheal intubation safer for these neonatal patients. In these neonates usually require elective postoperative mechanical ventilator support in early postoperative period in NICU.

Estuation period is a critical as intubation. Likewise, it requires to be careful and attentive.

It should be take care with regard to residual neuromuscular block and the neuromuscular blocker drugs should be reversed. In extubation period, we may encounter with side effects such as bradycardia, hypoxia, bronchospasm, which can be seen in induction of anesthesia. Intubation equipments and drugs should be available in the anesthesia theater for immediate intervention.

Post-conceptional age (PCA) is important factor in ex-premature babies, for day case surgical procedures. Most ex-premature babies are suitable for day case surgical procedures at greater than 60 weeks post-conceptional age (PCA). Prior to 60 weeks PCA, especially in premature infants less than 44 weeks PCA, postoperative apnea risk increased. In these neonates is recommended postoperative saturation and apnea monitoring in postoperative 24 hours period.

Pain in neonatal patients has for many years been ignored. However, the theory that newborns do not feel pain has become a subject that has lost its validity nowadays.

Recent studies have shown that neuroanatomical and neuroendocrine systems of premature newborns are sufficient for the transmission and perception of pain [37].

Untreated pain causes restlessness, increased oxygen consumption, ventilation/perfusion deficiency, and reduced food intake in early period of neonatal life. Long-term effects are learning disability and developmental retardation. Surgical trauma causes pain and a hormonal stress response that is directly related to the severity and urgency of surgery. Opioids (such as fentanyl, ultra-short acting remifentanil or traditional longer acting morphine) reduce the stress response and catecholamine release in response to painful stimuli. In addition, opioids provide effective pain control so decrease the pulmonary vasoconstrictor responses to painful stimuli in NICU.

In recent years, intravenous paracetamol has begun to be used in the treatment protocol of pain in neonates [38].

6. General anesthesia and developing brain. A special highlight for neonatal anesthesia

One of the most interesting topics in the last 20 years is the general anesthetic effect on the developing brain and neurocognitive functions.

Animal studies show that exposure to general anesthetics (especially these acting through the NMDA and GABA receptors) during the critical period of neuronal development in the developing brain leads to an apoptotic cell death and neurocognitive impairment especially in immature brain [39, 40]. It is reported that this effect to be related to drug dosages and exposure time.

Long-term neurobehavioral effects of sedative and anesthetic agents should be supported by long-term human studies. In recent years, early results of international, multidisciplinary, prospective clinical trials such as GAS and PANDA have begun to be published [41, 42].

In these studies and in Wilder et al. study, it has been reported that multiple exposures to anesthesia, rather than single exposure to anesthesia, pose a risk factor for later development learning disability in children [41–43].

However, to withhold sedation and anesthesia when necessary, would result in ethical consequences, in addition will trigger many negative consequences of painful stimulation in neonatal patients.

7. Conclusion

Approximately 1.5 million neonates receive general anesthesia each year for a surgical procedure according to literature data on neonatal patients [44].

In recent years, it has seen significant improvements in pediatric and neonatal anesthesia practice such as patient safety, advanced monitoring methods and new anesthesia equipments. Nevertheless, the neonatal period is still challenging for the anesthesiologist.

Anesthetic approach in neonatal population has to take into consideration the many immature vital organ functions as well as the effects of the underlying disease processes, which can frequently lead to severe physiological derangements.

Therefore, reliable anesthesia management is possible with a good understanding of the anatomical, physiological and pharmacological differences of the neonatal period.

Also, basic understanding of risk factors in neonatal anesthesia is a starting point for the reduction of risk. A careful preoperative examination of the child and the child's medical record, careful and close perioperative monitoring and follow-up and effective pain treatment would reduce mortality and morbidity.

The basics of safe anesthetic management in neonatal patients are summarized in this chapter, based on feature of neonatal period. The approach in neonatal emergency surgical procedures has not been mentioned in this chapter, since it was described another chapter.

Author details

Esra Caliskan

Address all correspondence to: duru5654@gmail.com

Department of Anesthesiology and Reanimation, Baskent University Faculty of Medicine, Ankara, Turkey

References

[1] Gregory GA, Brett C. Neonatology for anesthesiologists. In: Davis PJ, Cladis FP, Motoyoma EK, editors. Smith's Anesthesia for Infants and Children. 8th. Chapter 17 ed. Philadelphia: Elsevier Mosby; 2011. pp. 512-553 ISBN: 978-0-323-06612-9.ch3

[2] Brusseau R, McCann ME. Anaesthesia for urgent and emergency surgery. Early Human Development. 2010;**86**:703-714. DOI: 10.1016/j.earlhumdev.2010.08.008

[3] Dierdorf SF, Krishna G. Anesthetic Management of Neonatal Surgical Emergencies. Anesthesia and Analgesia. 1981;**60**:204-214 ISSN: 0003-2999

[4] Thomas J. Reducing the risk in neonatal anesthesia. Pediatric Anesthesia. 2014;**24**:106-113. DOI: 10.1111/pan.12315

[5] Davidson AJ. Editorial: In search of the big question. Pediatric Anesthesia. 2012;**22**:613-615. DOI: 10.1111/j.1460-9592.2012.03808.x

[6] Buttterforth JF, Mackey DC, Washnick DC. Pediatric Anesthesia. Morgan & Mikhail's Lange Clinical Anesthesiology. 5th. Chapter 42 ed. United States of America: McGraw-Hill Medical Publishing; 2013. pp. 849-873

[7] Cote CJ. Neonatal anaesthesia. Southern African Journal of Anaesthesia and Analgesia. 2010;**16**:6-11. DOI: 10.1080/22201173.2010.10872624

[8] Finnemore A, Groves A. Physiology of the fetal and transitional circulation. Seminars in Fetal & Neonatal Medicine. 2015;**20**:210-216. DOI: 10.1016/j.siny.2015.04.003

[9] Motoyama EK, Finder JD. Respiratory physiology in infants and children. In: Davis PJ, Cladis FP, Motoyoma EK, editors. Smith's Anesthesia for Infants and Children. 8th. Chapter 3 ed. Philadelphia: Elsevier Mosby; 2011. pp. 23-79. ISBN: 978-0-323-06612-9.ch3

[10] McCann ME, Soriano SG. Progress in anesthesia and management of the newborn surgical patient. Seminars in Pediatric Surgery. 2014;**23**:244-248. DOI: 10.1053/j.sempedsurg.2014.09.003

[11] Jain A, McNamara PJ. Persistent pulmonary hypertension of the newborn: Advances in diagnosis and treatment. Seminars in Fetal & Neonatal Medicine. 2015;**20**:262-271. DOI: 10.1016/j.siny.2015.03.001

[12] Cote CJ. Pediatric Anetshesia. In: Miller RD, editor. Miller's Anesthesia. 7th ed. Philadelphia: El Churchill Livingstone; 2010. pp. 2559-2597. ISBN: 978-0-443-06959-8.ch

[13] de Wildt SN. Profound changes in drug metabolism enzymes and possible effects on drug therapy in neonates and children. Expert Opinion on Drug Metabolism & Toxicology. 2011;**7**:935-948. DOI: 10.1517/17425255.2011.577739

[14] Brett C, Davis PJ. Anesthesia for general surgery in the neonate. In: Davis PJ, Cladis FP, Motoyoma EK, editors. Smith's Anesthesia for Infants and Children. 8th. Chapter 18 ed. Philadelphia: Elsevier Mosby; 2011. pp. 554-588. ISBN: 978-0-323-06612-9. ch3

[15] Allegaert K, Velde MV, Anker JV. Neonatal clinical pharmacology. Paediatric Anaesthesia. 2014;**24**:1-14. DOI: 10.1111/pan.12176

[16] Anderson BJ. Pharmacology in the very young: Anaesthetic implications. European Journal of Anaesthesiology. 2012;**29**:261-270. DOI: 10.1097/EJA.0b013e3283542329

[17] O'Brien F, Walker IA. Fluid homeostasis in the neonate. Paediatric Anaesthesia. 2014;**24**:49-59. DOI: 10.1111/pan.12326

[18] Tourneux P, Libert JP, Ghyselen L, et al. Heat exchanges and thermoregulation in the neonate. Archives de Pédiatrie. 2009;**16**:1057-1062. DOI: 10.1016/j.arcped.2009.03.014.

[19] Friedman M, Baumgart S. Thermal regulation. In: MacDonald MG, Seshia MMK, Mullett MD, editors. Avery's Neonatology: Pathophysiology and Management of the Newborn. 6th ed. Philadelphia: Lippincott Williams & Wilkins; 2005. pp. 445-455

[20] Pearce B, Christensen R, Voepel-Lewis T. Perioperative hypothermia in the pediatric population: Prevalence, risk factors and outcomes. Journal of Anesthesia and Clinical Research. 2010;**1**:102. DOI: 10.4172/2155-6148.1000102

[21] Lerman J. Pharmacology of inhalational anaesthetics in infants and children. Paediatric Anaesthesia. 1992;**2**:191-203. DOI: 10.1111/j.1460-9592.1992.tb00200.x

[22] LeDez KM, Lerman J. The minimum alveolar concentration (MAC) of isoflurane in preterm neonates. Anesthesiology. 1987;**67**:301-307

[23] Short JA, Gordon JK. Preoperative assessment and preparation for anaesthesia in children. Anaesthesia and Intensive Care Medicine. 2015;**16**:381-388. DOI: 10.1016/j.mpaic.2015.06.003

[24] Ivanova I, Pittaway A. Principles of anaesthesia for term neonates: An updated practical guide. Anaesthesia and Intensive Care Medicine. 2014;**15**:103-106. DOI: 10.1016/j.mpaic.2014.01.008

[25] Pittaway A. Principles of anaesthesia for the term neonate. Anaesthesia and Intensive Care. 2008;**12**:95-98. DOI: 10.1016/j.mpaic.2016.11.002

[26] Weiss M, Dullenkopf J, Fischer E, et al. Prospective randomised controlled multi-centre trial of cuffed or un-cuffed endotracheal tubes in small children. British Journal of Anaesthesia. 2009;**103**:867-873. DOI: 10.1093/bja/aep290

[27] Cambell S, Graham W, Engelhart T. Equipment and monitoring – What is in the future to improve safety? Pediatric Anesthesia. 2011;**21**:815-824. DOI: 10.1111/j.1460-9592.2011.03553.x

[28] Bachiller PR, McDonough JM, Feldman JM. Do new anesthesia ventilators deliver small tidal volumes accurately during volume-controlled ventilation? Anesthesia and Analgesia. 2008;**106**:1392-1400. DOI: 10.1213/ane.0b013e31816a68c6

[29] Garcia-Fernandez J, Tusman G, Suarez-Sipmann F, Llorens J, Soro M, Belda JF. Programming pressure support ventilation in pediatric patients in ambulatory surgery with a laryngeal mask airway. Anesthesia and Analgesia. 2007;**105**:1585-1591

[30] Intravenous Anesthetics. Morgan & Mikhail's Lange Clinical Anesthesiology. 5th. Chapter 9 ed. United States of America: McGraw-Hill Medical Publishing; 2013. pp. 175-189

[31] Paterson N, Waterhouse P. Risk in pediatric anesthesia. Pediatric Anesthesia. 2011;**21**:848-857. DOI: 10.1111/j.1460-9592.2010.03366.x.

[32] Sale SM. Neonatal apnoea. Best Practice & Research Clinical Anaesthesiology. 2010;**24**:323-336. DOI: 10.1016/j.bpa.2010.04.002

[33] Meretoja OA. Neuromuscular block and current treatment strategies for its reversal in children. Paediatric Anaesthesia. 2010;**20**:591-604. DOI: 10.1111/j.1460-9592.2010.03335.x

[34] Mitanchez D. Glucose regulation in preterm newborn infants. Hormone Research. 2007;**68**:265-271

[35] Sümpelmann R, Becke K, Crean P, et al. European consensus statement for intraoperative fluid therapy in children. European Journal of Anaesthesiology. 2011;**28**(9):637. DOI: 10.1097/EJA.0b013e3283446bb8

[36] Datta PK, Pawar DK, Baidya DK, Maitra S, Aravindan A. Dextrose-containing intraoperative fluid in neonates: In randomised controlled trial. Pediatric Anesthesia. 2016;**26**:599-607

[37] Lee SJ, Ralston HJ, Drey EA, Partridge JC, Rosen MA. Fetal pain: A systematic multidisciplinary review of the evidence. JAMA. 2005;**24**(294):947-954

[38] Härmä A, Aikio O, Hallman M, Saarela T. Intravenous Paracetamol decreases requirements of morphine in very preterm infants. The Journal of Pediatrics. 2016;**168**:36-40. DOI: 10.1016/j.jpeds.2015.08.003

[39] Sinner B, Becke K, Engelhard K. General anaesthetics and developing brain. An overview. Anaesthesia. 2014;**69**:1009-1022

[40] Sun L. Early childhood general anesthesia exposure and neurocognitive development. British Journal of Anaesthesia. 2010;**105**:i61-i68. DOI: 10.1093/bja/aeq302

[41] Davidson AJ, Disma N, Graaff JC, et al. Neurodevelopmental outcome at 2 years of age after general anaesthesia and awake-regional anaesthesia in infancy (GAS): An international multicentre randomised controlled trial. Lancet. 2016;**387**:239-250. DOI: 10.1016/S0140-6736(15)00608-X

[42] Miller TL, Park R, Sun LS. Report of the fourth PANDA symposium on "anesthesia and neurodevelopment in children". Journal of Neurosurgical Anesthesiology. 2014;**26**:344-348. DOI: 10.1097/ANA.0000000000000109

[43] Wilder RT, Flick RP, Sprung J, et al. Early exposure to anesthesia and learning disabilities in a population-based birth cohort. Anesthesiology. 2009;**110**:796-804. DOI: 10.1097/01.anes.0000344728.34332.5d

[44] Nasr VG, Davis JM. Anesthetic use in newborn infants: The urgent need for rigorous evaluation. Pediatric Research. 2015;**78**:2-6. DOI: 10.1038/pr.2015.58

Permissions

All chapters in this book were first published in PNS, by InTech Open; hereby published with permission under the Creative Commons Attribution License or equivalent. Every chapter published in this book has been scrutinized by our experts. Their significance has been extensively debated. The topics covered herein carry significant findings which will fuel the growth of the discipline. They may even be implemented as practical applications or may be referred to as a beginning point for another development.

The contributors of this book come from diverse backgrounds, making this book a truly international effort. This book will bring forth new frontiers with its revolutionizing research information and detailed analysis of the nascent developments around the world.

We would like to thank all the contributing authors for lending their expertise to make the book truly unique. They have played a crucial role in the development of this book. Without their invaluable contributions this book wouldn't have been possible. They have made vital efforts to compile up to date information on the varied aspects of this subject to make this book a valuable addition to the collection of many professionals and students.

This book was conceptualized with the vision of imparting up-to-date information and advanced data in this field. To ensure the same, a matchless editorial board was set up. Every individual on the board went through rigorous rounds of assessment to prove their worth. After which they invested a large part of their time researching and compiling the most relevant data for our readers.

The editorial board has been involved in producing this book since its inception. They have spent rigorous hours researching and exploring the diverse topics which have resulted in the successful publishing of this book. They have passed on their knowledge of decades through this book. To expedite this challenging task, the publisher supported the team at every step. A small team of assistant editors was also appointed to further simplify the editing procedure and attain best results for the readers.

Apart from the editorial board, the designing team has also invested a significant amount of their time in understanding the subject and creating the most relevant covers. They scrutinized every image to scout for the most suitable representation of the subject and create an appropriate cover for the book.

The publishing team has been an ardent support to the editorial, designing and production team. Their endless efforts to recruit the best for this project, has resulted in the accomplishment of this book. They are a veteran in the field of academics and their pool of knowledge is as vast as their experience in printing. Their expertise and guidance has proved useful at every step. Their uncompromising quality standards have made this book an exceptional effort. Their encouragement from time to time has been an inspiration for everyone.

The publisher and the editorial board hope that this book will prove to be a valuable piece of knowledge for researchers, students, practitioners and scholars across the globe.

List of Contributors

Abdulkerim Temiz
Başkent University, Faculty of Medicine, Department of Pediatric Surgery, Turkey

Marissa Vadi, Chelan Nour, Patrick Leiter and Harmony Carter
Loma Linda University School of Medicine, Loma Linda, CA, USA

Chengzhan Zhu
Department of Hepatobiliary and Pancreatic Surgery, The Affiliated Hospital of Qingdao University, Qingdao, China
Shandong Key Laboratory of Digital Medicine and Computer Assisted Surgery, The Affiliated Hospital of Qingdao University, Qingdao, China

Bingzi Dong
Department of Endocrinology and Metabolism, The Affiliated Hospital of Qingdao University, Qingdao, China

Qian Dong
Pediatric Surgery Department, The Affiliated Hospital of Qingdao University, Qingdao, China
Shandong Key Laboratory of Digital Medicine and Computer Assisted Surgery, The Affiliated Hospital of Qingdao University, Qingdao, China

Kenneth W. Gow and Matthew Dellinger
Seattle Children's Hospital and the University of Washington, USA

Shelly Haug, Sara Farooqi, Anamika Banerji and Andrew Hopper
Loma Linda University Children's Hospital, Loma Linda, CA, USA

Ayse B. Ozer and Sibel Ozcan
Faculty of Medicine, Department of Anesthesiology Intensive Care, Firat University, Elazig, Turkey

Asifur Rahman
Department of Neurosurgery, Bangabandhu Sheikh Mujib Medical University, Shahbag, Dhaka, Bangladesh

Eva Miranda Marwali
Pediatric Cardiac Intensive Care Unit, National Cardiovascular Center Harapan Kita, Jakarta, Indonesia

Beatrice Heineking and Nikolaus A. Haas
Department of Pediatric Cardiology and Pediatric Intensive Care Medicine, University Hospital of Munich, Ludwig Maxmilians University, Munich, Germany

Esra Caliskan
Department of Anesthesiology and Reanimation, Baskent University Faculty of Medicine, Ankara, Turkey

Index

www.ingramcontent.com/pod-product-compliance
Lightning Source LLC
LaVergne TN
LVHW060548210926
848485LV00005B/1279